WITHDRAWN

rebuild

rebuild

Five Proven Steps to Move from Diagnosis to Recovery and Be Healthier Than Before

ROBERT ZEMBROSKI, DC, DACNB, MS

HARPER WAVE

An Imprint of HarperCollins*Publishers*

This book contains advice and information relating to health care. It should be used to supplement rather than replace the advice of your doctor or another trained health professional. If you know or suspect you have a health problem, it is recommended that you seek your physician's advice before embarking on any medical program or treatment. All efforts have been made to ensure the accuracy of the information contained in this book as of the date of publication. This publisher and the author disclaim liability for any medical outcomes that may occur as a result of applying the methods suggested in this book.

REBUILD. Copyright © 2018 by Robert Zembroski, DC, DACNB, MS. All rights reserved. Printed in the United States of America. No part of this book may be used or reproduced in any manner whatsoever without written permission except in the case of brief quotations embodied in critical articles and reviews. For information, address HarperCollins Publishers, 195 Broadway, New York, NY 10007.

HarperCollins books may be purchased for educational, business, or sales promotional use. For information, please email the Special Markets Department at SPsales@harpercollins.com.

FIRST EDITION

Designed by Bonni Leon-Berman

Library of Congress Cataloging-in-Publication Data has been applied for.

ISBN 978-0-06-269920-6

18 19 20 21 22   LSC   10 9 8 7 6 5 4 3 2 1

To all those affected by chronic disease or unresolved health issues who are looking for real answers in a world of confusing medical options.

This book is dedicated to you.

Contents

Foreword

I have had the privilege of knowing Dr. Robert Zembroski for the past eight years, and I have found him to be an inspiration. His successful victory over cancer is only part of his remarkable story. He is a person who "walks the talk." Through his expertise and advocacy, he has helped his patients achieve amazing results with improving their health.

So this begs a question: What does his book, *Rebuild*, uniquely offer to the reader?

I have reviewed hundreds of health-related books over the past thirty years during my career as a medical researcher, health educator, and opinion leader in nutrition and functional medicine. Most of these books discuss diet and exercise programs to help prevent disease.

Dr. Zembroski's book, however, is focused on the description of his tried-and-proven approach to return to vital health after illness or injury. Dr. Zembroski can speak from experience, not only from his own successful battle with cancer and his path back to optimal health, but also from the clinical application of his program by his many patients who have successfully regained their health after illness.

Rebuild reads like a manifesto of the remarkable.

It demonstrates that miraculous things can happen when a person commits to the right program, designed to return to the best of health and vitality.

The use of case histories from Dr. Z's practice provides the connection to reality of the health message delivered in this book. The reader can feel the passion and pursuit of excellence that Dr. Z brings to his practice. He is clearly an expert in translating the science of healing and recovery into a program that can be successfully applied by people seeking to recover their health.

As I read the book, I reflected on the conversations I have had with

Dr. Z over the years, and I asked myself, "What makes certain people special?" My answer is that every person is special, but some have had life experiences that bring their "specialness" to a higher degree of visibility. Such is the case with Dr. Z, who has leveraged his own remarkable experience in successfully fighting back from cancer into an opportunity to share what he has learned with others in order to improve their ability to recover good health.

The quality that makes Dr. Z special comes through loud and clear in this book. It motivates readers to want to do better, to take charge of their lives, and to commit to something that they may have thought was too difficult before reading this book.

It is my belief that the biggest obstacle most people face when making meaningful changes in their health is the inability to see beyond the sacrifice of the required changes to the payoff of improved health and vitality. This is where coaching and a positive support system come into play.

Dr. Z has written a book that provides reinforcement and step-by-step encouragement to push through the moments of doubt when a reader may ask, "Is it worth it?" His story demonstrates that yes, it *is* worth it, and it can happen to anyone following his program with commitment.

It has been a great pleasure to get to know Dr. Z over the years. It is hard to know exactly how many people will change their health for the better by following Dr. Z's program. From my years of experience, I expect that the number of success stories will be absolutely transformative.

—**Jeffrey Bland**, PhD, FACN, FACB, President and Founder, Personalized Lifestyle Medicine Institute, Seattle, Washington (www.plminstitute.org), author of *The Disease Delusion*

rebuild

Introduction

Recovering from Disease:
A New Perspective

Can you recover from heart disease, cancer, diabetes, obesity, auto-immune issues, and other chronic conditions and actually be healthier than you were before you got sick? Can you rebuild your body during a health crisis and then prevent recurrence? Can you melt unwanted toxic fat off your body as you gain lean muscle and restore your health? The answer to all these questions is an emphatic "yes!" By using the tools in *Rebuild*, you will come out of your health crisis not only a victor but also healthier, leaner, and more energetic than you have felt in years.

In *Rebuild*, I explain the link between an unhealthful lifestyle and the creation of disease. I lead you through the steps you must take to re-build yourself after disease, while you are being treated for a condition, and afterward, to prevent recurrence. You will also learn how to sustain your newfound health for a lifetime and discover the dangers of an un-healthy body composition—the ratio of fat to muscle. An unhealthy body composition is a driving force in the development and return of cancer, heart disease, diabetes, and other chronic ailments. This book presents the latest research in an easy-to-read format so that you can create a lifestyle that will help you not only look great but also have lots of energy and feel good about yourself.

My Story
Known to my patients as "Dr. Z," I am a physician, specialist in functional medicine, board-certified chiropractic neurologist, clinical nutritionist,

and transformational speaker. My clinical practice of twenty-four years is focused on helping people resolve health issues by finding the root causes of their problems, an approach known as functional medicine. Whether it's hormone-based problems, a chronic disease, neurological problems, or weight issues, I take a functional approach—looking at the whole person—to search for clues. I dig deep for facts that enable me to understand the mechanisms of each issue. That way, I can help you reverse the cause and rebuild yourself back to normal function. I know that what I'm sharing with you works because it has worked for countless patients, and it worked for me.

At the age of thirty-eight, after a few years of feeling intense stress and neglecting a healthful lifestyle, I was diagnosed with non-Hodgkin's lymphoma, a life-threatening blood cancer. The diagnosis took me by surprise. The first symptoms had been mild; I started losing muscle weight and developed a low-grade fatigue that no amount of caffeine and B vitamins would help. As the symptoms became more severe—including intense head pain and being awakened by gushing night sweats—I knew I was in trouble. I had blood work and X-rays done to find the reasons for my symptoms. On August 18, 2006, a radiologist and friend announced, "You have a five-inch tumor in your chest." My heart nearly stopped beating, and voices around me sounded muffled. As I walked out of the doctor's office that day, I realized that by not taking care of myself, I had compounded my health problems.

Right before I started treatment, the doctors told me, "We're giving you the strongest stuff we have." They were not kidding. Within a two-year period, I had seven months of the most toxic chemotherapy—including a chemical similar to mustard gas and a noxious substance known as "Red Death"—and four weeks of radiation.

During the first three months of chemotherapy, the symptoms and side effects were devastating. I developed the nasty side effects that many people develop: I suffered from peripheral neuropathy (burning and tingling) in my fingertips, uncomfortable constipation, burning eyes, and fatigue. My beard stopped growing, my eyebrows fell out, and so did the little bit of hair I had on my head (hair is overrated anyway). Midway through the chemo cycle, I developed nosebleeds that became a regular occurrence every morning. My left lower leg became very swollen, and the skin surrounding my left ankle turned an amber reddish-brown from the drug called Red Death. I also lost all sense of taste except for the sweet and tangy taste of tomato sauce. Since I'm a foodie, having everything taste like cardboard was a bummer.

When I first started chemotherapy, I wasn't told the importance of getting a port put in (a device inserted under the skin where the drugs are infused); as a consequence, the drugs were given to me through a catheter pushed into my veins that caused them to flatten and turn brown. On top of that, one of the chemo drugs affected my bladder, delaying the sensation of urgency when I had to urinate. When I finally felt like I had to go . . . I *really* had to go.

During this period of time, I began wading through research to understand my disease and figure out what I could do to improve my health even during cancer care. The more I learned, the more I applied to myself. As a result, my appetite and strength returned rather quickly, and I began to recover. Future scans revealed "activity" in my chest that I was told was benign. With much excitement, I was back in my practice full-time, working out at the gym, eating well, and now driven to know more about the factors that create disease.

As it turned out, I recovered quickly only to find out I was gearing up for round two. Follow-up scans revealed that the lesion in my chest wasn't benign; it was cancer that had not been completely eradicated by the first round of chemo. The excitement that had been building in me was quickly replaced with frustration. I began a second cycle of drugs that were just as toxic as the first. But this time, I was armed and ready for battle. I had engineered a "rebuild" plan to mitigate the side effects of the chemo and keep myself relatively healthy so I could function normally in my practice, work out, socialize, and feel human.

Despite the toxicity from the drugs, I continued on my rebuild plan. It was so effective that I was called "the freak" by my doctors because they couldn't understand how I was doing so well physically and mentally while being treated with "the strongest stuff." I was still seeing patients full-time, working out, and living a somewhat normal life during my care.

When those treatments were over, the cancer was diminished but not eradicated. At that stage, my prognosis looked grim. In a meeting with my doctors at a well-known cancer hospital, we discussed a stem-cell transplant from my brother. The preparation for the transplant involved more chemo to suppress my immune system. As I contemplated the upcoming procedure and its potential health risks, I realized—based on my education and experience—that a stem-cell transplant would not work for me.

I developed a Plan B. I challenged the doctors to remove the tumor, a procedure they claimed never to have done before in cases like mine. But I persisted. Two years from the day of my diagnosis, a surgeon cracked open my chest from throat to belly and removed the mass of scar tissue where once a giant ball of cancer cells had been growing. That operation—and my persistence—saved my life. However, the cumulative effect of nearly two years of chemo, radiation, and major surgery left me with new challenges.

Yes, I was cancer-free, but the cancer treatment had taken its toll. Blood work revealed a low red blood cell count, low platelets, and low white blood cells. My thyroid had been affected, which created low levels of thyroid hormones and the symptoms associated with hypothyroidism, including cold hands and feet, slow metabolism, and dry skin. Hormone testing revealed low testosterone and low vitamin D levels. A special test to check my metabolism and energy production revealed that the drugs had also caused malabsorption of B vitamins. On top of discolored skin on my lower left leg from the Red Death and the collapsed veins in my arms, I suffered from weakness in the muscles of my lower left leg, which made fast walking or running a problem.

With my health crisis behind me, I asked my providers what I should do to prevent recurrence, and they responded with the sage advice, "Don't eat junk, and stay healthy." Wow! That was so profound and helpful. Since my doctors couldn't give me more advice, I knew I had to find the information to help myself going forward. I wanted to learn what had caused my disease so I could prevent its recurrence. I also wanted to learn how to rebuild my body after the side effects of the cancer therapies. My goal was to create the ultimate healthy body—one that was disease-free and lean.

I dove into the best research and applied my findings to myself. The facts were there: I had created my own disease. For a few years prior to my diagnosis, I had not taken proper care of myself. Circumstances involving my busy practice, coupled with some standard life problems and setbacks, created extreme levels of stress. This disrupted my sleep and led me to eat unhealthful foods and neglect my exercise regimen. After reading research on nutrition, nutritional biochemistry, genetics, cancer, endocrinology (the study of hormones), chronic disease, and exercise physiology, I refined my program for myself with one thing in mind—to rebuild.

In following this plan, I have improved my low blood counts and restored my thyroid, testosterone, and vitamin D levels. My energy is back to normal, and I have no residual tingling in my limbs—a major problem that plagues many people who have received certain chemotherapy drugs. Frantically pulling off the highway at the next exit to empty my bladder is a problem of the past. Although the discolored skin remains, the weakness in my left leg no longer interferes with my physical activity. Currently, I am lean, with 10 percent body fat.

My personal experience, coupled with countless hours of research, ignited a passion to help others rebuild from their health issues so they don't have to go through what I experienced. Facing the Grim Reaper is not fun, to say the least! Neither is enduring debilitating and scarring procedures. Worrying about a recurrence or worsening of your condition is emotionally draining. And I'm sure those of you who are being or have been treated for a serious illness feel the same way.

The Keys to Health

Most physicians will say that what you eat and how much you exercise has a nominal effect, if any, on the creation of disease or ill health. Many health "authorities" also say that disease is inherited, or that it originates from some unknown source we have no control over. But the scientific research is clear: most chronic disease does not come from our genetic makeup alone. In most cases, it can be traced back to specific aspects of what we do to ourselves—our lifestyle, our habits, and our daily rituals.

Your health crisis didn't emerge out of thin air. Most of the diseases we now call "Western diseases" are caused by the interaction between your internal environment—which you control—and your genes. In many cases, health can be traced back to specific aspects of diet, lack of exercise, emotional stress, poor sleep habits, and toxins.

In other words, our environment and the choices we make set the stage for the diseases we develop.

If our choices affect disease progression, then these choices can be modified. The major factor that you can modify to your benefit is your body composition, a mixture of elements that create a synergy of normal function and health, and different types of tissues, such as fat and muscle. My reading through countless research studies and dissecting the scientific literature showed one clear message: an unhealthy body composition correlates with the creation of many leading Western diseases.

To have a healthy body composition, you need to consume an abundance of nutrients from a variety of foods, as well as exercise to burn fat, tone muscle, and regulate the hormones that, in turn, control fat and muscle.

One major problem, however, is the colossal amount of misleading information out there on what foods to eat and not eat, and what exercise program is best. We've all seen the health books that tout some new fad or plan. Others promote some gimmicky workout or fat-burning supplement. How many times have we seen a smiling celebrity on a book cover promising we'll "lose twenty-one pounds in seven days"? Then the next trend grabs our attention, and off we go again. Three months later, we've regained all the pounds we lost on our diet—and often more.

Before going any further, I'd like to clarify the definition of the word *diet*. Somewhere along the line, the real meaning of diet was subverted. It is commonly misunderstood as a jail sentence of eating gruel. The word conjures up images of short durations of restriction and starvation, where you have to give up foods you like for boring and tasteless "health food." You decide to "go on a diet" to get rid of fat, lose weight, or improve your health because you have just been diagnosed with some chronic health issue. The decision seems less painful because you know the "diet" is for a finite amount of time.

Instead, the word *diet* actually just refers to the type of food you eat regularly. Some people choose to eat only plant-based foods; others eat foods high in animal protein and low in carbohydrates. Many people eat anything and everything. What you are putting into your body— *that's* your diet.

Most restrictive diets fail because they are too extreme. The approach of "going on a diet" doesn't work because it creates only a famine mind-set. Then you indulge in rebound feasting on the processed and unhealthful foods that created the overfat body composition and helped cause your disease in the first place. ("Overfat" means carrying too much subcutaneous and visceral fat, even at a BMI—body mass index—that would otherwise not be classified as overweight.) Instead, dieting should be seen as a *lifestyle*.

In my experience of working with countless patients to help them rebuild from disease, changing one's diet typically means reducing calories. Yet calorie restriction in most diet books means nutrient restriction. If you are overfat and looking to improve your body composition, be careful you don't starve yourself of vital nutrients that come from nutrient-dense whole foods, as nutrient deficiency is a major cause of all disease. The key to getting rid of inflammatory harmful fat is eating plenty of low-calorie, nutrient-dense foods throughout the day.

The body composition diet in this book goes far beyond getting rid of fat and reducing weight. It is a research-based plan that leads to excellent health and a strong and lean body. The best thing about this approach is that you can create a custom plan that uniquely suits your metabolism and your specific health issues.

Considering the negative mind-set around the word *diet*, I wanted to make the definition more appealing. I decided to use DIET as an acronym standing for words that provide a positive approach to your health: Decide, Indulge, Enjoy, and Transform.

When restoring your health, the first thing you have to do is DECIDE. As I say to my patients, the first step to rebuilding from any health issue is *making a decision*. Make the decision to do what it takes to rebuild from your illness and prevent its recurrence. Once you make the decision, INDULGE in a variety of nutrient-dense and tasty whole foods that will communicate with your cells to turn on genes that create normal function, while at the same time shutting off genes that set the stage for disease. Indulging in a variety of healthful foods will force your body to burn fat and build lean muscle. Doing that enables you to ENJOY the fruits of your effort with more energy, vibrancy, and health. Enjoy looking and feeling better. Finally, watch yourself TRANSFORM physically and aesthetically. Transform yourself into the physically fit and healthy person you deserve to be.

Does this sound more appealing? I will show you how to set this plan into action in the pages that follow.

Still, changing the foods you eat to rebuild yourself is not enough. According to the prevailing research, there are five steps that should be taken to be victorious in rebuilding yourself.

First, you must eliminate all processed foods while replacing them with nutrient-dense, low-calorie whole foods. This is how you will recalibrate the way your body communicates with your genes, allowing you to shut off the disease process and improve your internal physiology.

Second, you must move more. You need to adopt an exercise regimen, including high-intensity interval training (HIIT), that will restore normal function and help you quickly lose the fat and get lean.

Third, you have heard that stress kills . . . and it does. Whatever the stressors are in your life, the next step is to change your perspective and rebuild your thinking about those stressors. The best approach is to find a coach—not your son's soccer coach or your daughter's field hockey coach, but someone with experience who can help you navigate and manage the stressors that drive you into harm's way.

Fourth, you need to be aware of and eliminate major toxins not only in your foods but also in your environment—things that you may be inhaling, swallowing, or smearing on your skin. You may be aware of the four thousand known toxins and carcinogens found in a single cigarette. But did you know that in dairy products, there are also harmful compounds that fuel cancer and autoimmune diseases? You will be surprised to learn which toxins from the foods we eat and the substances we are exposed to on a daily basis contribute to the development of disease.

Fifth and last, sleep is extremely important to rebuild your health. Sleeping regulates critical hormones and the immune system needed to rebuild yourself. Sadly, we shock ourselves awake with latte-frappu-crème-macchiato-whatevers, which are loaded with caffeine, sugary syrups, dairy, and soy—disastrous cocktails of inflammation. We also sedate ourselves before bed with a glass of wine, or two, or three, which can alter the sleep cycle and set the stage for a health crisis.

The only permanent way to rebuild yourself from disease, and to become lean and strong, is to have a vision for what you really want. You also need to set new standards for yourself while at the same time making realistic changes. That means laying out attainable goals. Setting your sights only on the finish line can be overwhelming. Instead, you can take small, incremental steps, similar to a runner looking ahead to the next telephone pole during a marathon. Unless you focus on your progress, your old, unhealthful habits can sneak back in. *Rebuild* helps you celebrate small wins while on your journey to becoming healthy, which is an important way to move forward.

Why Functional Medicine?

My victory over cancer, and certainly the restoration of my health, was achieved by using medical treatment combined with my own education and critical thinking. If I had not taken a stand with my doctors to advocate for my own health, I would have followed the "standards of care" for my diagnosis, and likely would not have lived to tell my story . . . or to help you by writing this book. All through my ordeal—the chemo hell, radiation, surgery, and the miserable side effects—I never lost sight of victory.

I pushed the oncologist, surgeon, and nurses to think about me as an individual, to think "outside the box" when devising my treatments. Finally, I convinced them to do a surgery that they never would have considered if I had not insisted. It took a tremendous amount of personal research, initiative, and effort to get them to listen to me and try something that was not part of the usual protocol for my diagnosis. Perhaps the reason I was finally able to get through to them was that I am a doctor and I can speak their language. That made me realize how difficult, if not impossible, it must be for someone who isn't a health professional or doesn't have the knowledge to suggest something different.

My quest to find something better, something more holistic, began with a meeting—or rather, a non-meeting. I wanted to find out how to rebuild myself, so I called a meeting with my doctors. On that day I looked around, and I was by myself . . . nobody showed up. Why? The reality is that most doctors are not trained to handle "postwar" treatment and rehabilitation. Sadly, there are no standard-of-care guidelines to help you rebuild from and prevent recurrence of heart disease, cancer, diabetes, autoimmune diseases, and other chronic ailments. The specialists in crisis care had each done their piece, but they had nothing to offer me in my quest to rebuild myself. Every one of my doctors felt responsible for their individual contribution; nobody felt responsible for the whole.

This should not be surprising. Our current health care system is not one of health care; rather, it is crisis care based on an old algorithmic way of thinking. Dr. Jeff Bland says it nicely in his book *The Disease Delusion*: "Name the disease and prescribe the cure." Chronic diseases and conditions are usually treated with hard-hitting pharmaceuticals. This old model of treating people often fails to restore health to those battling disease. Because all health problems and diseases are multi-dimensional, with many underlying roots, attempting to tackle human ills with a magic bullet just doesn't work.

Fortunately, through the genius of Dr. Bland, there is a new model of health care that is spreading over the globe: functional medicine. Functional medicine is a methodology of uncovering why disease happens. It provides an understanding of how to reverse conditions while at the same time restoring health. Like an archaeologist digs for fossils or clues, a specialist in functional medicine digs for physical clues to understand the origins of your disease. The functional medicine approach also understands that the body functions as an orchestrated network of interconnected systems, and disease is created from an imbalance in those systems. Once the physical clues are found in the dysfunctional internal terrain—the physical condition or state of the inside of the body—a plan is engineered to help resolve the physiological dysfunctions through individual treatment. This method is health-centered, not disease-centered.

The realization that functional medicine could help me—and my patients—recover from illness drove me to get additional training, reshape my clinical practice, write this book, create educational material and videos, and go on the lecture circuit. Why? Because of my personal experience, I am committed to doing all I can to create options for other people facing critical or chronic disease, so that they don't have to face what I've faced or feel as lonely and disconnected as I felt. My own experience also enabled me to look at patients differently, to listen more closely, to be more attentive, and to really discover and document what people need to understand in order to avoid the bad lifestyle choices that lead to disease. *Rebuild* is a culmination of my experience treating my own health and the health of my patients using the principles of functional medicine.

You can find more resources beyond the book by tuning in to my YouTube channel (Dr Z TV); finding me on social media (facebook .com/Zembroski, twitter.com/DrRobZembroski); and visiting my website (www.drzembroski.com). I would love to hear from you, and I would love to share your wins, your personal rebuild story, and your new outlook on life with others. By following the five rebuild actions (re-actions) I describe in Part II, I know you can come back from whatever health crisis you are facing and be better—stronger, leaner, healthier—than you were before.

Here's to your victory.

I
It Can't Happen to Me

OKAY, YOU'VE BEEN DIAGNOSED with heart disease, cancer, diabetes, autoimmune disease, or some other unresolved chronic condition. You've been through a slew of tests and diagnostic procedures—poked, prodded, stitched up, and drugged. Let's not forget the long office visits in cold exam rooms trying to piece together everything you've been told while your internal monologue is saying, "Is this for real? Is this really happening?" You may have been running into dead ends in a maze of providers as you search for effective and affordable answers to your questions.

Now what?

For most people, becoming your own disease detective while dealing with a serious health issue can be too much to handle, especially on top of all your other responsibilities. Furthermore, medical jargon is often confusing and potentially stressful if you don't have a clinical background.

In addition to your chronic health issue(s), you may be suffering from medical apathy—a learned helplessness that comes from seeing doctors who haven't helped you. Many people get stuck in a medical holding pattern and feel frustrated, lonely, and disconnected. Perhaps you have been told by different "specialists" and "-ologists" that you have been dealt a bad hand, that your condition is genetic, or that you're just going to have to live with it. Perhaps you have a big folder full of test results, but still no answers. In some cases, you may have the wrong diagnosis. You have exhausted the best of what conventional medicine has to offer—more medications—and are now looking for real answers to your unresolved health issues.

How often have you sat across from a doctor and felt as though you haven't been listened to or acknowledged as you try to figure out what's wrong with your health? You—and your symptoms—may have been brushed off, as if what you feel and say don't matter. The lack of acknowledgment in that seven-minute visit is extremely frustrating. As a patient myself, I experienced the "medical cold shoulder" before the actual discovery that I had cancer.

Perhaps you've been bounced around from doctor to doctor, trying to navigate all the (sometimes conflicting) information being thrown your way. Deciding which option is best for you isn't easy, especially when you're feeling far from *your best*. Don't get me wrong—there are wonderful practitioners out there. Unfortunately, it is more and more common for patients to feel brushed aside, confused, and in the dark as they're trying to restore their health and get their life back.

Here's my advice: If your doctors are not willing to work with you, fire them. Hire new people to help resolve or control your condition, and use the information in this book to be your own advocate. Remember, statistics are about *groups of people*, not you. The information in this book will help you become your own statistic.

While studying the latest research on the mechanisms of disease, I realized how difficult it must be for people without the necessary time, knowledge, or background to find and interpret useful information, and to be able to use it to create a personalized protocol to rebuild. My journey through a health catastrophe pushed me further into the research and allowed me to break it down into easy-to-understand language for you. I wrote this book so others could benefit from what I learned during my rebuild.

Many people diagnosed with a disease do not have the resources to understand their illness, rebuild from it, and prevent a recurrence. You do—you have this book. Your first step is understanding your disease or chronic health issue and what caused it. That is covered in chapter 1. Chapter 2 asks you to assess your health to identify a baseline from which to rebuild. And for those of you who want more information on a topic, I have included details in the form of "Z Notes" placed throughout the book to provide additional science and/or further research. You can also choose to skip over those sections and continue reading.

1

Anatomy of Disease

In centuries past, the leading causes of death were the result of poor sanitation and infectious diseases. Countless people died from smallpox, yellow fever, malaria, and dysentery, among many other causes. Since the accidental discovery of penicillin, and the manufacturing of vaccines and other forms of biotechnology, these infectious diseases are not the prevailing reason for our current suffering (though they still exist). Today, a poor state of health, for many, is self-inflicted. I know that's tough to hear, but it's true.

You may have been told that the cause of or reason for your chronic disease or condition is unknown, or that it runs in your family. In this chapter, I provide an explanation of how certain diseases develop, but it's important to understand first that the main reason behind your cancer, heart disease, diabetes, obesity, or other chronic condition is probably *not* your inherited genes.

Before you scan the list of chronic diseases looking for your health issue, let's define *chronic*. A chronic illness is a long-lasting condition that does not self-remedy and for which there is no vaccine. It usually requires ongoing medical attention and often treatment with pharmaceuticals. It may remain stable, or it may worsen over time. Sometimes the symptoms of a chronic disease go dormant for a time and then reappear with a vengeance.

Chronic disease develops due to alterations in some aspect of your physiology. Networks within the body short-circuit and cause a breakdown of cells, tissues, or even an entire organ. When the disease progresses, you often develop symptoms. The onset of symptoms leads to a diagnostic evaluation, which then leads to naming the pathology (deviation from normal cells and tissues) or giving it a diagnosis. The symptoms dictate what treatment is recommended, whether drugs, surgery, or some other form of therapy.

Here is a list of the major conditions classified as chronic diseases. Some are potentially life-threatening, while others can impair your daily activities or just make you miserable.

- Autoimmune diseases
- Cancer
- Diabetes
- Digestive disorders
- Heart disease
- Neurological conditions
- Obesity

Z NOTE: Obesity is now considered a chronic disease. Rather than an actual "disease," it is a chronic metabolic and inflammatory condition that can create more serious diseases, such as most of those in the list above. Obesity is typically classified based on a measurement called body mass index (BMI), a value derived from your height and weight that can be an indicator of an unhealthy body composition. BMI is a screening method to categorize your weight, but it does not reveal the amount of fat you have on your body. In the pages that follow, you will find simple calculations that will tell you how overfat you are.

According to the Centers for Disease Control (CDC) and World Health Organization (WHO), chronic disease is the leading cause of death and disability in the United States, accounting for 87 percent of all U.S. deaths, or roughly 1.7 million people, annually. An estimated 50 percent of all Americans have a chronic health condition, and one in four have multiple chronic conditions. The journal *Public Health Reports* projects chronic conditions to rise in the next thirty years. Not surprisingly, health care costs are expected to rise in tandem. The Milken Institute projects that by the year 2023, there will be a 42 percent increase in cases of chronic disease, costing this country $4.2 trillion in treatment fees and lost economic output.

Disease: Inherited or Self-Inflicted?

Dr. Jeffrey Bland, known as the "father of functional medicine" and author of *The Disease Delusion*, has said, "Inherited doesn't mean inevitable." Let me explain.

Genes are sets of instructions programmed for specific functions that control health and patterns of disease. Genes are distinct portions of a cell's DNA that make everything the body needs, especially protein. The proteins produced by genes are the building blocks for everything that allows the body to work properly. As a computer responds to a programmer, genes respond to signals. These signals come from your internal environment, which is determined mainly by the foods you eat, the amount of exercise you get or how much you move, the stressors you experience, your sleep, your exposure to toxins, and your thoughts. If your genes are getting signals from habits that encourage normal function (such as a diet of healthful foods, moderate exercise, and enough sleep), you remain healthy. But if your genes are getting their signals from toxic, processed, inflammatory foods; lack of exercise; chronic unresolved stress; and a lack of sleep, those signals tell the genes to switch on the production of disease.

No single gene causes the development of chronic illness. When the dance between your environment and your gene network goes awry, your physiology begins to deteriorate to the point of dysfunction, what we call disease. Disease can be acute, rapid onset, and short-lived; but chronic disease lasts for a long time. Basically, your unhealthy internal terrain has influenced your genes over a long period of time, and that influence gradually causes the making of a disease.

DISEASES ARE RELATED

An unhealthy internal terrain sets the stage for any number of conditions that lead to disease—sometimes more than one. For example, heart disease is not an isolated pathology that develops within a small artery of the heart. It is created from the combined influence of abnormal blood sugar, the immune system, and distress in the liver. Cancer is not one disease but an accumulation of smaller diseases that interact in a network to create a tumor. The network is made up of high insulin levels, weakened immune cells, poor liver detoxification, abnormal hormone levels, low levels of vitamin D, and DNA damaged by free radicals and nutrient deficiency. Autoimmune diseases develop from a reaction in the gut when certain proteins interact with gut bacteria, an unbalanced immune system, stress hormones from the adrenal glands, and an unhealthy body composition (too much fat and not enough muscle).

A free radical is a simple molecule with a missing electron. To become whole again, free radicals interact with, and steal, electrons from other cells or tissues in the body. Doing so leaves those cells or tissues damaged. This process, called oxidation, has been linked to many chronic diseases.

Z NOTE: Oxidation takes place when free radicals attack and damage the low-density lipoprotein (LDL) particle; think of hail denting the hood of a car. A common theme, threaded throughout the research, states that free radicals from a processed and nutrient-deprived diet, high blood sugar, and smoking are the initiators and main drivers for coronary artery disease, a preventable, lifestyle-based, and often fatal disease.

As you can see, the chronic condition from which you want to rebuild stems from many different systems of the body. Therefore, if you are rebuilding from heart disease, read the diabetes section as well. If you are rebuilding from cancer, read the information on diabetes and obesity. Our current health care system is based on treating the ill with a pill, rather than looking at the broader causes of why diseases develop. We also have specialists who treat just one organ system, rather than treating the whole person to uncover why disease has developed. That's where functional medicine differs from conventional medicine. Functional medicine looks at the whole person as an interconnected system—not a series of independent variables.

Symptoms of a chronic disease can be insidious, or they can come on abruptly, as in a sudden heart attack. Sometimes you get a warning signal that something is wrong. For example, those with developing heart disease may get chest pain (angina) and shortness of breath. In extreme circumstances, the first sign of a major disease—like advanced coronary artery disease —is sudden death due to abrupt heart failure. If you have symptoms in one part of the body, it could mean there's a problem in another part; this is sometimes called referred pain. As you rebuild yourself, it's important to listen to your body and keep track of your symptoms. If you have any, make sure you describe them in detail to your doctor(s).

LEADING CAUSES OF DEATH VS. ACTUAL CAUSES OF DEATH

In the United States, heart disease is the number one killer of men and women, and cancer is the runner-up. Approximately 610,000 people die each year from heart disease, and roughly 589,000 die from cancer. Right behind them are medical errors, stroke, respiratory issues, and diabetes. Yet while these conditions are what we die from, they are only the end results of issues long stewing within us.

A landmark study in the *Journal of the American Medical Association* (*JAMA*) revealed the most prominent causes of mortality in the United

States were tobacco use, poor diet (soon defined, keep reading), and physical inactivity, accounting for 80 percent of the factors that create disease. We have *complete control* over these factors. If you don't smoke, then you need to focus only on poor diet and physical inactivity. Simple, right?

Mortality data reported to the CDC were published in a more recent study found in *JAMA*. Smoking, poor diet, and physical inactivity are still the top killers. However, current trends say a poor diet and inactivity will soon overtake smoking to become the leading causes of early mortality.

The good news is that modifying your personal choices will profoundly affect your health. This is also borne out by research: a large population-based study published in the *Archives of Internal Medicine* showed that people who ate healthful foods, routinely exercised, avoided smoking, and controlled their body composition had an 80 percent lower probability of developing and dying from chronic illnesses. An 80 percent lower probability sounds like a get-out-of-jail-free card to me. Just as heartening is the fact that changes in your lifestyle will help you rebuild from disease and prevent any recurrences. This is why I wrote this book.

I WON'T LIE: rebuilding your health takes discipline and determination; sometimes it's hard work. That's because rebuilding your health is a process, not an event. However, the support protocols (what I call "supportocols") in *Rebuild* are not difficult to implement, and restoring your health is not as complicated as you may think. If you follow the steps in this book, they will help you rebuild your body's internal environment. It worked for me, and it has worked for countless patients who have found themselves dealing with a health crisis.

The following sections explain how the top chronic diseases develop, so you can better understand your condition when you begin your personal rebuild. It's important to also understand that all diseases have common roots in an unhealthy internal terrain. For example, having too much body fat not only is linked to all chronic diseases but is one of the primary drivers of the development of disease. Another common link to all chronic disease is inflammation. As such, I'd advise that you read about each condition even if you don't think it pertains to you, as the root cause is likely relevant to your overall health.

Z NOTE: What is inflammation? Under normal circumstances, the inflammatory response, created by the immune system, is needed to fight foreign invaders and heal injuries. We can feel and see inflammation when there is pain, redness, and heat—a sore throat, a cut, a sprained ankle, even a sunburn. Inflammation is a sign that the immune system is actively fighting infection and/or mending cells and tissues. This type of immune response should be short-lived. However, the body runs into trouble when the immune system runs out of control, creating chronic inflammation. Unmanaged, this type of inflammation can result in cancer, atherosclerosis and coronary artery disease, autoimmune disease, and obesity. The extent of chronic inflammation is influenced by diet, physical inactivity, exposure to toxins, too much stress, and genetics.

Z NOTE: A new study estimates that more than 400,000 Americans are dying each year due to hospital errors. Yes, you read that correctly: 400,000 deaths from mishaps and improper care provided in hospitals. Data published in in the *Journal of Patient Safety* put medical errors as the third leading cause of death in the United States. Errors that cost thousands of lives included improper diagnosis and inappropriate treatment; a procedure done incorrectly; poor communication among doctors; and improper advice and treatment recommendations. John James, PhD, the author of the article, proposed a great strategy to help reduce the incidence of serious harm and death: a national bill of rights for hospitalized patients that would allow them to be more integrated into their personal care so they could take the lead in reducing their risk of serious harm or death. Politics, bureaucracy, and red tape would undoubtedly make this challenging, but it is a suggestion worthy of pursuit. In the wise words of Sophocles, "All men make mistakes, but a good man yields when he knows his course is wrong, and repairs the evil. The only crime is pride."

Cardiovascular Disease

Heart disease remains the leading cause of morbidity (state of poor health) and mortality (death) in the United States with more than 90 million Americans living with some form of cardiovascular disease. Roughly 800,000 people die of heart disease each year; 2,200 people die each day, an average of 1 death every 40 seconds. Almost 800,000 people in the U.S. have heart attacks each year, with coronary artery disease claiming more than 380,000 lives. An estimated 50 percent of males and 30 percent of females over the age of forty will develop coronary artery disease. Although *cardiovascular disease* is an umbrella term encompassing different disorders of the heart and the peripheral blood vessels, coronary artery disease is the most common condition.

Modern medicine has created multiple ways of treating coronary artery disease, including coronary stents, bypass surgery, and drugs to lower cholesterol (statins). Cholesterol has become synonymous with heart disease; for decades we have been told that cholesterol is the single reason for its development. Promotional campaigns by pharmaceutical companies are designed to convince us that the only way to reduce the chance of developing heart disease is to lower cholesterol with the use of statins. Let's take an in-depth look at what cholesterol really is and why it is essential to health.

THE STICK-AND-CLOG THEORY

Cholesterol—a natural fat found in the body—has long been blamed for hardening arteries and the development of coronary artery disease. The pharmaceutical establishment and mainstream media—through pictures and pamphlets—show depictions of cholesterol sticking to and clogging arteries, like melted butter solidifying and sticking to the pipes of your kitchen sink.

Unfortunately, the theory of cholesterol sticking to the arteries has been proven false. According to *Circulation*, the journal of the American Heart Association (AHA), and the *New England Journal of Medicine*, atherosclerosis (clogging of the arteries) is an ongoing inflammatory condition, not the accumulation of fat on the artery wall. If cholesterol does not stick to your arteries, then what *does* it do?

Cholesterol is one of a family of compounds called lipids (fats). It is an essential component of the myelin sheath, the fatty covering that insulates nerve fibers (axons). It is essential for the synthesis of vitamin D and steroid hormones (testosterone, progesterone, pregnenolone, androsterone, estrone, estradiol, corticosterone, and aldosterone), as well as the production of bile for digestion; in fact, every cell in the body needs it to function normally. Cholesterol is produced from fragments of fats, proteins, and carbohydrates by several organs—the liver, gut, adrenal cortex (the glands above your kidneys), ovaries, and testes. Cholesterol from food can also be absorbed by the body, but only to a small extent. Cholesterol prevents pro-inflammatory fats from causing damage to cells. In addition, it acts as an antioxidant that neutralizes free radicals—key ingredients in the formation of atherosclerosis.

We know fat and water don't mix. Blood is a watery system; therefore, cholesterol needs a way to travel through the blood via some transport vehicle. Lipoproteins shuttle cholesterol through the blood. You are probably familiar with the terms LDL and HDL. LDL (low-density lipoprotein) is a protein that brings cholesterol into tissues and arteries. HDL (high-density lipoprotein) shuttles cholesterol away from the heart and arteries to be recycled by the liver. Both HDL and LDL have beneficial jobs in the body. Is there such a thing as "good" or "bad" cholesterol? No. Cholesterol is just cholesterol. LDL and HDL are just the lipoproteins that transport it.

> **FACT:** Fifty percent of those who suffer a heart attack or stroke have normal cholesterol levels. That's right: according to the *New England Journal of Medicine,* 50 percent of those who suffer a heart attack or stroke have LDL cholesterol levels below the current recommendations for treatment. Despite all the brainwashing to consume cholesterol-lowering drugs, the real question is this: Why would something naturally found in the body turn against us? We need to stop targeting cholesterol and focus on inflammation.

MECHANISM OF CORONARY ARTERY DISEASE

Coronary artery disease was once thought of as a "stick-and-clog disease." The AHA now recognizes that coronary artery disease is an inflammatory response created by a hostile environment in the wall of the artery. This process is called *atherosclerosis.* It is characterized by a thickening and hardening of the vessel wall in large and medium-size arteries.

Coronary artery disease develops in stages:

1. Due to a number of reasons—a processed-food diet consisting of white refined flours and sugars and partially hydrogenated vegetable oils, deficiency in antioxidants and vitamin C, smoking, high and uncontrolled blood sugar, high blood pressure, and bacterial infection—the endothelium (a single-cell-thick layer lining the inside of the artery) can become damaged. This allows the passage of LDL cholesterol and white blood cells into the wall of the artery.

2. LDL brings cholesterol into the arterial wall, where it is oxidized (damaged by free radicals). White blood cells, called macrophages, recognize the oxidized LDL and proceed to gobble it up along with its cholesterol.

3. After consuming the damaged LDL, the macrophages turn into foam cells, which spit out inflammatory chemicals and enzymes, causing swelling and damage to the protective layers of cells in the wall. This swelling and damage is called a vulnerable (unstable) plaque and causes a narrowing of the artery and restricted blood flow.

4. The vulnerable plaque has a thin fibrous cap. As the inflammation continues, white blood cells release eroding enzymes. Those enzymes break down the fibrous cap, making the artery prone to rupture. Debris released from the arterial wall forms a thrombus (a mass of blood cells, platelets, and fibrin)—a clot that blocks the artery.

5. The pulsing expansion of the artery from the pumping of the heart causes mechanical stress in the area of the vulnerable plaque. During moments of physical activity or stress, expansion of the artery can cause the vulnerable plaque to erupt, leading to an immediate blockage in the artery, resulting in a sudden lack of blood flow to some part of the heart. This is a heart attack. If the thrombus blocks a cerebral artery (an artery to the brain), it causes a stroke.

(In chapter 8, Testing the Disease Terrain, you will read about a revolutionary panel of biomarkers found in blood work that provides information regarding the inflammation in your arteries. This critical test panel goes far beyond the old standard tests of liver function: cholesterol, LDL cholesterol, HDL cholesterol, and triglycerides. This is not to say you shouldn't have your cholesterol checked as a general screening, but the test does not determine the health of your heart.)

Z NOTE: Cholesterol-lowering drugs (statins) go beyond lowering your cholesterol levels. Statins block inflammation. They function by modifying the orchestrator of inflammation—a genetic switch known as NF-kB. This switch turns on the process of inflammation and its production of pro-inflammatory compounds called cytokines, chemical messengers that communicate with and control the function of other cells. NF-kB and cytokines are involved in all chronic diseases.

What can you do to avoid coronary artery disease? The endothelium (lining of the artery) can be damaged by nutrient-depleted processed foods, smoking, high blood pressure, too much belly fat, thyroid weakness, stress hormones, chronic inflammation, infection, and high blood sugar (hyperglycemia). It's important to make a connection between heart disease and high blood sugar and diabetes. Atherosclerosis is a complex dysfunction with multiple causes, including high blood sugar and too much insulin. Unmanaged blood sugar can cause tissue damage by several mechanisms; one is the addition of a sugar to a protein in a process called glycation. These sugarized proteins are called advanced glycation end products (AGEs). Research published in *Diabetes Care* has demonstrated the detrimental effects of these AGEs on blood vessels. AGEs impair the endothelium, and the glycated proteins cause the passage of white blood cells into the wall of the artery. Both are crucial steps in the development of coronary artery disease.

Z NOTE: As previously stated, atherosclerosis is an inflammatory disease caused by multiple factors, including bacterial toxicity. In the section titled The Leaky Gut Connection (see page 64), you will learn of a destructive and dangerous compound that is released when specific bacteria in the gut die. Lipopolysaccharides (LPS) are toxins released from the broken-down cell wall of dead bacteria; they interact with the lining of the intestine to create increased gut permeability (leaky gut) and systemic inflammation. According to *Cellular Microbiology* and *Human Physiology*, LPS plays critical roles in the development of atherosclerosis. For one, LPS may initially cause the induction of atherosclerosis by damaging the endothelium.

LPS—through inflammatory cytokines—was shown to increase the accumulation of fats in the artery and increase the migration of white blood cells into the arterial wall, thus furthering the progression of inflammation and disease.

DAVE'S STORY

Roughly three years before my "heart event," I had embarked on a new health plan, eliminating all harmful foods—including fried calamari, my favorite junk food—and began an exercise regimen of exercising six days a week, doing weight training, biking, and functional training using the TRX straps. I felt good. However, during one of my workouts, I felt an odd pressure in my chest, which got my attention. I called my general practitioner, who told me to go to the ER. I listened, but then ran some errands and headed home. I was thinking, "I'm healthy, nothing to worry about." Sound familiar? But on the way home the feeling came back, stronger. I took my doctor's advice and headed to the ER. Without delay, diagnostic testing was done to assess what was happening.

It took me by surprise to hear that I needed stents. There was no time for a second opinion; I was told "time is muscle"; stents were my only option. After the procedure, my doctors told me my healthful diet and exercise had allowed me to sail through without pain or complications.

Ironically, at my most recent physical six months earlier, my blood work had shown great numbers, and I received a glowing report from my doctor. That was good to hear, but it's why my need for three stents came as such a surprise. Although I was on the right path, three years of "good" had not been able to overcome sixty-three years of "less-than-good"—eating too much junk food (that fried calamari) and not working out regularly.

Following the procedure, I went to cardio recovery, but the pace was so slow that I felt I was losing conditioning. I wanted to get back to my regular workouts as soon as I could. Many patients there were repeat offenders of the same procedure, and it was not a very stimulating environment.

The focus of my medical treatment was to stay on a number of meds for months and on statin drugs for the rest of my life. I had to fight the doctors to reduce my dosages and to take me off each drug as soon as it was safe (in their minds). I also told them I had no intention of staying on strong statins for the rest of my life. I was sure my diet/exercise/healthy-emotional-life plan would eventually eliminate the need for the statin.

I believe that proper diet and exercise, including a positive attitude, were the keys to accelerating my recovery. I continue to eat well and exercise, despite my doctors' thinking that people don't stick to plans like that; they think I should just stay on the medications they prescribed. I also realized that the tests done during standard physicals are indirect measures of health at best. Despite my glowing reports, the tests did not reveal the state of my cardiovascular system. Therefore, my answer was to stay in charge of my own recovery and health. Years after my stent procedures, I continue to stay on my diet/exercise/emotional-life plan. I'm not taking any meds, and I feel great. At seventy-three years old, I'm enjoying new adventures; I just achieved a personal best with a deadlift of 330 pounds. My advice to you is to find new challenges and strive for your personal best. Check back with me in thirty years.

DR. Z SAYS . . . Dave made an abrupt lifestyle change to overcome sixty-three years of not taking care of himself. Fortunately, he got in the game and saved himself from further internal damage. As with all inflammatory conditions, once they start, they can gain momentum, requiring you to slam on the brakes—with nutrient-dense foods, short bursts of exercise, and, often, targeted supplements—in order to stop the disease process and rewind back to a healthy state.

Right before he heard "time is muscle"—meaning that the longer the heart goes without adequate blood flow (ischemia), the more damage (necrosis) to the heart muscle is created—Dave had gotten a "glowing report" from his doctor. What was done to determine that Dave was in excellent health—the standard fifteen-minute physical exam, unspecific blood work, blood pressure taken in one arm, jumping on a scale, and having someone listen to his heart? Unfortunately, for the majority of people, health evaluations are both antiquated and inadequate. For more on this, see chapter 8, Testing the Disease Terrain, where I outline specific tests you should have done to give you a more detailed picture of the health of your internal terrain.

STROKE

A stroke is essentially a heart attack in the brain. Similar to the mechanism of coronary artery disease, a stroke is caused by a sudden arterial blockage and subsequent reduction of blood flow to some part of the brain. When that flow is interrupted, brain cells no longer receive nutrients and oxygen, and they die. When you are rebuilding from a stroke, you will likely need various forms of physical therapy. However, proper nutrition is still the key to recovery. Throughout this book, I will circle back to nutrition and the importance of whole foods, because—as I said earlier, but it bears repeating—research shows that a poor diet is the number one cause of all chronic disease.

According to the *Journal of Nutrition and Metabolism*, malnutrition and nutrient deficiency are not only serious risk factors for having a stroke; poor nutrition appears to exacerbate brain damage after a stroke and lessen likelihood of successful recovery. Longer hospital stays were also attributed to malnutrition—we know how toxic hospital food is—and malnutrition also worsened impairments due to the actual stroke itself, including an inability to use a limb, depression, or difficulty swallowing. The research found a deficiency of protein and nutrients—including folate; vitamins B_6, B_{12}, and D; zinc; and antioxidant vitamins A, C, and E—were all associated with increased risk of recurrence and poor recovery after a stroke. If you are rebuilding, physical rehab is very important to help prevent atrophy (shrinkage) of your affected limbs. Adopting the supportocols I've outlined in *Rebuild* will give you the best chance for recovery, as well as help prevent permanent impairment.

Z NOTE: Autoimmune diseases are linked to heart disease. For example, rheumatoid arthritis greatly increases your risk for developing atherosclerosis and coronary artery disease. Autoimmune diseases are a group of inflammatory disorders characterized by aggressive immune reactions to different tissues and organs of the body. Systemic autoimmune disorders include rheumatoid arthritis (RA), multiple sclerosis (MS), systemic lupus erythematosus (SLE), and primary Sjögren's syndrome (pSS). The link between atherosclerosis and autoimmune disease is inflammation, driven by specific white blood cells. These same cells drive the process of inflammation in the walls of the arteries.

To summarize, in heart disease, inflammation is the culprit, not cholesterol. The factors that trigger and then drive inflammation include a diet of nutrient-absent and processed foods, smoking, hypertension, high blood sugar, abdominal obesity, psychosocial factors, a lack of consumption of fruits and vegetables, excessive alcohol, physical inactivity, and bacterial toxicity. These are all modifiable factors that are under your control. Later in this book I will explain how.

Cancer

Cancer is a disease of uncontrolled cellular growth, a result of alterations not only to the genetic information within the cells but also to the signals those cells receive from the body. Normally, all cells have stages of development, internal cell mechanisms for regulating cell growth, and eventually a programmed death. This is the natural life cycle for a cell. With natural growth and proliferation, a cell needs checkpoints to make sure its operations work properly. When those checkpoints lose their ability to regulate normal growth, cancer develops.

The checkpoints are specific genes called oncogenes—genes that can transform a cell into a cancer cell—and tumor-suppressor genes—genes that control cell growth and division. They are like the yin and yang of gene regulation. When genes are damaged or mutate, they lose control over cell division, creating uncontrolled cell growth. Unfortunately, due to their compromised checkpoints, mutated cells have no limit on cell division. Unmanaged cell growth eventually leads to the development of a tumor. However, there are genes that can repair the damage causing uncontrolled cell growth. One example is a gene called p53.

The p53 gene is a guardian of your genes. It has two unique functions: it can help repair corrupted DNA, and it can act as a tumor suppressor to slow or stop tumor growth. When DNA gets impaired, p53 puts the brakes on cell function long enough for the cell to repair itself. If the defect can't be repaired, p53 causes the cell to commit suicide—a process known as apoptosis. This natural termination of defective cells is a protective program to prevent the cells from passing on faulty DNA. However, p53 itself can become broken and cease to function normally. This can lead to abnormal cell growth, thus causing the formation of cancer.

Once genes are damaged and can no longer stop cell growth and/or cause the faulty cell to commit suicide, cells with DNA mutations rapidly proliferate until they become a tumor. Once a tumor reaches the size of one millimeter, it needs its own blood supply to provide nutrients for its survival. This tiny tumor spits compounds into the blood that cause neighboring blood vessels to sprout new blood vessels in a process called angiogenesis; these eventually reach the tumor and supply it with nutrients. With this nourishment, the cancer cells continue to rapidly divide, increasing the size of the tumor until it becomes detectable.

With continued growth, cells from the tumor can become invasive and leave their initial growth site to migrate to other parts of the body. This is called metastasis, the process by which cancer cells from a primary site spread to a new location, where they develop into a secondary tumor. Metastasis is a poorly understood process, and for many patients, metastases remain undetected until long after the initial cancer diagnosis. In my research on the process of metastasis, I learned that we have more control over it than we think. According to a study published in *Nature Reviews*, metastasis is an inefficient process. After cancer cells are shed off the primary tumor, they have to survive an attack from the immune system and also circumvent mechanical factors, such as the size of the blood vessels they must travel through. If cancer cells make it to a distant organ, they also have to survive the internal environment of that organ.

To put this into perspective, a study in the *New England Journal of Medicine* states that only a tiny minority (0.01 percent or fewer) of cancer cells entering circulation actually develop into metastases. Simply stated, if ten thousand cancer cells are shed from the primary tumor, only one will survive. A rogue cancer cell, or a group of clones that break off a tumor, rarely survives in the body unless something favors its survival. What is it about the internal environment of the body that would favor the survival of this cell, thus allowing it to grow into a secondary, health-threatening tumor? Similarly, what is it about the internal terrain of the body that prevents the vast majority of cancer cells to set up a home in some other organ?

The immune system presents another obstacle. The immune system is a complex and intricate arrangement of white blood cells that all have some role in defending against a possible threat. As the body's watchdog, it has evolved to scout, search, and destroy bacteria and viruses, as well as unwanted cells, including cancer cells.

T lymphocytes—a type of white blood cell—play a pivotal role in killing cancer. One specific type of T lymphocyte is called a natural killer (NK) cell. Its job is to find and kill cancer cells and cells infected by viruses. When the immune system is fully charged, NK cells find and attach to cancer cells, then kill them in two ways. In the first, they inject chemicals into the cancer cell, which causes an influx of free radicals, called an "oxidative burst," that damages the machinery in the cell and causes its death. The second way NK cells destroy cancer involves the death receptor pathway. (Sounds cool, doesn't it?) Here, the NK cell comes into contact with a cancer cell and activates a ligand (an ion or molecule that acts as a flag) on the surface of the cell, which then sends a signal into the cancer cell instructing it to activate its self-destruct program. As a result, the cancer cell dies.

But we run into a problem when our immune system ceases to target and kill cancer cells. When we compromise the immune system via stress, eating processed foods, overexercising, and overloading our bodies with toxins, cancer gains a survival advantage and puts us in danger.

To summarize, cancer develops as a result of a series of cellular changes caused by errors or dysfunction in the genes that control specific cellular processes. Researchers recognize that the biology of a tumor is made up of not one cell type, but a collection of different mutated cells. This is why there will never be a single magic bullet to cure cancer. It will require different therapies based on the individual and the makeup of his or her genetically unique cancer.

CAUSES OF CANCER

According to work published in *Pharmaceutical Research*, only 5 to 10 percent of all cancer cases can be traced to genetic defects, while the overwhelming majority are born of unhealthful lifestyles. You may have heard that certain lifestyle habits can contribute to the development of cancer, but not really know what that means. Listed within each one of the following habits or behaviors are more detailed reasons for its connection to the development of cancer.

Nutrient-Deficient Processed Foods
Nutrient deficiency causes DNA damage and poor cellular repair, poor detoxification of hormones and environmental toxins, high blood sugar and insulin, and chronic inflammation.

Physical Inactivity
Lack of exercise can increase estrogen levels and inflammatory hormone-producing fat, weaken the immune system, and cause high blood sugar and insulin levels.

Unhealthy Body Composition (Being Overfat)
Fat produces cancer-promoting compounds called adipocytokines. Fat can also increase estrogen levels and cause inflammation that can trigger cancer and drive the cancer process.

Chronic Stress
Reactions to stress cause surges of hormones, including cortisol, adrenaline, and norepinephrine. These hormones suppress the immune system, cause inflammation, and ignite and fuel all stages of tumor development.

Smoking, Toxins, and Other Environmental Pollutants
Chemicals from smoking, processed foods, and the environment can act like hormones, damage DNA, and cause vitamin deficiencies.

Poor Sleep

Lack of sleep disrupts many cellular, metabolic, and physiological functions, ultimately increasing inflammation; preventing DNA repair; increasing hormone abnormalities, including cortisol; and causing immune suppression.

Most cancers (90 to 95 percent) are due to both eating processed foods and not eating enough nutrients—in other words, a poor diet. However, current media hype says cancer is just bad luck. According to that theory, for some unknown reason, all your specialized cancer-fighting processes simply break down. If this is the case, why are so many businesses raising money to stave off "bad luck"? People are led to believe that they have no control over their health. That, in turn, allows them to continue their unhealthful lifestyles.

You *do* have control over your health. If you disrespect your genes, they will turn on you and cause disease. Respect them, and your health will be amazing. Rebuilding from cancer and preventing a future crisis requires that you eat nutrient-dense foods; exercise with short moments of intensity; put your stressors in check; eliminate environmental and food-based toxins; and get enough sleep.

Z NOTE: Nutrient deficiency causes cancer. The damage a nutrient-deprived diet inflicts on a cell's DNA mimics the effects of radiation. Dr. Bruce Ames, professor emeritus of biochemistry and molecular biology at the University of California, Berkeley, found that deficiencies of the micronutrients folate, vitamin B_6, vitamin B_{12}, niacin, vitamin C, vitamin E, iron, and zinc cause DNA damage that will contribute to the formation of cancer. Deficiencies of folate, vitamin B_6, and vitamin B_{12} in particular were found to cause breaks in certain parts of chromosomes in the same manner as radiation would.

Countless studies have shown that vitamins, minerals, antioxidants, and other bioactive compounds from fruits and vegetables reduce the incidence of all cancers, and those who don't eat enough nutrient-dense fruits and vegetables have a much higher cancer rate. In chapter 3, you will learn about the importance of food and the nutrients within certain food groups that will further enhance your ability to rebuild yourself.

Eating right has an additional crucial benefit: it dissolves the link between cancer and body fat, blood sugar, and inflammation. There are two types of body fat, also known as adipose tissue: subcutaneous fat, which forms the layer just beneath the skin; and visceral fat, the dangerous fat deep inside the body that surrounds the organs. Visceral fat and the hormones it produces are like a petri dish for the development and progression of cancer. Visceral fat is involved in numerous mechanisms that promote tumor development. Both fat and tumors are low in oxygen, a state called hypoxia. When both fat cells and cancer cells lack oxygen, they release a protein called hypoxia-inducible factor 1 (HIF1). HIF1 from fat cells is known to cause dysfunction in the immune system, and contributes to all stages of cancer development, including cell growth, proliferation, and metastasis. When released by a tumor, HIF1 causes surrounding blood vessels to sprout new blood vessels to provide nutrients to the developing tumor. Visceral fat will also release a protein called fibroblast growth factor 2 in the body, which can cause a non-cancerous cell to turn into a cancerous one.

There is a connection between cancer and high blood sugar as well. A high-sugar, low-nutrient diet causes high blood sugar levels, which eventually trigger the release of high amounts of insulin to deal with the excess sugar. Insulin acts on a cell much like a key in a lock, causing a gate in the cell to open and allow blood sugar in. In a normal state, when your blood sugar elevates, insulin helps get the sugar into your liver and muscles, where it is stored as an energy source called glycogen; the excess is stored as fat.

However, when your diet contains too much sugar for your body to handle, your cells eventually *reject* insulin, a condition known as insulin resistance. This causes excess sugar to remain in the blood, leading to an increase in both subcutaneous and visceral fat. The visceral fat eventually becomes a hormone-producing organ that causes more insulin resistance, inflammation, and the production of the hormone estrogen. Here is where the danger lies. Research published in the journals *Integrative Cancer Therapies* and *Diabetology & Metabolic Syndrome* shows the role of the hormones insulin and insulin-like growth factor 1 (IGF1) in enhancing cancer growth and tumor development. Insulin and IGF1 were shown to increase cancer proliferation and prevent cancer cells from activating their programmed cell death.

Fat is also a metabolically active organ, producing many proteins and inflammatory compounds called adipocytokines. These include interleukin 6 (IL-6), tumor necrosis factor (TNF), and leptin—all chemical messengers created by fat cells. IL-6 is an inflammatory agent that has many effects, including regulating different malignant cancers (prostate, lung, and breast). IL-6 is known to increase cancer cell proliferation, survival, and invasion into other tissues. IL-6 was also shown to suppress the components of the immune system needed to fight cancer and tumor activity. Thus, being overfat causes a metabolic mishap that leads to insulin resistance, inflammation, and the development of cancer.

REBUILD DURING CANCER CARE

Can you rebuild yourself while you are undergoing chemotherapy? Yes. To do so, you need to know exactly which chemotherapy drugs you are getting, what side effects to expect, why those side effects occur, and what you can do to combat them.

The term *chemotherapy* means to fight disease with chemicals. Pharmaceutical agents destroy the cancer both by direct damage and by interrupting the cancer cells' ability to replicate. Chemo also destroys healthy cells, especially cells that reproduce quickly, including those found in the gut, hair follicles, sperm, eggs, and the lining of the mouth. Chemo drugs cause injury to all cells, tissues, and organs, resulting in a variety of unpleasant side effects that can range from mild to devastating. As you go through conventional cancer care, knowing what to expect in terms of side effects will allow you more control when combating those side effects. If you are rebuilding yourself during your cancer care, here is a list of potential side effects, which may be temporary or permanent:

- Fatigue due to anemia (low red blood cell and hemoglobin counts). Chemo can damage bone marrow, reducing the number of red blood cells.
- Immune system suppression due to neutropenia (low white blood cell count). Bone marrow suppression or damage can also cause neutropenia.
- Low platelet count.
- Nausea and vomiting.
- Loss of appetite and diminished capacity to taste.
- Nutrient malabsorption. Chemo drugs can destroy the cells of the stomach lining (parietal cells) responsible for secreting hydrochloric acid, which is essential for activating pepsinogen, an enzyme needed to digest protein. Chemo can also damage the cells that produce a protein called the intrinsic factor, which is needed for the absorption of vitamin B_{12}. This can also contribute to anemia.
- Painful mouth sores (mucositis).
- Constipation. Destruction of the cells lining the colon can disrupt bowel function, impairing movement of waste through the bowel and decreasing mucus secretion. This will cause constipation. Chemo can also interfere with nutrient and protein absorption in the gut, leading to muscle loss (sarcopenia) and wasting syndrome (cachexia).
- Peripheral neuropathy (nerve pain and tingling in the hands and feet). This can be extremely painful and disabling.
- Hair loss. Nothing will stop this.
- Brain fog.

- Heart damage or failure. The chemo drug Adriamycin (known to many patients as Red Death) is a toxic drug that destroys muscle cells of the heart.
- Infertility.
- Early onset of menopause or menopausal symptoms in women.
- Weight loss/weight gain from changes in metabolism.
- Hearing loss.
- Respiratory disorders, including pulmonary fibrosis.
- Kidney and bladder dysfunction.
- Eye irritation.
- Secondary cancers. Why? Because these drugs damage DNA. Anticancer drugs attach to DNA just like any other toxin. When a chemical becomes attached to DNA, it is called a DNA adduct. Each time a cell divides, the DNA adduct is passed along, thus increasing the chance of DNA damage and the production of a secondary cancer. (You can read more about DNA adducts on page 334.)
- Swelling (lymphedema).
- Blood has difficulty clotting.
- Difficulty swallowing.
- Fluid accumulation in the abdomen (ascites).
- Foot drop (dragging of the foot while walking), caused by nerve damage.
- Infections from immune suppression. Chemo will destroy your white blood cells, resulting in a low white blood cell count, or neutropenia. Weekly blood testing will determine if you need Neulasta, a drug that increases your white blood cell count.
- Mental confusion.
- Joint and muscle pain.
- Shortness of breath.
- Skin conditions and reactions.
- Insomnia.

- Urinary incontinence.
- Depression.

This list creates fear and concern, for sure. Who wants to hear about the possibility of developing permanent nerve pain, heart damage, or a secondary cancer? Fortunately, the supportocols in *Rebuild* will mitigate the side effects of the chemo and lessen your suffering. The tools in this book will also keep you strong so you can continue your day-to-day activities. Chemotherapy causes malnutrition and nutrient deficiencies, particularly of vitamin C, folate, and vitamin B_6. Eliminating unhealthful processed foods, bread, dairy, and sugar and eating plenty of nutrient-dense foods will help you avoid these deficiencies and boost the effectiveness of chemotherapy. Radiation (radiotherapy) as a cancer treatment also has its list of complications, including malnutrition, nutrient malabsorption, and deficiencies. Patients receiving radiation therapy to the head, neck, and abdomen frequently experience symptoms ranging from painful mouth sores and swallowing, to nausea, vomiting, abdominal pain, and diarrhea, all of which can lead to an inability to ingest and digest food.

However, the uninformed oncology community has warned patients going through cancer care to refrain from taking nutraceuticals (supplements), as they might interfere with the toxic effects of chemotherapy drugs. Research conducted by Dr. Charles Simone and published in the journal *Alternative Therapies* found this not to be the case. Dr. Simone and his researchers collected data from 280 peer-reviewed studies that included 5,081 patients who took supplements while undergoing chemotherapy. Their findings revealed that nonprescription antioxidants and other supplemental nutrients did not interfere with the cytotoxic effects of chemo. They actually found the opposite to be true: vitamins A, C, D, E, and K; beta-carotene; selenium; cysteine; and B vitamins enhanced the cancer-killing effects of chemo while protecting normal tissue. Patients taking these nutrients had fewer side effects and, most important, increased survival rates compared with those who took no nutrient supplements.

I can attest to the truth of this research based on my own personal experience with chemo, as well as the experiences my patients have had while rebuilding during their cancer care. With proper nutrition and targeted supplements, you can significantly mitigate the debilitating impact of chemotherapy and prepare your body to rebuild after treatment. Once your cancer care is completed, you will also experience a speedier recovery, as well as improved health and fitness.

REBUILD FROM BREAST CANCER

The global impact of breast cancer is enormous, and growing. Since human genes have remained constant for eons, the only plausible reason for this epidemic is dysfunction of the internal terrain. According to the CDC and the American Cancer Society, breast cancer is the second leading cause of cancer deaths among women, after lung cancer. In 2017, an estimated 252,710 new cases of invasive breast cancer were diagnosed among women, and 2,470 cases were diagnosed in men. In addition, 63,410 cases of in-situ breast cancer were diagnosed in women. Most serious, approximately 40,610 women and 460 men were expected to die from the disease.

Contrary to the common assumption that breast cancer is genetic, a study published in the *Journal of Epidemiology Community Health* states, "Genetic inheritance is an infrequent, but not the main, cause of breast cancer." The consensus is that breast cancer susceptibility, or genetic cancer predisposition, is associated with only 4 to 8 percent of breast cancer cases. These estimates are uniform across the spectrum of medical studies. Research published in the *New England Journal of Medicine* found that only 7 percent of women from families with a history of breast cancer had BRCA1 mutations. BRCA1 and BRCA2 are the well-known genes associated with the development of breast cancer. They are tumor-suppressor genes that produce proteins to help repair damaged DNA. If these genes mutate or become damaged, they fail to produce the right proteins, and the damaged DNA may not be repaired. This can lead to more mutations and, eventually, the development of breast cancer. According to research published in the journal *Carcinogenesis*, mutations of the BRCA1 and BRCA2 genes account for only 5 percent of breast cancer cases in the United States annually.

Here is a key question: If genes cause breast cancer, why is it so rare for adolescent girls to develop breast cancer? Why does it show up in women in their thirties, forties, and fifties? Basically, genes like BRCA1/BRCA2 or the p53 gene don't just fail. The body's internal environment causes those genes to stop functioning as they were intended. Remember, our cells have checks and balances to regulate cell growth, create differentiation, and even trigger the death of malfunctioning cells. Breast cancer, along with other tissue cancers, stems from a malfunction in these control mechanisms that leads to uncontrolled cellular growth and tumor formation.

The regulation of estrogen, insulin, and insulin-like growth factors—hormones that can play a role in the development of breast cancer—are all controlled by diet, exercise, and stress levels. Eating nutrient-deficient, high-calorie foods and dairy; carrying too much body fat; smoking; drinking excessive alcohol; vitamin D deficiency; and environmental exposure to pollutants like bisphenol A (BPA) from plastics increase the risk for breast cancer, as does a high intake of unhealthful fats during hormone replacement therapy (HRT). HRT has been clinically proven to induce cell proliferation. According to research published in *Perspectives in Cancer Research*, "Chronic administration of estrogen [a primary component of HRT] results in tumor formation." Yet despite the research, HRT is still prescribed.

You may have heard that breast cancer is driven by estrogen. How does that happen? Estrogen is a hormone essential for normal sexual development, and it helps control a woman's menstrual cycle—a process that prepares the body for reproduction. Estrogen is also important for a woman's heart and bones, as well as the development of the breasts and reproductive organs. Many of the cells in the body, both healthy and potentially cancerous, have estrogen receptors on them. These receptors stimulate cell growth when they come in contact with estrogen. Raising your lifetime levels of estrogen, as well as the length of time your cells are exposed to estrogen, increases your risk of developing breast cancer.

Your body composition plays a role here: too much body fat can raise your estrogen levels. Fat tissue creates an enzyme called aromatase, which can transform other hormones into estrogen. Believe it or not, cancer cells can also produce aromatase, thereby increasing estrogen levels. It would seem that cancer may have been initiated and then driven by the high levels of estrogen from both the fat and the cancer itself. In chapter 3, you will read about foods that can shut down the production of aromatase, reducing your estrogen levels and thus your chance of developing breast cancer.

High blood sugar levels have a connection with breast cancer, too. Insulin and the hormone IGF1 are the other major hormones implicated in breast cancer. Similar to estrogen, insulin and IGF1 have strong anabolic (growth) effects, resulting in increased cell growth and proliferation. A study published in the *Journal of Clinical Oncology* sheds light on the link among type 2 diabetes, insulin, and breast cancer. The authors of the study discovered that breast cancer cells have an abundance of insulin and IGF1 receptors, which, once turned on by insulin and IGF1, cause the rapid growth of breast cancer. Type 2 diabetes and high insulin levels are the direct result of an unhealthful diet.

One more important factor in breast cancer is vitamin D. This is produced in the body when UV radiation from the sun comes in contact with the skin. The sun's energy turns a form of cholesterol in the skin into a pre–vitamin D, which is then processed in the liver and sent to the kidneys, where it becomes the active hormone 1,25-dihydroxyvi-tamin D_3 (calcitriol). (See section on vitamin D in chapter 3 for more information.) Every single tissue in the body has receptors for vitamin D, as vitamin D is required for more than just healthy bones. It regulates genes that control cell growth and development in various tissues of the body, including breast tissue.

Calcitriol (the active form of vitamin D) was found to turn off cell proliferation and tumor growth. Studies published in the *Indian Journal of Pharmacology* found that vitamin D and the vitamin D receptor shut down tumor growth in the breast and interfered with the anabolic effects of insulin and IGF1 on breast cancer cells. Sound too good to be true? Another study, published in *Annals of Epidemiology*, found that raising blood levels of vitamin D from 30 ng/ml to a therapeutic level of 40 to 60 ng/ml would prevent 58,000 new cases of breast cancer (and 49,000 new cases of colorectal cancer) each year.

Diabetes

Diabetes mellitus is a condition of high blood sugar resulting from either inadequate insulin production (type 1 diabetes) or lack of cellular response to insulin (type 2 diabetes). Some of the symptoms of diabetes include increased thirst and hunger, frequent urination, impotence in men, and numbness or tingling in the hands and feet (peripheral neuropathy).

Type 1 diabetes (also known as juvenile diabetes and insulin-dependent diabetes) is caused by an autoimmune reaction; the immune system destroys the beta cells of the pancreas, resulting in extremely low insulin levels. Type 1 diabetes has always been regarded as having an unknown cause. Its development has been blamed on viruses, German measles, mumps, and, of course, genes. While viruses and bacteria can spark the immune process, the foods we are introduced to early in life may also cause autoimmune diseases. The journals *Diabetes* and *PLOS ONE* found that the protein casein in cow's milk and the protein gliadin—a component of gluten in grains—caused an immune response that destroyed the cells of the pancreas, causing them to fail to produce insulin and triggering type 1 diabetes.

Type 2 diabetes (also known as adult-onset diabetes) is characterized by high blood sugar as a result of cells failing to respond to the hormone insulin. Normally, when your blood sugar goes up, the pancreas produces insulin, which triggers cells to take in the sugar. When cells don't respond to insulin, blood sugar elevates, causing the pancreas to release more insulin and contributing to the development of hyperinsulinemia (high levels of insulin in the blood). Type 2 diabetes is now a global epidemic. Statistics from the International Diabetes Federation (IDF) show that 387 million people have diabetes; those numbers are projected to rise to 592 million by 2035. Currently, diabetes costs this country $310 billion in annual health care expenditures. According to the IDF, cardiovascular disease is the major cause of death in diabetics, accounting for 50 percent of all diabetes-related fatalities.

Both types of diabetes have an inflammatory component in their cause. Type 1 is the direct result of an immune reaction destroying the insulin-producing cells of the pancreas. Type 2 is caused by cells rejecting the function of insulin due to an unhealthful diet and too much body fat. As stated previously, body fat releases inflammatory compounds called adipocytokines, which are known to contribute to insulin resistance. Uncontrolled high blood sugar can also cause inflammation from the creation of sugar-derived compounds called advanced glycation end products (AGEs). These crystallized proteins increase free radicals and turn on NF-kB—the orchestrator of inflammation. This causes the production of numerous inflammatory cytokines, which rapidly accelerate the disease process occurring in atherosclerosis, cancer, and diabetes.

This brings us back to the point that chronic diseases are not separate entities, but are connected through a dysfunctional internal terrain. The link between diabetes or high insulin and cancer was shown in a study published in *Integrative Cancer Therapies*. The study found that insulin enhances cancer cell growth by allowing a steady flow of nutrients, including glucose and amino acids, to cancer cells. Insulin was also found to increase unwanted hormones and to activate receptors on the surface of cells responsible for accelerated cell growth and proliferation.

Type 2 diabetics with increased belly fat and other markers of insulin resistance have a higher incidence of colon cancer. Likewise, insulin has in recent years been implicated in the onset of colon cancer. A low-fiber diet and consumption of red meat have historically been blamed for the development of colon cancer, but mounting evidence suggests that insulin and IGF1 are the primary drivers. Research published in the *Journal of Nutrition* and the *American Journal of Clinical Nutrition* consistently showed high levels of insulin and IGF1 in people with colon cancer. Other studies indicate that a diet high in sugar and simple starches stimulates insulin production and the growth of colon cancer cells.

On the list of physical ailments and diseases that stem from diabetes is sleep apnea, a serious disorder in which you periodically stop breathing while you sleep. Chronic sleep apnea is associated with higher rates of heart disease, high blood pressure, brain fog, and serious fatigue. Poor sleep increases your risk for heart disease, cancer, and immune suppression (more on sleep in chapter 6). Sleep apnea is typically associated with being overfat, which sets you up for low-grade inflammation and insulin resistance. Studies published in the *Journal of Applied Physiology* and the *American Journal of Respiratory and Critical Care Medicine* suggest that sleep apnea is independently associated with poor control of blood glucose and insulin levels. If you want to get rid of that bothersome CPAP machine, you need to rebuild your body: get rid of the excess fat, and get your blood sugar and insulin under control.

Z NOTE: If you feel tired after you eat, you may have a problem regulating your blood sugar. This may be due to insulin resistance and/or high or low cortisol levels. See chapter 8, Testing the Disease Terrain, for more information on specific tests to have done when you are rebuilding from insulin resistance and the complications of diabetes.

Supportocols to lowering your blood sugar naturally:

- First, eliminate bread and refined baked goods, dairy, and all refined sugar from your diet.
- Eat five servings of plant-based nutrient-dense foods a day. This will ensure normal blood sugar levels and provide you with nutrients and fiber that regulate glucose metabolism and the output of insulin.
- Exercise with periods of intensity. High-intensity interval training (HIIT) will quickly improve insulin sensitivity and help your muscles pick up sugars from the blood. (See chapter 4.)
- Rebuild your blood sugar with magnesium, vitamin D, and EGCG (a plant-based compound in green tea).
- Drink plenty of water.
- Let's not forget stress. Stress triggers the body to increase your blood sugar to prepare you for fight-or-flight action. If you have diabetes, the stress reaction can make your blood sugar worse. You will learn all about the stress reaction in chapter 5.
- Get seven to eight hours of sleep a night. Not enough sleep creates hormonal changes during the day that cause you to crave high-sugar foods—the reason behind diabetes. See chapter 6 for more on sleep.

DIABETES AND ALZHEIMER'S DISEASE

It's important to bring up another chronic disease associated with diabetes—Alzheimer's disease. This is a deteriorating neurological condition characterized by the formation of beta amyloid plaques, abnormal clusters of protein that build up between nerve cells in the brain. These clusters clump together, causing failed electrical signals, nerve atrophy, and, eventually, nerve death. This reaction turns on the immune system, which triggers the inflammatory response, causing further destruction to the nerve cells and brain. The symptoms of Alzheimer's include dementia, forgetfulness, confusion, and eventual brain failure and death.

Alzheimer's is also an inflammatory condition, similar to diabetes, that I call "inflammatory diabetes of the brain." In fact, Alzheimer's is now being considered type 3 diabetes. Research published in the *Journal of Alzheimer's Disease* links abnormal blood sugar, insulin, and IGF1 as major causes of beta amyloid proteins and plaque production. The amyloid plaques that develop in the brain, as well as chronic insulin resistance, both increase the harmful cytokines IL-6 and TNF, which cause nerve-signaling dysfunction and nerve damage. Data from *Frontiers in Aging Neuroscience* show that low-grade inflammation is linked to the cognitive dysfunction seen in Alzheimer's disease.

Growing evidence shows that the development of Alzheimer's disease is also linked to an unhealthful diet of processed foods. Chronic exposure to nitrosamines (carcinogenic compounds) contributes to the development of insulin resistance, a fatty liver, and Alzheimer's disease. Nitrosamines are found in processed cured meats and bacon, cheese, and milk products, as well as tobacco smoke, chewing tobacco, and the vapor from e-cigarettes. Data from *Mutation Research* show that nitrosamines found in processed meat also increase the risk of developing cancer of the stomach, esophagus, and nasopharynx.

Z NOTE: Food for thought—literally. Although diabetes does not cause Alzheimer's disease, they have the same root: an unhealthful diet full of refined white sugars and processed foods that cause a yo-yo effect with your blood sugar and insulin. The link between a poor diet and Alzheimer's again voids the notion that chronic disease is all in your genes.

Overfat and Obesity

According to the CDC, 69 percent of the adult population is overfat and 35 percent is obese. Why is this significant? Excessive body fat, especially visceral fat (the fat surrounding your organs), can release hormones, modify your appetite, increase inflammation, and increase your risk of developing diabetes, high blood pressure, heart disease, cancer, sleep apnea, arthritis, reproductive issues, and gallbladder problems, to name a few. Obesity is not only taking a toll on health; it is affecting the economy: the annual cost to deal with obesity-related conditions is roughly $147 billion. Simply stated, being overfat and/or obese is dangerous and expensive.

Being overfat and/or obese is a catch-22. There are specific metabolic steps that create obesity, as well as metabolic changes in the body that create disease caused by the excessive body fat. Being overfat or obese results from a chronic imbalance between energy intake and energy expenditure. Too much energy in and not enough energy out creates fat.

As discussed earlier, there are two types of fat: subcutaneous (under the skin) and visceral (inside the body surrounding the organs). Subcutaneous fat may be a nuisance and make buying nice jeans difficult, but visceral fat increases your risk of developing the most serious diseases. Visceral fat serves as a reserve of energy for the body, but it can also produce hormones and cause chronic inflammation.

JC'S STORY

Here's a quick backstory on JC: the general manager of a high-end car business, he is a workaholic with erratic eating habits—late-night eater, fast eater, and, under stress, binge eater. (Sound familiar?) Consequently, JC had become obese and suffered from low energy, sleep apnea, knee pain, and difficulty urinating. As he pushed through the day, his energy puttered out from chronic stress and poor nutrition. Let's not forget his interrupted sleep from the apnea, which required him to hook up to a CPAP machine every night before going to bed.

When JC came to see me, he was fed up and frustrated with the state of his health. He had also watched his father slowly deteriorate and pass away from Parkinson's disease. Fearing he might follow in his father's footsteps, JC was highly motivated to rebuild himself back to health. Following a comprehensive workup, including blood work, hormone profiling, and a body composition evaluation, we diagnosed the following: low testosterone, low vitamin D, high blood sugar, high hemoglobin A1c (a long-term blood sugar marker), low cortisol levels throughout the day, and 37 percent body fat.

There were multiple mechanisms at play: Eating nutrient-deficient, high-calorie foods elevated his blood sugar and insulin. With little physical activity and poor eating habits, his body composition shifted to one of excessive fat. His elevated body fat and blood sugar caused decreased signaling from the hypothalamic-pituitary region of the brain to the testes, resulting in low testosterone levels. High blood sugar and insulin levels can cause sleep apnea and enlargement of the prostate, which contributed to his difficulty urinating. Finally, his low cortisol levels (a condition known as adrenal fatigue) were a consequence of his high-stress work environment and also certainly due in part to not eating enough nutrient-dense foods.

Based on his test results, I worked with him to create a personalized food plan of five to six small meals of nutrient-dense foods to be eaten throughout the day, not just late at night or when it was convenient. I stressed that eating during the day allowed his body to use the nutrients and calories from the foods—rather than eating a lot of food late, which would shift his body into storing the unused calories (energy) as fat.

I emphasized also that the more nutrient-dense foods he ate, the more fat he would lose. At first, he couldn't grasp the concept. *More food = less body fat?* The principle was counterintuitive to what he'd been told all his life. However, eating more calories creates more body fat. Eating nutrients, not calories, causes the body to get rid of fat.

The food plan was supplemented with specific nutraceuticals to improve adrenal function, in turn increasing energy, regulating blood sugar, and increasing testosterone levels. I had custom orthotics made to support his feet, thus reducing the mechanical issues in his knee that were causing him pain.

Following his plan, JC has lost 120 pounds of body fat to date. His cortisol and testosterone levels are back to normal. Functionally speaking, he has little knee pain, more energy, and no difficulty urinating, and with more time, I expect he will no longer depend on his CPAP machine.

FAT AND CANCER

Studies have shown that excessive body fat and obesity are associated with hormone-dependent cancers (such as breast and prostate cancers), along with cancers of the esophagus, pancreas, colon and rectum, and kidney. A cancer prognosis is also adversely affected by a patient's excessive body fat. We have already covered the link between body fat and cancer (see page 38), but let's dig deeper into the scientific causes: estrogen and inflammation.

It's disturbing to think that estrogen, a natural hormone found in both women and men, is a cancer-causing agent. As mentioned earlier, fat tissue produces the enzyme aromatase, which converts other hormones into estrogen. Under normal circumstances, estrogen undergoes a process called oxidative metabolism, in which liver enzymes modify and change estrogen into three different forms: 2-hydroxyestrone, 4-hydroxyestrone, and 16-alpha-hydroxyestrone. The form 2-hydroxyestrone has a protective effect against estrogen-induced cancers in specific organs, including the breast and prostate. On the dark side, the form 16-alpha-hydroxyestrone, and to a lesser extent 4-hydroxyestrone, *promotes* breast and other cancers. Breast tissue also produces higher levels of 16-alpha-hydroxyestrone and lower 2-hydroxyestrone, a combination that increases the risk of developing cancer. (Additionally, when these estrogen forms get damaged by free radicals, they can in turn damage DNA, leading to cell mutations and the formation of cancer.)

So what can you do to reduce the 16 and raise the 2? Cruciferous vegetables, such as kale, broccoli, cauliflower, and Brussels sprouts, contain a compound called indole-3-carbinol (I3C) that steers estrogen into creating 2-hydroxyestrone and simultaneously shuts down the production of 16-alpha-hydroxyestrone. (You will read more about the benefits of cruciferous vegetables and I3C in chapter 3.)

Individuals with excessive body fat have higher estrogen levels, and the tissues of obese/overweight and overfat women are exposed to more estrogen stimulation than the tissues of women who are lean. In men, there is evidence that increased body fat and estrogen act as fuel for prostate cancer. That's because on the surface of prostate cells, there are receptors called estrogen receptor alpha (ERalpha) and estrogen receptor beta (ERbeta). ERalpha promotes cell proliferation, and ERbeta shuts it down, either directly or by blocking the effects of ERalpha. Although other growth factors are involved, like insulin and IGF1, research is pointing to estrogen as a trigger for prostate cancer.

Studies have also shown that being overfat is associated with cancers of the kidney, gallbladder, esophagus, and colon. Going further than that, a study published in the *New England Journal of Medicine* reported that increased body fat is associated with increased death rates for *all* cancers. Studies in the *Journal of Clinical Investigation, Frontiers in Bioscience,* and *Trends in Molecular Medicine* reveal the influence interleukin 6 (IL-6) and tumor necrosis factor (TNF), two of the inflammatory adipocytokines produced by body fat, have on the cancer microenvironment. TNF was found to initiate tumor growth and proliferation, and to increase angiogenesis (blood vessel development; see page 36), tumor invasion into tissues, and tumor metastasis. It was also shown to make cancer cells resistant to chemotherapy and radiation.

If a cancer doesn't respond to the different chemotherapies thrown at it, chances are good that inflammation is blocking the effects of the treatments. At the same time, chemo is killing healthy cells and tissues, setting the patient up for the miserable side effects associated with toxic cancer drugs (see page 42). Things get worse: IL-6 helps keep cancer cells alive by deactivating their built-in suicide program, and was also shown to increase cancer cell growth and proliferation, and contribute to insulin resistance, another trigger for the growth of tumors.

Being overfat can also increase your risk of developing cancer by suppressing a component of the immune system needed to kill cancer: natural killer (NK) cells (see page 37). A study published in *Autoimmunity Reviews* discovered that the soup of inflammation created in fat tissue lowered the number of NK cells.

FAT AND DIABETES

Adipose tissue is a highly complex and active organ, producing inflammatory chemical messengers and hormones that have many effects in the body; one of those is insulin resistance. Many studies have documented that visceral fat is closely associated with type 2 diabetes. When you eat too many sugars and carbs, the excess energy from these food sources gets stored as fat. Over time, the fat cells swell like oversized water balloons, then release IL-6, TNF, and free fatty acids (fat released from adipose tissue and transported in the bloodstream). Fatty acids are similar to glucose (blood sugar) in that both are used as fuel for the body. When the body contains too much fat, there are too many circulating free fatty acids. These block the actions of insulin, leading to the onset of type 2 diabetes. It's a vicious metabolic cycle that perpetuates itself.

FAT AND HEART DISEASE

IL-6 from fat travels into the liver, causing the production of another harmful protein called C-reactive protein (CRP). Numerous studies have shown that baseline levels of CRP are highly predictive of future heart attack, stroke, and sudden cardiac death. CRP can also be used as a marker to predict future coronary events in those who have already had a heart attack.

Adding salt to the wound, TNF plays an important role in damaging the lining of the arteries, which is the first step in the development of atherosclerosis and coronary artery disease.

FAT AND AUTOIMMUNE DISEASE

Toxic fat is also associated with autoimmune conditions including Crohn's disease, rheumatoid arthritis, systemic lupus erythematosus, Hashimoto's thyroiditis, multiple sclerosis, type 1 diabetes, and psoriatic arthritis. The question is, how? In recent decades, a dramatic increase in cases of autoimmune disease has paralleled the major growth of obesity. Fat can suppress the function of natural killer cells, increasing susceptibility to infection and cancer. Fat tissue will also inhibit the function of a specialized white blood cell called a regulatory T cell, which acts like a mediator in the immune system to prevent excessive immune responses. When regulatory T cells fail to function, the unruly division of the immune system goes after the body's own cells and tissues, a condition known as autoimmunity.

Among the inflammatory adipocytokines produced by body fat is the hormone leptin. It plays a major role in regulating appetite and energy expenditure. When fat cells get bigger and more toxic, they spit out more leptin, which has the adverse effect of promoting inflammation, while at the same time suppressing regulatory T cells. Research in *Autoimmunity Reviews* found a link between the foods that cause obesity—the Western diet, including synthetic salts, processed sugars, and unhealthful fats—and abnormalities in gut bacteria, resulting in reduced function of the regulatory T cells.

Now that you see how detrimental excessive body fat is on the body and its link to serious disease, here is a more detailed list of the conditions linked to being overfat:

- Asthma
- Autoimmune diseases
- Back pain
- Cancer
- Gallstones
- Gout
- Heart disease
- High blood fats and triglycerides
- High blood pressure
- Infertility
- Osteoarthritis
- Osteoporosis
- Sleep apnea
- Stroke
- Type 2 diabetes
- Ulcers

Do you see why improving your body composition is so important?

Autoimmune Disease

The American Autoimmune Related Diseases Association estimates that up to 50 million Americans suffer from autoimmune disease, and those numbers are rising. Researchers have identified roughly eighty to one hundred different autoimmune diseases, which cause decreased quality of life, high health care costs (estimated at $100 billion annually in the United States), and loss of productivity. Rebuilding from an autoimmune disease requires an understanding of how and why these diseases develop.

The main function of the immune system is to defend against foreign invaders, things like viruses and bacteria. Our defenses are made up of specialized white blood cells and organs that directly assault invaders and produce antibodies to fight off infection. But sometimes the immune system becomes overactive and targets the body's healthy cells, tissues, and organs rather than infections and viruses—basically, it fails to sense the difference between self and non-self. When this reaction occurs, it is known as autoimmunity. Autoimmune diseases are complex dysfunctions of the immune system involving an imbalance of the Th1, Th2, and Th17 immune cells. Let me explain further.

The immune system is composed of five types of white blood cells; lymphocytes are one type. Lymphocytes can be divided into three groups: B cells, T cells, and natural killer (NK) cells. B cells produce antibodies that neutralize viruses and bacteria. T cells produce chemical messengers called cytokines that help direct the immune response. Within the group of T cells are white blood cells called T helper (Th) cells, which can be further divided into Th1 and Th2 cells. Th1 cells are involved with immunity against viruses and parasites, while Th2 cells direct the immune system to get rid of unwanted bacteria and environmental irritants or allergens. Less than a decade ago, a new set of T helper cells was identified: Th17 cells. Th17 cells play an important role in defending against bacterial and fungal infections at mucosal areas of the body, such as on the skin and in the intestinal tract. NK cells are the white blood cells that kill cancer, as well as cells infected by viruses.

JUNE'S STORY

June was suffering from symptoms associated with the autoimmune disease scleroderma, including significant pain in both knees, Raynaud's disease in her fingers, major sensitivity to cold temperatures, and joint pain that made it difficult to walk for extended periods of time. She also had chronic heartburn and acid reflux, insomnia, fatigue, and gastrointestinal distress with loose stools and diarrhea that occurred just about every day. Her thyroid had been removed due to cancer, and she had also had a complete hysterectomy. June also complained of slowly progressing weight loss that she and her doctors couldn't figure out. She was taking numerous medications, including Synthroid (synthetic thyroid hormone), Dexilant (a proton pump inhibitor), Benadryl, and Zantac, and she ate Tums like candy to help soothe her irritated gut.

While the autoimmune disease caused annoying chronic symptoms, the most distressing health issue for her was the irritable bowel and midday diarrhea that had haunted her for years. She was told by a scleroderma specialist that her GI distress was due to her autoimmune disease; she was told to "just live with it."

After our lengthy consult, June had three major goals to improve her health: she wanted to gain weight, reduce her pain, and figure out why she had daily diarrhea. After reviewing her history, including past blood tests, I suggested more detailed blood work and hormone profiling. Not satisfied that her gut issues were caused by scleroderma, I recommended stool testing to rule out any pathogens that could have been responsible for her midday digestive distress. As we waited for the results of the new tests, June was scheduled for a weekend trip to Chicago with her niece; she was reluctant to go due to her chronic knee pain, and feared her symptoms would put a damper on their trip. Days before the trip, I urged June to eliminate bread, dairy, and processed sugar from her diet. Knowing that grains with gluten are the single greatest cause of autoimmune disease, I encouraged her to fight the urge to eat any crumb of bread or grain or other food containing gluten. She agreed, and to her surprise, she had much less discomfort while she enjoyed the day with her niece.

June's test results came in with expected findings: low estrogen and progesterone levels, adrenal fatigue, and high inflammatory markers. But after twenty years of suffering, June learned the culprit of her gastrointestinal issues: the parasite *Blastocystis hominis*, found via stool testing. June immediately began taking a product containing the probiotic *Saccharomyces boulardii*. Within six weeks, her suffering ended: her gut issue was resolved. With a food plan and supplements, June has put on healthy weight and now has minimal joint pain. She says she feels fantastic.

HOW AUTOIMMUNE DISEASES DEVELOP

Autoimmune diseases develop from an abnormal immune response to cells and tissues of the body, which occurs when there is an imbalance of Th1 and Th2 cells and the cytokines (chemical messengers) they release. Generally speaking, Th1 cytokine production is inflammatory and responsible for the autoimmune reaction in the body, while Th2 cytokine production is more involved in allergic responses and generally considered anti-inflammatory. If Th1 cells are overactive, they can suppress Th2 cells. When Th2 cells are overactive, they can suppress Th1. In people with autoimmune dysfunction, there is usually a dominance of Th1 or Th2 cytokine production.

Th1-dominant conditions include:

- Celiac disease
- Crohn's disease
- Grave's disease
- Hashimoto's thyroiditis
- Multiple sclerosis
- Posterior uveitis
- Psoriasis
- Rheumatoid arthritis (Higher levels of inflammation associated with rheumatoid arthritis greatly increase the risk of developing atherosclerosis and cardiovascular disease. See the section Testing for Arterial Inflammation in chapter 8 on page 340 to determine your level of inflammation and your risk for atherosclerosis and heart disease.)
- Type 1 diabetes

Th2-dominant conditions include:

- Allergic dermatitis
- Asthma
- Cancer
- Eczema
- Irritable bowel syndrome (IBS)
- Lupus
- Sinusitis
- Ulcerative colitis

The onset of autoimmune disease can be triggered by foods you have eaten, including foods containing the protein gluten and/or the dairy protein casein; leaky gut syndrome; viral and bacterial infections; major stressful events; pregnancy; changes in hormones; heavy metal toxicity; vitamin D deficiency; insulin resistance; and obesity.

THE LEAKY GUT CONNECTION

Before we look deeper into the specific causes of autoimmune disease, here is a little anatomy and physiology of the gastrointestinal (GI) tract. The GI tract is a thirty-foot-long tube, running from the mouth to the anus, that separates the outside world from the body's internal environment. It is designed to digest food and absorb nutrients, electrolytes, and water. It is also a barrier that prevents harmful substances, unwanted bacteria, parasites, and toxins from getting into the bloodstream.

In addition to its extreme importance to health and survival, the GI tract even has a mind of its own, as well as a specialized defense system. The gut's brain—the enteric nervous system—is located in the tissues lining the esophagus, stomach, small intestine, and large intestine (colon). It is a massive network of neurons capable of carrying out complex activities without any influence from the brain and spinal cord. It records and responds to chemical stimuli and mechanical conditions involved in digestion and peristalsis—the wavelike muscle movement that pushes food through the GI tract. The enteric nervous system also produces and regulates neurotransmitters identical to those within the central nervous system, including serotonin, dopamine, nitric oxide, and acetylcholine. The gut's "brain" can act independently of the brain; it is also responsible for producing your "gut feelings."

In addition to digestion and absorption of nutrients, another crucial function of the GI tract is to safely traffic unwanted bacteria, toxins, and food particles that may injure the body in some way. The GI tract possesses the largest immune tissue in the body, the gut-associated lymphoid tissue (GALT). The GALT stores B and T lymphocytes (see page 37), which defend against invaders, including bacteria, viruses, fungi, parasites, and other microorganisms.

To maximize the absorption of nutrients, the surface of the intestines is covered with tiny fingerlike projections called villi, which are lined with epithelial cells, a single layer of specialized cells that separates the GALT from the outside environment. The tissue of the epithelium is composed of sheets of cells joined together at tight junctions; it performs the vital function of blocking unwanted proteins and microorganisms from entering the bloodstream.

The gut microbiota is a complex community of up to one thousand different species of "good" bacteria. Among the many critical roles it plays is working synergistically with the immune system. It also makes vitamins, including vitamins B and K; enhances the muscular activity that moves waste through the intestines; and assists in the digestion of food and absorption of nutrients. These beneficial gut bugs also help eliminate toxins and break down plant-based foods to produce butyrate, an energy source for the GI tract. Butyrate is a short-chain fatty acid that acts as an anti-inflammatory and reinforces the gut's defense barrier by increasing its antimicrobial proteins. Research published in the *Journal of Medical Microbiology* shows that butyrate decreases intestinal permeability by increasing the strength of the tight junctions between the epithelial cells, thus preventing unwanted leakage through the wall of the gut into the bloodstream.

Where is all this going? Numerous illnesses can occur when the protective functions of the gut are diminished, either by the overgrowth of gut bacteria or compromised function of the epithelium and its tight cellular junctions.

In reading the scientific literature on the causes of autoimmune disease, I was consistently directed back to a condition called leaky gut syndrome. Leaky gut is a condition in which the tight cellular junctions of the epithelium are weakened and fail to prevent the passage of unwanted substances through the walls of the intestine and into the bloodstream. While I'm sure there are others, there appear to be three major reasons for leaky gut: the consumption of foods containing gluten; an overgrowth of harmful gut bacteria, known as dysbiosis or small intestinal bacterial overgrowth (SIBO); and surges of the stress hormone cortisol. Regardless of the cause, leaky gut has been linked to countless diseases, including celiac disease, a host of neurological diseases, and many autoimmune diseases.

Eye-opening research published in *Physiological Reviews* found that the protein gluten compromises the epithelium and its tight cellular junctions. Gluten, found in many grains, is a nasty protein that interacts with bacteria in the gut to produce a compound called zonulin. Zonulin is the biological key that opens these tight junctions. Once open, they allow unwanted foreign proteins, bacteria, and toxins to exit the intestines into the body, causing an immune response and systemic inflammation.

Leaky gut has been linked to celiac disease, a well-known autoimmune condition characterized by an aggressive immune response in the gut, which ultimately destroys the villi lining the walls of the intestines. Since the villi are responsible for nutrient absorption in the intestines, the body is unable to properly process nutrients, which can result in malnutrition. Left unresolved, celiac disease can lead to additional complications, including anemia, osteoporosis, infertility, miscarriages, epilepsy, and stunted growth. The treatment for celiac disease is the complete elimination of grains and other foods containing gluten.

But celiac disease isn't the only condition related to gut dysfunction. Here is a list of diseases proven or suspected to be associated with leaky gut syndrome:

Autoimmune diseases
- Celiac disease
- Crohn's disease
- Hashimoto's thyroiditis
- Rheumatoid arthritis
- Type 1 diabetes
- Systemic lupus erythematosus

Cancer
- Brain cancer
- Breast cancer
- Ovarian cancer
- Pancreatic cancer

Neurological disease
- Multiple sclerosis
- Lou Gehrig's disease (ALS)
- Autism (neurodevelopmental disorder)
- Schizophrenia (brain disorder)

Z NOTE: Hashimoto's thyroiditis is a condition of decreased thyroid function due to an autoimmune attack on the thyroid. The inflammation occurring from the immune reaction often leads to an underactive thyroid gland, a condition known as hypothyroidism. Among the many symptoms associated with hypothyroidism are chronic low-grade depression, unintentional weight gain, poor stamina, low energy levels, and fatigue.

According to the American Thyroid Association, an estimated 20 million Americans have some form of thyroid dysfunction, and roughly 60 percent of those are unaware they have it. Having a weak thyroid and low levels of thyroid hormones can cause some of the metabolic issues that contribute to the development of heart disease, cancer, diabetes, and obesity. The links between Hashimoto's thyroiditis and the other chronic diseases are autoimmune response and inflammation. If you've been diagnosed with hypothyroidism, dig deeper to find out if there is an autoimmune dysfunction behind it.

Several other autoimmune diseases are intimately connected to leaky gut and the toxic proteins that often lead to colon cancer. Crohn's disease and ulcerative colitis, the two most common inflammatory bowel diseases, are chronic conditions characterized by severe inflammation of the GI tract. A study published in the *American Journal of Gastroenterology* has shed light on how leaky gut causes these diseases. The inflammatory adipocytokine tumor necrosis factor (TNF) is a possible reason. Leaky gut causes inflammation; in turn, inflammation perpetuates leaky gut.

Gluten, zonulin, and overgrowth of toxic bacteria can disrupt the function of the tight junctions, thus causing leaky gut. The microbial population living in the intestines is made up of roughly one thousand different species, including both friendly bugs and potentially harmful or toxic bacteria, coexisting in unity. For multiple reasons—including the use of antibiotics, synthetic hormones, antacids, H2 blockers, and/or proton pump inhibitors; the consumption of alcohol; stress; and a high-calorie, low-nutrient diet—friendly bacteria are reduced and harmful bacteria become the majority. This overgrowth of "bad" bacteria is called bacterial dysbiosis.

When dysbiosis occurs, the elevation in harmful bacteria poses a serious threat to a person's health. For example, when potentially harmful bacteria such as *E. coli* die, the bacterial cell wall disintegrates, releasing large toxic compounds called lipopolysaccharides (also known as endotoxins). These toxins are known to disrupt tight junctions in the gut, thus increasing gut permeability. In fact, researchers have found that even the smallest dose of endotoxin compromised the integrity of the GI mucosal barrier, leading to leaky gut. Lipopolysaccharides are extremely toxic and have been implicated in the onset of serious diseases, including Parkinson's, Alzheimer's, irritable bowel syndrome, and cardiovascular disease. Lipopolysaccharides are also linked to the formation of mood disorders such as depression and the neurobehavioral dysfunction autism.

How are stress and cortisol linked to leaky gut? Stress is a threat to the internal equilibrium. It involves a stressor—a threat or demand—and the ensuing stress response, a neurological and hormonal event that prepares the body to deal with the stressor. During the stress response, the hormone cortisol is released to increase blood sugar for the brain and the availability of energy-rich substances to repair tissues. The adrenal glands release the hormone adrenaline, which increases your heart rate and blood pressure, and gives you a surge of energy meant to help you run from the threat. In times of stress, these hormones activate mast cells (a type of white blood cell) in the intestinal tract, causing them to release the inflammatory compounds TNF (tumor necrosis factor) and IFN (interferon gamma). These inflammatory immune chemicals have been shown to open the tight junctions, increasing intestinal permeability.

Z NOTE: The Western diet, characterized by the consumption of processed foods, factory-farmed meat, dairy, refined grains, and high-sugar foods and drinks, is a major cause of endotoxemia (high levels of lipopolysaccharides in the blood) and dysbiosis. Research published in the journal *Gastroenterology* states that eating a typical Western diet for one month caused a 71 percent increase in blood levels of lipopolysaccharides—*71 percent.* Both the lipopolysaccharides and the unhealthful food sources caused increased gut permeability and systemic inflammation. It was also found that the consumption of omega-3 polyunsaturated fatty acids (good dietary fats) reduced lipopolysaccharide production, gut permeability, and systemic inflammation.

KRISTINA'S STORY

Kristina's health had begun to decline two years prior to her first visit with me. It started with chronic respiratory issues, where breathing became a physical chore requiring the use of a nebulizer several times a day. Over time, she developed hives, first on her hands and feet, then spreading to the rest of her body. The hives—an immune reaction—would flare up in times of stress, as well as after Kristina had eaten certain foods, including grain and dairy.

In addition to her hives, Kristina was dealing with headaches, joint pain, and chronic low energy. Her lack of stamina arose from her immune dysfunction, the nutrient-poor diet, and avoidance of food out of fear of triggering a severe reaction.

The hives became unbearable; she woke every night incessantly scratching her skin to the point of bleeding. Multiple doctors and many vials of blood later, Kristina was diagnosed as suffering from an extreme elevation of immunoglobulin E (IgE) antibodies. IgE antibodies are produced by the immune system in response to some type of foreign protein. They activate specific white blood cells called basophils and mast cells, which, in turn, produce inflammatory agents— including histamine, leukotrienes, and cytokines—responsible for her allergic reactions. The only treatment she was offered at that time was antihistamines, which provided no relief.

Experiencing medical apathy, Kristina continued to search for the cause of her condition. She heard about functional medicine and eventually got to my clinic. During our first consultation, it was clear that Kristina had some issue in her gut that was either the cause of her extremely elevated IgE or an agitator for her immune dysfunction. Having seen an extreme case of elevated IgE before, I had her tested for Hyper IgE Syndrome (HIES) and the genetic dysfunctions that cause it—mutations to the STAT3 and DOCK8 genes. Fortunately, Kristina did not have mutations of either gene. We continued to dig.

With the suspicion that her extremely elevated IgE antibodies were due to faulty gut function, stool testing was performed to check for dysbiosis (small intestinal bacterial overgrowth, or SIBO). Kristina's stool testing revealed significant overgrowth of harmful bacteria, including *Odoribacter*, *Prevotella*, *Pseudoflavonifractor*, and *E. coli*.

Kristina immediately eliminated all refined flours, breads, and grains containing gluten; dairy; and refined sugar. She loaded her diet with healthful protein and fat, and plenty of plant-based foods. I put her on two different probiotics to balance her bacterial flora, a medical food to help heal the gut, and nutrients to rebuild the lining of the gut to prevent further permeability issues and immune reactions. Within a few weeks, Kristina's hives dramatically diminished and she could sleep through the night without scratching her skin away. She was ecstatic.

Despite the fact that there are as many as one hundred autoimmune disorders, by some estimates, they all appear to have similar causes. Leaky gut and intestinal permeability caused by the reaction between gluten and an overgrowth of gut bacteria top the list. Additional causes of autoimmune dysfunction include:

- Chronic stressors
- Estrogen surges
- Heavy-metal toxicity
- Insulin surges
- Pregnancy
- Vitamin D deficiency

As you can see, autoimmune diseases develop for different reasons, but for the most part these causes are under our control—under *your* control. Taking action to eliminate the causes of leaky gut—including omitting all refined grains and grains containing gluten from your diet, regulating bacterial overgrowth, and controlling your stress levels— should begin immediately.

How do you know if you have increased gut permeability and leaky gut? Self-diagnosis is difficult, and your family doctor may not know the mechanisms and health consequences of a leaky gut. However, it may be worth having a functional medicine specialist help you evaluate your gut condition. My motto is "Test, not guess."

TESTS FOR LEAKY GUT

1. Intestinal Permeability Assessment (Genova Diagnostics, www .gdx.net): The most definitive test for leaky gut is the lactulose and

mannitol test. It is simple: You consume premeasured quantities of lactulose and mannitol, two nonmetabolized sugars, and collect a urine sample six hours later. If these sugars find their way into your urine, you have leaky gut.

2. Intestinal Antigenic Permeability Screen (Cyrex Laboratories, www.cyrexlabs.com): An antibody assessment of the intestinal barrier integrity, as well as the levels of lipopolysaccharides and zonulin in the blood.

3. GI Effects Comprehensive Profile (Genova Diagnostics, www.gdx .net): A comprehensive evaluation of gastrointestinal function, providing clinical information on digestive performance, gut inflammation, gut microbiota, and parasitology. As an add-on to the GI Effects evaluation, Genova can also test for zonulin to assess intestinal permeability.

In addition to the diseases linked to gluten, zonulin, and lipopolysaccharide toxicity, other signs and symptoms may point to leaky gut and warrant undergoing these specialized tests. These symptoms include reactions to certain foods, stomach pain, indigestion, gas, heartburn, unexplained fatigue, fibromyalgia, skin issues (hives, eczema, acne, rosacea, psoriasis, rashes), brain fog, asthma, irritable bowel syndrome, mood swings, depression, allergy symptoms, and weight gain.

REBUILDING FROM LEAKY GUT

At this point, if you have identified with any of the chronic health issues listed in this chapter or you are rebuilding from a chronic disease and/ or leaky gut, follow all the supportocols described between the covers of this book, beginning with the following:

· Eliminate all foods containing gluten (especially grains) and inflammatory fats and oils. Eliminate legumes, as they can (and will) cause the bacteria in the gut to produce gas and bloating, uncomfortable symptoms to have as you're trying to heal a leaky gut. Legumes also contain lectins, proteins found in a variety of foods, including dairy and grains, that can provoke a toxic response in some people, causing damage to the intestinal wall and contributing to leaky gut.

- Eliminate alcohol, caffeine, and all processed refined sugars.
- Rebuild your microbiome. Instead of killing off the bad bugs, nourish the healthy bacteria to increase their diversity, which will naturally suppress the harmful bacteria. To do this, diet is the key. Eliminate processed foods and add fermented foods, such as pickles, sauerkraut, tempeh, miso, and kimchi, which act as a prebiotic (food for the bacteria). Other plant-based foods that are extremely beneficial to good gut bacteria are sweet potatoes and other root vegetables, jicama, leeks, onions, Jerusalem artichokes, and dandelion greens.
- Consider the following nutrient supplements to help repair the gut lining:
  - **Digestive Enzymes.** Enzymes are critical in breaking down the foods into individual nutrients so the body can absorb them. In those with leaky gut, nutrient absorption and utilization will help repair the tight junctions of the epithelium, contributing to the resolution of leaky gut. Digestive enzymes will also clean up the gut by removing bad bacteria, damaged cells, and toxins.
  - **Probiotics.** For any diet, supplementing with probiotics helps replenish beneficial bacteria to the gut. Good bacteria will overcome the harmful bacteria, support healthy communication between the gut's immune system (GALT) and the intestinal tract. Probiotics will reduce inflammation and help the breakdown of foods we eat. Note: When first taking probiotics to heal your gut, you may experience some bloating, cramping, or diarrhea as the bacteria move into the gut and begin repair. If you get symptoms, they will pass shortly.
  - **L-Glutamine.** L-glutamine is the most abundant free amino acid in the body and is involved in different metabolic and biochemical

processes in different organs, including the gut. It is an anti-inflammatory nutrient that influences the gut's immune response, enhances gut barrier function, maintains the gut epithelia, and fights against bad bacteria. Impressively, glutamine has also shown protective effects in the gut from the endotoxin lipopoly-saccharides.

- **Licorice Root.** Deglycyrrhizinated licorice (DGL) is an herb that improves stomach-acid production and helps maintain and support the lining of the stomach and intestine. DGL supports the lining of the gut by increasing mucin—a viscoelastic mucous gel that acts as a protective barrier for the intestinal epithelia.

- **Zinc-Carnosine.** Zinc and carnosine are nutrients that have multiple functions in human biology. Zinc acts as a coenzyme to defend against free-radical damage, and it is an immune modulator that can reduce inflammation. Carnosine, a powerful antioxidant, can boost the effects of zinc. Together, zinc-carnosine has been shown to stabilize the gut lining, reduce gut permeability, and stimulate healing and repair in the GI tract.

Z NOTE: It's estimated that 60 to 70 million people suffer from some form of gastrointestinal disease or disorder, including abdominal pain, esophagitis, ulcers, gastroesophageal reflux disease (GERD), nausea, vomiting, constipation, diarrhea, *Clostridium difficile* infection, pancreatitis, and colorectal cancer. For many, the first-line therapy for peptic ulcers, esophagitis, and GERD is the use of proton pump inhibitors (PPIs).

PPIs work by shutting down the proton/potassium pumps found in the parietal cells of the stomach, thus reducing the production of stomach acid. The theory is that acid reflux or heartburn is caused by excess stomach acid, so shutting down the pumps that produce the acid will reduce overall acidity, prevent the formation of ulcers, and reduce the burning pain associated with heartburn. However, research from the *Journal of*

Gastroenterology and *Proceedings of the Nutrition Society* has confirmed that *low* stomach acid (a condition called hypochlorhydria)—*not* an overproduction of acid—is to blame for GERD. Hypochlorhydria can be caused by an *H. pylori* infection; a hiatal hernia (where the muscular upper valve of the stomach pushes through the diaphragm); overgrowth of harmful bacteria in the gut; and poor carbohydrate digestion. PPIs don't treat any of these causes and should not be used by those with gastric reflux.

PPIs also come with a host of detrimental side effects. For one, they will change the pH of the gut, causing dysbiosis and an overgrowth of harmful bacteria. They impair the body's ability to absorb vitamins and minerals, including vitamin B_{12}, vitamin C, magnesium, calcium, and iron. And that's hardly all—PPIs damage the lining of the arteries, reducing the production of nitric oxide, which then restricts the dilation of arteries and subsequently blood flow. PPIs have also been shown to negatively affect kidney and cognitive functions.

Before someone convinces you to take these damaging drugs, instead consider removing all refined grains and bread, dairy, and refined sugars from your diet, getting tested for bacterial overgrowth, and taking digestive enzymes containing betaine HCl (hydrochloric acid).

Summary

If you want to rebuild from and prevent recurrence of a chronic disease, you should know that it is caused not by a single gene, but rather by the interaction between your genes and the internal environment they inhabit. Since human genes have remained constant for eons, the major changes driving chronic diseases are our personal choices, habits, and food sources. An unhealthy body composition is the trigger for the development and progression of heart disease, cancer, diabetes, and autoimmune diseases, among others. Within this diseased internal terrain, the inflammatory process fuels chronic disease as gas fuels a fire. Excessive body fat is a burning inferno of inflammatory compounds, including IL-6, TNF, and leptin, which all play a role in worsening the disease.

The research clearly shows that chronic diseases develop from a diet of nutrient-deprived processed foods, unresolved stressors, environmental toxins, lack of exercise, and poor sleep. When any or all of these factors are out of alignment with your genes, disease is the result. The tried-and-true supportocols outlined in this book will help you rebuild from your health crisis and avoid future complications.

But first, you need to assess your baseline health and habits so you know where your weaknesses lie and where to focus your time and energy. How do you do that? Easy: Read on.

2

Assessing Your Health

You are born with something you take for granted—your health. Health is really an abstract; it's not something you can purchase, hold, wear, drive, taste, or get a buzz from. It's not something you think about until it is threatened or taken away. Most people don't think disease will happen to them, but it can, and it does. A serious disease usually takes years to develop, and the internal environment that created the disease was stewing for all those years. Once the disease takes root, it spirals out of control, and the decline in your health builds momentum until you develop symptoms and, eventually, find a diagnosis.

The information in *Rebuild* will allow you to make the best choices as you take personal responsibility for recovering from disease. I realize that many people are looking for a quick fix; they're fine with taking pills to sustain their current state of health rather than putting in the effort to rebuild from a disease and prevent its return. Maybe you have chosen that path because it's all you know. Maybe it's what your trusted doctors are recommending, or maybe you think taking care of yourself is boring, restrictive, or just too hard. Whatever the reason, the outcome of choosing most shortcuts is more suffering. The real shortcut to good health is following a plan customized for you, your unique body, and the unique conditions of your disease.

Rebuilding yourself is simple; it's just not an overnight fix. You need to be disciplined and motivated. Ask yourself: *What choice do I have, and what are the consequences if I don't rebuild?* To restore your health, you must adopt the rebuild actions, because the internal terrain of the body is seriously complex.

For some people, the harmful habits and poor choices they make to satisfy momentary pleasure far outweigh the potential hazards and consequences they will face down the road. We have all done it—gone to the doctor for an annual physical and sighed in relief as we get a "passing grade." That gives us permission to continue down our current path, reasoning, "I must be doing okay, no need to really change. There are people in far worse condition than I am."

Often, a health-threatening diagnosis is still not enough to flip the emotional switch away from unhealthful habits. People continue to smoke even when diagnosed with lung or bladder cancer, emphysema, or congestive heart failure. For them, the pressures of addiction and the "reward" of smoking far outweigh the realities of living with a serious disease or the threat of death.

The same is true of those who eat processed, nutrient-deficient, and/or sugary foods. I work with diabetics—many of whom are overfat and/or dealing with neuropathy in their feet, discolored skin, or other complications of the disease—who can't seem to give up sugar. Usually there is some underlying issue: an emotional block that runs deep, causing the continuation of self-destructive ways even in the face of a serious health issue.

Unlike a T-shirt, you can't replace your health when it's worn out; you have to rebuild the one body you have. Instead of maintaining good health, we tend to take action only when we get sick. Once diagnosed, we make all kinds of promises and resolutions. Good, do that. Make a resolution to do what it takes to rebuild yourself back to good health. Tony Robbins, a world-renowned life coach, has said, "To resolve is to cut off any possibility except for the thing you commit to." It's time you commit to rebuilding yourself back to health with a sustainable plan.

To help you create that plan, it's important that you answer these questions for yourself. Please answer the questions honestly, as this is a baseline, or starting point, to help you focus where you need to.

1.   From which major health condition(s) do you need to rebuild?

\
\

2.   What medical procedures have you gone through, and what medications were prescribed? Did you have, or are you having, any side effects from the medications? What are they, and how do they make you feel emotionally?

\
\
\
\

3.   What health care practitioners have you consulted for this problem? What did they tell you about your current state of health and what to expect in the future?

\
\
\
\

4. Before your diagnosis, what were your eating habits? How much bread, refined grains, dairy products, and refined white sugar did you eat? When did you eat your biggest meal each day? What did that meal typically consist of? How often did you eat packaged foods?

_____

_____

_____

_____

5. Before your diagnosis, how much did you exercise, and what did you do? How would you rate your fitness level? Do you suffer from exercise ADD (an inability to focus on a consistent ritual of movement and exercise)?

_____

_____

_____

_____

6. How much stress do you deal with, and how often? Are your stressors physical or emotional? How long have you been under stress?

_____

_____

_____

_____

7. Do you smoke? How much per day, and for how many years? What are your triggers? When you smoke, do you drink alcohol at the same time?

_____

_____

_____

_____

8. How many alcoholic beverages do you drink per day/week/month? Have you ever had a problem with alcohol? Have you ever been told by someone else your drinking habits were unhealthy? Does alcohol prevent you from functioning in your home life or work?

_____

_____

_____

_____

9. Do you eat any foods or drink beverages containing artificial sweeteners, such as NutraSweet (aspartame) and Splenda (sucralose), or add artificial sweeteners to your coffee or tea? How much artificial sweetener do you consume on a daily/weekly basis?

_____

_____

_____

10. On average, how many hours do you sleep per night? If you have trouble falling asleep, describe how you physically feel when trying to fall asleep? If you wake in the middle of the night, what are you feeling when you are awake? Is there anything you do that helps get you back to sleep? If you get sleepy during the day, what do you do or take for a pick-me-up? If you take a sleep aid, does it work, and how does it make you feel the next day physically and mentally?

_____

_____

_____

11. If you could go back in time, what would you change about your lifestyle and habits in the past that may have contributed to your current state of health?

_____

_____

_____

_____

12. Did you ever expect to have this type of problem at your current age? Why or why not?

_____

_____

_____

13. How does your current state of health affect your family, work, and activities you enjoy?

_____

_____

_____

_____

14. What are you currently doing to improve your health? Do you need help with that?

_____

_____

_____

_____

15. On a scale of 1 to 10, with 10 being the highest, rate your commitment to rebuilding from your disease or chronic health issue and preventing its recurrence. Is there anything that will prevent you from using the tools in this book to rebuild yourself?

_____

_____

_____

_____

You now have a choice: muddle through the broken "bandage and manage" health care system that pulls you along and helps you survive rather than thrive, or elect to rebuild your body and mind to create a new outlook on your health and life.

Hopefully, you choose the latter.

I want you to focus on thriving, rebuilding, and getting healthy, strong, and lean, and to stop focusing on your disease or your current body composition. To keep you motivated, focus on where adopting new rituals and habits—your new supportocols—will get you, not on what you have to do to get there.

Rebuild is your road map to rebuilding from a disease or chronic health issue and preventing its recurrence. As your disease/health coach, I'll provide the information you need to know about your condition and the simple steps you need to take to feel empowered as you create your personal plan. It's time to make a comeback and be better than you were before—not just to survive, but to be victorious.

II

Time to Re-act

PERHAPS YOU HAVE BRUISES and scars as permanent badges of honor for all you have gone through in combating disease or some other chronic health issue. But how about the mental scars? Replaying in your head all that you have gone through, you may wonder what you need to do *now* to restore your health and prevent your disease or health issue from returning.

Maybe, as part of your treatment, you find yourself walking out of the hospital or a doctor's office holding a bag of pills and pages of warnings and side effects.

Maybe you just finished your last day of chemo, and after saying good-bye to your supportive oncology team, you find yourself standing outside the doors wondering, "Now what?"

Maybe you're asking yourself, "How did this happen? How did I get so far off track?"

Maybe you wish you could go back in time to alter your path. You wish you had been more mindful about your eating habits, exercise, stress management, and the onslaught of toxins you were inhaling and ingesting daily.

It's time to rebuild. Unfortunately, most practitioners have very limited time to spend with you, and many are not trained or equipped to provide you with the resources and support you need to rebuild yourself back to health. As a result, you are left to your own devices—but in my experience, patients who receive the necessary support are much more likely to adhere to their treatment regimens and their rebuild protocols and practice self-care than those who have to go it on their own.

So today, you and I become partners, a team. I have been through the battle and come out victorious. I'm sure we have gone through the same or similar procedures and experienced similar emotions along the way. As a clinician *and* a patient, I realize it's much easier to get through the crisis and restore your health when you have support and the right protocols—what I call supportocols. *Rebuild* has the supportocols you need to restore your health, prevent recurrence, and maintain your good health long after your health crisis is over. The supportocols in *Rebuild* will be baked into your new pattern of choices and habits. They will become your new standards of being and your new daily rituals.

Rebuilding is about not only restoring your health from your diagnosed condition but also reconstructing your mistreated internal terrain in which the disease developed.

By following the supportocols provided in this book, you will recalibrate the communication between your genes and your internal terrain to create a state of normal function and health.

The supportocols outlined in this section are also designed for those actively going through treatment for a current health crisis. In addition to helping you through your crisis, they will simultaneously improve your overall health and body composition, eliminating excess fat and leaving you lean. This is your chance to come back better than you were before.

Five Re-action Steps to Rebuild

Where do you start? You must take five necessary Rebuild Actions—what I call Re-actions—to rebuild yourself and restore your health.

RE-ACTION #1: EAT FOR YOUR GENES.
Since eating is the biggest constant in life, the most effective re-action is to make sure you eat the best foods to help you rebuild your health. Think of food as information that talks to your genes and tells them what to do. Poor nutrition can tell normal genes to create disease. To send the right message to your genes, you must eliminate high-calorie, nutrient-deficient foods from your diet and instead eat a variety of tasty nutrient-dense whole foods. These include healthful proteins, fats, and plant-based foods of all colors. Chapter 3, which covers Re-action #1, is the most information-dense chapter in *Rebuild*, so take your time going through it. I have also outlined how to create a personal food plan, a diet unique to your specific needs and metabolism.

RE-ACTION #2: EXERCISE WITH PERIODS OF INTENSITY.
High-intensity interval training (HIIT), an all-out burst of full-effort physical activity followed by a short period of rest, is hands-down the best way to rebuild yourself through exercise. HIIT triggers a chain re-action of beneficial genetic and biochemical events that regulate blood sugar, burn fat, reduce inflammation, and increase immune function. This begins the process of reversing disease and restoring normal function to the body. HIIT is easier than you think and requires a lot less time than the traditional modes of exercising you may be familiar with.

RE-ACTION #3: HIT THE BRAKES ON THE STRESS RESPONSE.

The stress reaction and the release of stress hormones (cortisol, adrenaline, and norepinephrine) drive disease, including cancer, heart disease, and autoimmune diseases, among others. Chronic and unmanaged stress sets off toxic chemical reactions in the body, which can ignite and promote the formation of disease. When your body's stress hormone levels are elevated for prolonged periods, it can suppress your immune system, reducing your ability to fight bacteria, viruses, and chronic illness. It is crucial that you control your stressors to lessen the harm an extended stress reaction may cause. You also need to carve out time in each day to unplug.

RE-ACTION #4: REBOOT YOUR INTERNAL CLOCK.

You need to get your *zzz*'s. Sleep is a period of inactivity, a suspension of consciousness, that occurs every day. It is an anabolic state, building up the nervous, immune, and muscular systems. Sleep is a complex process of internal rebuilding and recuperation, which are essential to your health and well-being. Lack of sleep has been linked to the most serious diseases, including heart disease, cancer, and diabetes. Sleep deprivation can severely impair your immune system and create inflammation—the driving force behind all chronic health issues and disease.

RE-ACTION #5: REDUCE CONTAMINATION.

Many people unwittingly expose themselves to toxins that create internal conditions favorable to the development of cancer and other chronic diseases. Rebuilding and allowing your body to heal after a disease requires you to stop using tobacco, eliminate environmental toxins such as pesticides and household chemicals—and yes, cut back on alcohol. "Drink in moderation" is too vague, too open to interpretation. I think the word *moderation* itself should be used in moderation. It's much clearer to say, "Drink alcohol sparingly as you rebuild yourself."

• • •

Listen, I get it: we all want an easy life full of delicious food, good company, and joy. Buying into the belief that you have no control over your life and health (or that you do have control but "Man, it's going to be a boring journey") is a sure way to set yourself up to develop or prolong disease. The good news—and I hope you begin to see it this way—is that you *do* have control. In the following chapters, I explain how to modify your personal habits and make the best choices as you begin your personal rebuild.

3

Re-action #1
Eat for Your
Genes

What is food? It provides not only the calories we need to produce energy but also the vitamins, minerals, and phytochemicals (plant chemicals) that control intricate cellular machinery and the raw material needed to make healthy bones, muscles, and other tissues of the body.

But perhaps more important, food is *information*. The nutrients in food serve as signals or commands that talk to our cells and regulate essentially all bodily functions. The signals that come from nutrient-dense whole foods turn on the genes that maintain normal function in the body, while the signals sent by processed foods act as alarms, turning on genes that set the stage for disease.

Macronutrients and Micronutrients

When you know what you're putting into your body, you can make better decisions at the grocery store. All foods—from a burger to a mixed-greens salad—are composed of three parts: macronutrients, micronutrients, and water. What do each of these components do?

MACRONUTRIENTS include three components with which you're likely familiar: carbohydrates, protein, and fat. Macronutrients provide the energy, measured as calories, needed to maintain life. Without them, we would suffer from malnutrition, starvation, and eventually death. Our bodies need energy to operate. From breathing to digesting food to moving and exercising, our bodily functions are fueled by calories derived from food. Carbohydrates, protein, and fats all provide energy, but in different amounts: 1 gram of carbohydrate provides 4 calories of energy, 1 gram of protein provides 4 calories of energy, and 1 gram of fat provides 9 calories of energy. Macronutrients play a second important role as well: they help regulate both the hormones that make us fat and the hormones that get rid of fat.

> **DR. Z SAYS . . .** You can do the math. Let's say a food contains 10 grams of carbs, 0 grams of protein, and 0 grams of fat per serving. That means it contains 40 calories (10 grams x 4 calories per gram = 40 calories).
>
> Now let's look at fat. If a food contains 0 grams of carbs, 0 grams of protein, and 10 grams of fat, that means it contains 90 calories (10 grams x 9 calories per gram = 90 calories).

MICRONUTRIENTS are vitamins, minerals, and trace elements. They provide no energy in the form of calories, but they are necessary for life. Without micronutrients, we would suffer from deficiency diseases.

WATER is the largest component of the human body, making up about 50 to 70 percent of your body weight. It has many important functions, including regulating body temperature, serving as a vehicle for nutrient absorption, maintaining blood volume, and acting as a medium for all biochemical reactions.

> What is a calorie? It is a unit of energy. In a lab setting, a calorie is the amount of heat it takes to raise the temperature of 1 gram of water by 1 degree Cel-

sius. Most of us think of calories as a number on a food label that can make us fat. While eating excessive calories can make you gain weight, understanding the effect of consuming calories from nutrient-dense foods versus those from nutrient-poor foods will make changing your body composition a lot easier.

CARBOHYDRATES

Carbohydrates (commonly known as carbs) are the macronutrient we need the most, because they are the cleanest-burning fuel in the body. They provide glucose, the main energy source for cells. Carbs also are needed to power the brain and nervous system, the heart and muscular system, and the kidneys, and to help keep the intestines healthy. Unused carbs are stored in the liver and muscles until the body needs them.

Simple and Complex Carbohydrates

The most common forms of carbohydrate are starches, fibers, and sugars. These are grouped into two categories: simple and complex. Carbohydrates are classified as simple or complex based on their chemical structure and how quickly they are digested and absorbed by the body.

Drawing a distinction between simple and complex carbs is important. Too much misinformation has been passed around about the two types of carbs because many diet books treat them as if they are the same.

Simple refined carbs are quickly digested and absorbed by the body, causing a rapid rise in blood sugar. They usually have no real nutrient value, as they lack vitamins and minerals. Examples of simple carbs and foods that contain them include white sugar, fructose (the naturally occurring sugar in fruit), honey, regular soda, candy, and baked goods like cakes, cookies, and pies.

Complex carbs, also known as starches, are slowly digested and absorbed by the body and take longer to raise blood sugar levels. Foods that contain complex carbs are usually packed with vitamins, minerals, and fiber. Examples of foods that contain complex carbs include brown rice and brown rice pasta, steel-cut oats, sweet potatoes, carrots, squash, beets, and legumes.

You can probably guess which type is best for your body composition!

Glucose

Glucose (which is what we mean when we say "blood sugar"), the body's key source of energy, comes from carbohydrates. It is stored in the liver and turned into muscle energy called glycogen.

Glucose is found in all the sugars we consume, including fructose (the naturally occurring sugar in fruit), sucrose (refined white sugar), and lactose (dairy sugar). However, the body uses these types of sugar in different ways.

FRUCTOSE: Fructose is broken down in two ways. It either becomes glucose for energy, or it is converted into fatty acids. These fatty acids are turned into triglycerides and transported to the muscles and fat cells to make fat. Natural fructose, which is found in plants—fruits, vegetables, and some legumes—is the best type, because the plants contain fiber in addition to the sugar. According to research published in the *Journal of Nutrition*, dietary fiber decreases the speed at which the body absorbs fructose, which may help prevent spikes and dips in blood sugar, reducing the risk for type 2 diabetes. It will also help prevent you from gaining fat.

SUCROSE: Sucrose is derived from sugarcane and sugar beets, among other sources, and is most commonly recognized as the white sugar you might use for baking or stir into coffee. In the body, sucrose is broken down into glucose and fructose. The glucose is used for energy, and the fructose gets stored as fat.

Diets high in refined sugars, such as granulated (white) sugar and high-fructose corn syrup (HFCS), will make you fat. HFCS is made from cornstarch; most of the glucose in the starch is chemically altered to produce refined fructose. Notice that I said "refined"—that means it's not natural; it does not contain fiber. The processed-food industry uses HFCS in breads, cereals, yogurts, soups, condiments, sodas, energy drinks, breakfast bars, lunch meat, and just about any non-food "food" product.

LACTOSE: Lactose is the sugar derived from dairy products. In the body, it is broken down into glucose and galactose. Galactose is then converted into glucose and stored in the liver.

Lactose is familiar mainly because of lactose intolerance, a common condition in which a deficiency in lactase, the enzyme needed to digest lactose, makes it difficult for the body to process dairy products. The milk sugar reacts with the bacteria in your gut, causing bloating, pain, and diarrhea—familiar symptoms of the condition known as lactose intolerance.

If you are lactose intolerant, your body is telling you that you should not drink milk or consume other dairy products. Why is that? Milk is the food source for babies of certain species. Human infants drink human breast milk; calves drink cow milk; monkeys drink monkey milk. For most people, when we transition to solid food sources after weaning and no longer need to drink milk, the body stops producing lactase, the enzyme needed to break down milk sugar. (For a smaller percentage of the population, lactase activity persists into adulthood due to a genetic alteration, enabling them to digest milk as adults.) If you have a reaction to dairy products, it's because your body can't break down the lactose—and that "condition" is actually quite normal.

KIRK'S STORY

At our first discussion, Kirk C. handed me a huge folder loaded with test results. His complaints were abdominal bloating, pain, and diarrhea—which occurred eight times a day. He was afraid to leave the house, and his gut problem was affecting his job. He listed the tests he'd had done to try to identify his mysterious health problem: an endoscopy, colonoscopy, repeated blood work, barium studies of his stomach, stool testing, and, last but not least, a biopsy of his intestine. He had agreed to all that testing in a desperate hope of finding something to explain his misery. However, all the tests came back normal.

I then asked Kirk what he was eating. He stopped short, then said, "No doctor ever asked me that." My first thought was, *Why the heck* (I'm being nice here) *was he not asked what he was eating? Diet and lifestyle are the most important factors in reversing and preventing disease.* Given the list of doctors he had seen and the amount of testing they had done, I was surprised no one had asked him the simple question of what he was eating. Kirk told me his typical diet consisted of eggs and fruit in the morning, a sandwich and more fruit for lunch, and a variety of proteins with vegetables for dinner. Then he paused, and added, "Oh, yeah, I eat a pint of Ben and Jerry's ice cream before bed."

Health problem solved: he had a simple case of lactose intolerance. Kirk agreed to eliminate the dairy, and I recommended he take digestive enzymes to help his digestion, plus a multispectral probiotic to repopulate his gut with healthy bacteria. I changed his diet to include not just healthful proteins and carbs, but also plenty of green vegetables and legumes, which are all high in fiber. Eating this way helped to resolve the long-term inflammation he had in his gut from the dairy products. In just a few days, he had no more stomach troubles, and in less than three weeks, Kirk reported that he had more energy and felt the best he had in a long time.

Fiber

I mentioned fiber before, but exactly what is it? Fiber—both soluble and insoluble—is a type of carbohydrate that the body cannot digest. Soluble fiber attracts water, becoming gel-like during digestion, which slows down digestion. Insoluble fiber adds bulk to the stool and helps the food pass more quickly through the gut. As fiber passes through the gut, it also helps remove waste from the body. You can think of it as a scrubber that works inside your plumbing. A diet high in fiber helps regulate blood fats and blood sugar, and reduce inflammation. Foods high in fiber include fruits, vegetables, and whole-grain products.

PROTEIN

Protein is the building block of life, and is needed at all stages of growth and development, from birth to advanced age. It helps repair cells and tissues when they are damaged. It is also needed to build and maintain muscles and bones, to create hormones, and for the immune system to fight off infections.

When protein is digested, it breaks down into amino acids, which are classified as essential or nonessential. This is not as complicated as it sounds: nonessential amino acids are produced in the body; essential amino acids cannot be produced by the body, so they must be obtained from food. There are nine essential amino acids; food sources that contain all nine are known as "complete proteins." Examples of complete proteins include beef, bison, venison, chicken, turkey, fish and other seafood, and eggs.

You may have heard of high-protein diets, which promote the consumption of high levels of protein. As a result, they cause a drastic reduction in carbohydrate intake. When carbs are dramatically reduced in the diet, the body goes into a state called ketosis, in which it burns fat for energy. Normally we get energy from carbs, but when there is no energy coming from carbs, fat is broken down into ketones, which then supply us with energy. According to a study in the *American Journal of Clinical Nutrition*, high-protein, low-carb diets have been found to reduce hunger, decrease calorie consumption, and induce significant weight loss. Eating high amounts of protein causes a drop in the hormones that regulate appetite. So, when you eat more protein, you are less hungry, and therefore you eat less. But there is a catch. Most diets that promote high protein and low carbohydrate consumption may cause potential health problems down the road.

Most high-protein, low-carbohydrate diets don't permit a high intake of carbohydrates from fruits and starchy vegetables. By omitting those carbs from your diet, you risk not taking in enough B vitamins (including folate), vitamin C, and fiber. These nutrients are vital for your body. Those same high-protein diets also promote eating foods like dairy products, which may increase your risk for heart disease, autoimmune diseases, and certain cancers. Furthermore, individuals with kidney disease may have trouble eliminating the waste products of a protein-spurred metabolism. Yes, having more protein helps you lose fat. However, I don't agree with excluding carbs and other food sources, which provide vital nutrients. The trick here is to get rid of the fat with only short periods of ketosis. This is done by eating a variety of foods, including protein, fats, *and* carbs.

What about the folks promoting no-meat, no-fat diets? The theory that eating animal protein, and any kind of fat, will kill you does not line up with the facts, or even with common sense. Humans have been around for millions of years. According to research published in the *Annual Review of Anthropology*, eating animal products and fat provided vital nutrients and polyunsaturated fats necessary for the evolutionary development of a larger brain. And a study published in the *Journal of Nutrition* determined that routine access to animal-derived foods was the most likely reason for the development of the human race into large social beings. Early humans ate fruits, vegetables, and tubers, but they were also scavengers, eating the carcasses of animals killed by carnivores. Besides the leftover meat (the animal's muscle), they ate the brain and bone marrow, a source of fat for energy. In fact, eating the brains of animals provided early man with an omega-3 fatty acid called docosahexaenoic acid (DHA), which is essential for the development of the brain and nervous system. Early humans got most of their energy from consuming super-lean meats, which also provided fat-soluble vitamins like A, D, E, and K. Animal meat, organs, and brains were also concentrated sources of iron, calcium, sodium, zinc, and B vitamins, including B_1, niacin, B_6, B_{12}, and folate. Animal protein was necessary for early man's physical development and health, and remains so for us today.

You often hear that red meat is bad for your health, causing conditions like heart disease and colon cancer. Later on, I dissect the facts and present what the current research confirms: unprocessed red meat is not the cause of colon cancer. Think about it: not all red meat is the same. Available for your consumption are processed/factory-farmed red meat, grain-fed red meat, and grass-fed red meat. Clearly, distinctions need to be made among them so we can stop blaming our ill health on something we've consumed for millions of years.

Certain healthful, lean, free-range meats are loaded with omega-3 essential fatty acids and an abundance of nutrients. These meats, however, do not come from abused, factory-farmed livestock, injected with synthetic hormones to keep them lactating long after they give birth, shot up with antibiotics, and fed unnatural food sources such as corn and soy—not grass, but grains. Unfortunately, for most of us, our food supply is controlled by companies that put this crap into the meats. Buying free-range, grass-fed, organic meats that have no toxins is the best way to ensure a healthful source of protein.

Since we are on the topic of meat, I want to mention how to safely prepare it. Grilling is a traditional way to cook meat, and while nothing beats a grilled grass-fed burger, there are potential health risks associated with cooking meat at high temperatures. While high-heat cooking methods kill bacteria and other foodborne pathogens, the heat causes the protein in meat to produce compounds called heterocyclic amines, which can be carcinogenic (cancer-causing) when the meat is burned, blackened, or charred. To combat the production of these nasty compounds, grill meats on low heat and flip them frequently to avoid burning and charring.

Luckily, Mother Nature has created anthocyanins, compounds in fruits and vegetables that neutralize heterocyclic amines. (Anthocyanins are also responsible for certain fruits' and vegetables' purple hue.) In fact, according to the *Journal of Toxicological Sciences*, anthocyanins in purple sweet potato and red cabbage neutralized heterocyclic amines and their damaging effects in the gut. There are many ways to add red and purple fruits and vegetables to grilled meats to counteract the production of heterocyclic amines. Check out the Red Cabbage, Onions & Oranges recipe on page 423 for a simple side for your grilled and cooked meats, making them not only safer to eat but unbelievably delicious.

Not All Protein Is the Same

I mentioned previously how protein is broken down into amino acids in the body. These amino acids are then broken down into nitrogen, which is necessary for normal cellular function. Nitrogen balance refers to the amount of nitrogen taken into the body minus the amount excreted or lost. Ideally, we want to stay at a point where the amount of nitrogen in equals the amount of nitrogen lost. Because protein is the only macronutrient that provides us with nitrogen, a negative balance can be a sign of malnutrition and inadequate dietary protein. When rebuilding from a disease or while losing fat and working toward getting lean, you want to be in positive nitrogen balance. This means eating protein-based foods with all the essential amino acids. To stay in a positive nitrogen balance, you need enough amino acids from the right amount and type of protein. If you omit an amino acid from your diet, you will be in a negative nitrogen balance.

That being said, there is much confusion regarding which food sources provide the most complete protein, which again comes down to nitrogen balance. Do legumes and other plant-based foods have the same amount of protein as animal-based foods? Plant proteins are considered incomplete because, unlike animal proteins, they don't contain all nine essential amino acids. If you follow a plant-based diet or eat meat infrequently, you have to eat combinations of foods, such as rice or pasta with beans, to create a complete protein. Plants cannot meet your nitrogen needs unless you food combine.

What About Protein Powders?

Rebuilding from a chronic health issue or improving your body composition often increases your protein requirements. To increase your dietary protein, I recommend protein powders that are easier to digest and allow for quick absorption for a speedier rebuild. I also recommend using protein powders to get back into positive nitrogen balance after a workout. Here's why: When muscles are overloaded during a workout, microscopic tears happen in them—a normal response of your muscles when they experience stress—and they use up their proteins (nitrogen) during the workout. Too much training coupled with insufficient protein consumption will create a negative nitrogen balance and muscle protein breakdown.

In order for these muscles to repair and/or grow, there needs to be an accumulation of protein or nitrogen in the muscle. Eating high-quality proteins and supplementing with a healthful protein source after a workout puts you into positive nitrogen balance, thus promoting muscle growth and proper repair.

Because it takes time for the body to digest and absorb solid food, shakes provide an easy and quickly digested protein source for your body. Widely available protein powders include whey, egg white, soy, and casein.

WHEY PROTEIN has a great nutritional reputation, as it provides all the essential and nonessential amino acids, as well as branched-chain amino acids (which prevent muscle oxidation and breakdown). Whey comes from dairy, but it does not contain the lactose or other bioactive compounds found in dairy products. There are three different types of whey protein: isolate, hydrosylate, and concentrate. Whey protein isolate is roughly 90 to 94 percent pure protein. Whey protein hydrosylate is "predigested" and very expensive. Whey protein concentrate usually has trace amounts of lactose.

EGG WHITE PROTEIN was the popular choice before whey became available. Like whey, egg whites are an excellent source of protein to maintain or build lean muscle and recover from disease. Egg white protein is quickly digested and absorbed by the body.

SOY PROTEIN ISOLATE comes from soybeans and is the most popular vegetable-derived protein supplement. Others include hemp, pea, and brown rice. While the protein found in soy supplies all nine essential amino acids, it takes longer to digest and has a slow absorption rate.

CASEIN, like whey, is derived from dairy, making up roughly 80 percent of dairy protein. Like soy, it is absorbed slowly in the digestive system.

Protein is measured by its biological value—the amount of protein retained after absorption and used by the tissues of the body. The higher the value, the greater the bioavailability of the protein. A high biological value reflects a high level of amino acids from the protein source. According to the *Journal of Sports Science and Medicine*, the biological values of these four popular protein sources are:

- Whey—104
- Egg White—100
- Soy—74
- Casein—77

Whey and egg white protein have the highest values and the best bioavailability for use by muscles. However, you should be aware that all protein sources have potential side effects. Whey protein isolate and hydrosylate are both virtually lactose-free and should pose no problems for those who are lactose intolerant. If you have a reaction (bloating, nausea, or other GI issues) to whey protein, consider getting IgE food-allergy testing to see why you may be reacting. Egg protein can also cause an allergic response in susceptible individuals. Again, consider food-allergy testing to explain a reaction.

As a physician and nutritionist, I strongly recommend avoiding soy and casein, as both have been shown to cause health issues.

The digestion of the milk protein casein releases bioactive compounds, one of which is bioactive peptide beta-casomorphin 7 (BCM-7). BCM-7 acts like morphine in the body and is linked to type 1 diabetes, ischemic heart disease, and sudden infant death syndrome, as well as constipation, insomnia, allergies, and other inflammatory conditions.

Unfermented soy—the type used in protein powders, bars, and meal replacements—is also not as healthful as we have been led to believe. Unfermented soy (which has not been soaked or treated with magnesium chloride) most likely comes from GMO soybeans that have been engineered to resist the pesticide Roundup. GMOs have been linked to infertility, low-birth-weight babies, birth defects, allergies, and many other health problems. Unfermented soy is also loaded with antinutrients, which have been linked to digestive disorders, allergies, malnutrition, and suppression of the immune system.

My advice is to use whey or egg white protein in your post-workout smoothie or as added protein when rebuilding from a crisis—provided you have no allergies. Mix the protein with fruit and a scoop or two of your favorite greens powder—a multivitamin containing many servings of vegetables and superfoods in a water-soluble powder. The best time to take in this protein is within 30 minutes after your workout, since your body starts to heal the microtears in your muscles right away. Refueling your body right after your workout will help you stay in nitrogen balance and create a lean, healthy body composition. If you are rebuilding from a chronic health issue, adding protein shakes to your food plan is one more way to ensure you are getting enough digestible protein.

NOTE: Throughout the book, I mention the use of specific nutraceuticals, protein powders, powdered multivitamins, and different specialty nutrients, including indole-3-carbinol, coenzyme Q10, and others. To prevent you from searching for, buying and taking subpar supplement products, you can go to my online store at www.drzembroski.com for any of the research-based nutrients discussed throughout the book.

FATS

The third category of macronutrients is fats. Fats provide us with essential fatty acids—the type we must get from food. Fats are needed for growth and development, as well as the maintenance of healthy cell membranes. Fats provide cushioning for the organs and are needed for the body to absorb the fat-soluble vitamins A, D, E, and K. Fats can be solid or liquid at room temperature. Solid fats include animal fats, avocado, nuts, nut butters, and seeds. Liquid fats include fish oils, olive oil, grape-seed oil, avocado oil, coconut oil, and ghee (clarified butter); note that coconut oil and ghee may solidify at cooler temperatures.

As with many food groups, there are important distinctions between different types of fats—olive oil is not the same as butter, or margarine, or partially hydrogenated vegetable oil (an industrial fat produced in a processing plant). Industrial and "fake" fats are hazardous to your health. Understanding why some fats are good for you and some fats are bad for you will not only help you lose weight but also make it easier for you to rebuild from a health crisis.

Fats can be categorized as saturated or unsaturated (we'll get to the dreaded trans fat category later).

SATURATED FATS are "saturated" with hydrogen atoms. Most saturated fats are solid at room temperature, and unsaturated fats are liquid at room temperature. Animal fats are saturated; they include cream, butter, cheese, ghee, lard, eggs, and meats. A few vegetable products, such as coconut oil, palm kernel oil, and chocolate, also contain saturated fats.

UNSATURATED FATS have fewer hydrogen atoms and can be broken down further into two additional categories: monounsaturated and polyunsaturated. *Monounsaturated* fats are found in nuts and nut oils, olives and olive oil, grape-seed oil, avocados and avocado oil, and oats. *Polyunsaturated* fats are found in nuts, seeds, fish (sardines, tuna, wild salmon), olive oil, seaweed, green leafy vegetables, and algae. They contain omega-3, omega-6, and omega-9 fatty acids.

TRANS FATS (trans-fatty acids) are a type of unsaturated fat that can be classified as naturally occurring or artificial. Naturally occurring trans fats are found in animal-based foods like meat and dairy. These fats are formed when the bacteria in the stomach of the animal assist in the digestion of grass. Research has found that a moderate intake of naturally occurring trans fats does not appear to be harmful. One example of a healthful trans fat is conjugated linoleic acid (CLA), a popular weight-loss supplement. CLA has been shown also to assist in glucose and insulin regulation. However, the artificial industrial trans fats (hydrogenated fats) used in food processing are toxic and dangerous. They are found in snack foods, baked goods, deep-fried foods, fast food, junk vegetable oils, shortening, margarine, French fries, fried chicken, chicken nuggets, chips, taco shells, doughnuts, pizza dough, hot chocolate mixes, store-bought salad dressings, crackers, cookies, pastries, and commercial bread crumbs and croutons ... to name a few.

Junk-food companies use partially hydrogenated fats because they are less prone to going bad or rancid, which means they have a longer shelf life. But eating foods with a long shelf life may shorten *your* shelf life.

The chemical processing of liquid vegetable oil into trans fat is known as hydrogenation or partial hydrogenation. Partially hydrogenated vegetable oil is the main ingredient in margarine and vegetable shortening. Let's say you want to turn a bottle of corn oil, an unsaturated liquid fat, into margarine, a solid. By adding hydrogen atoms to the oil, or "partially hydrogenating" it, you make the oil solid at room temperature. Why is this bad? Partially hydrogenated fats, or trans fats, have been shown to lower HDL, the protein that carts fat out of the heart, and increase LDL, the protein that delivers fat to the heart. High LDL has been associated with an increased risk for cardiovascular disease. Hydrogenated fats increase lipoprotein-A, which is a heart disease marker that can increase inflammation and blood clotting, both factors associated with heart attacks and strokes. Trans fats also increase the risk for developing cancer, Alzheimer's disease, obesity, and diabetes.

JOHN'S STORY

John C. is a forty-eight-year-old man with a busy life, juggling four children and a demanding career. While he was becoming successful in business and raising a family, he neglected to focus on his health. When John was young, his mother died suddenly from a heart attack, and for years, her passing haunted him; he feared that he, too, would have a sudden heart attack at an early age.

A couple of years ago, John began pursuing tests to rule out (or in) coronary artery disease. He had the standard blood tests, stress tests, and calcium-score testing. His calcium score, cholesterol level, and blood sugar were all high. He realized he was developing coronary artery disease, and the race was on to stop the disease. John did his research and became educated on the causes of heart disease, along with the lifestyle and diet changes needed to stop its progression. His fear motivated him to change his diet the best he knew how. He began searching for someone who could offer the right solution, but also work with him long-term to see him through it all.

John was referred to me for nutritional advice and counseling. After reviewing his previous lab work, we decided to get more in-depth testing done. The results indicated insulin resistance and continued high blood sugar. In addition, his cholesterol, LDL, Apolipoprotein B, oxidized LDL, and C-reactive protein (CRP, an inflammatory marker) were high.

John also complained of feeling soft, and hated the excess body fat he was carrying. When discussing his diet, I realized that he was eating processed, nutrient-deficient foods such as pasta made from refined white flour, dairy, and too many high-calorie sugary foods. Also, he was not eating nearly enough plant-based foods to sustain normal function and reduce inflammation—the culprit behind coronary artery disease. John immediately became committed to seeing his condition improve, and we eliminated refined grains, dairy, and white sugar from his diet.

In the weeks that followed, John had never felt better. His body fat percentage dropped dramatically, and he soon was staring at a six-pack he had last admired in college. Follow-up blood work confirmed that John's diet and lifestyle changes were paying off. His CRP is now normal, having dropped from 5.4 to 0.6, and his oxidized LDL is back to normal as well.

Then and Now: How Our Diet Has Changed

Ample research shows that a poor diet—consisting of processed, nutrient-deficient foods—is a major contributor, if not the *leading* contributor, to the rise in chronic disease cases and related deaths in the United States. Heart disease, cancer, and type 2 diabetes, as well as conditions like high blood pressure, arthritis, and autoimmune disorders, are the end result of eating the standard American diet (SAD) of processed "meats," white sugar, dairy, and refined grains.

Let's go back in time for a moment and discuss how this contemporary diet is vastly different from that of our prehistoric ancestors. A study in the *European Journal of Clinical Nutrition* describes our ancestral menu as consisting of vegetables, fruits, roots, herbs, insects, various meat sources, and fish. In addition to the organs and muscle tissue of an animal, the bone marrow was eaten and the bones gnawed. Foods consumed in the very distant past were unprocessed and, until fire was discovered, eaten raw. This so-called primitive diet was nutrient-dense.

Fast-forward to the early 1900s, when industrial food processing was developed and processed foods entered our food supply. Food processing involved the large-scale milling of grains, refinement of sugar, and canning of foods. These methods caused a significant loss of nutrients in the foods being processed. Knowing this, companies decided to "enrich" and "fortify" foods by adding back certain nutrients. Recently, processed food companies decided to introduce synthetic chemicals to make foods glow, prevent spoilage, and make them addictive. The consequence of these artificial food chemicals is ill health. Why would you eat anything that says "artificial" on the label?

How does all of this relate to disease? Simply put, the consumption of processed foods works contrary to your genes—your DNA. The nutrients that come from unprocessed, whole foods—our prehistoric diet—carry information (consisting of vitamins, minerals, and phytochemicals) to your genes, which regulate cell, tissue, and organ function. Without this information, your cells, tissues, and organs begin to malfunction. This is called subclinical nutrient deficiency, which happens before symptoms occur. The longer you are nutrient-starved, the worse the tissue dysfunction becomes; eventually, the cells, tissues, and organs become diseased and begin to fail. The end result is heart disease, cancer, type 2 diabetes, high blood pressure, autoimmune disease, arthritis, and/or obesity.

By contrast, in recent years, extensive research has focused on disease control and prevention through the consumption of whole foods and the phytochemicals they naturally contain. Eating whole foods, as they are found in nature, provides us with all the nutrients that allow us to live disease-free, and to age without crippling conditions and premature death. What is this diet of whole foods? Read on.

Rebuild with Fruits and Vegetables

No other food source is more important for your health than plant-based foods. For years you have been hearing how important it is to eat plenty of fruits and vegetables, but you may not have heard many reasons why. To start, fruits and vegetables are very low in calories and fat. They are loaded with antioxidants, enzymes, phytochemicals, and important vitamins, including A, C, K, E, B_1 (thiamine), B_2 (riboflavin), B_6, folate, pantothenic acid, and niacin. The minerals contained in fruits and vegetables include potassium, phosphorous, magnesium, sodium, calcium, iodine, iron, zinc, copper, manganese, and selenium. These vitamins and minerals help to run intricate cellular machinery responsible for producing energy, burning fat, detoxifying, and healing, as well as maintaining pH, electrolyte balance, nerve and muscle function, cellular repair, and proper immune function—to name a few benefits.

I think it's important to mention some of the vitamins, minerals, and phytochemicals found in plant-based foods, as well as why eating them will help you get rid of body fat and allow you to rebuild your health and prevent any future recurrence of disease.

Vitamins for Rebuilding

Vitamins are organic compounds that can't be made in the body but are required for optimal functioning of various bodily processes, and therefore must be obtained through diet. Vitamins can act as co-enzymes in metabolic reactions and are effective antioxidants to combat free radicals. They are classified as either water-soluble or fat-soluble. Water-soluble vitamins dissolve in water and are not stored in the body, so they must be taken in daily. The family of B vitamins and vitamin C are water-soluble. In contrast, fat-soluble vitamins dissolve in fat before they are absorbed into the bloodstream and subsequently stored in the liver. Vitamins A, D, E, and K are fat-soluble.

Let's look at each vitamin in turn, and examine how it acts in the body and why it is so essential for good health.

VITAMIN A

There are three forms of vitamin A—retinol, retinal, and retinoic acid—primarily found in animal-based foods, including liver and fish. Beta-carotene, an antioxidant that is converted into vitamin A, is found in plant-based foods, including butternut squash, carrots, collards, kale, pumpkin, red pepper, spinach, and sweet potato. Vitamin A is important for immune function and good vision. It is also important for red blood cell production, gene expression, bone health, suppression of cancer, and normal iron metabolism. Vitamin A deficiency can cause night blindness, a condition in which your eyes cannot adjust to dim light; thick and scaly skin; and sterility.

B VITAMINS

The family of B vitamins assists the body in making energy from food. B vitamins are needed for maintaining a normal appetite, good vision, healthy skin, smoothly running neurological function, and red blood cell formation. There are eight B vitamins in the B-complex group: B_1 (thiamin), B_2 (riboflavin), B_3 (niacin), B_5 (pantothenic acid), B_6 (pyridoxine), folate, biotin, and B_{12} (cobalamin). All eight are involved in producing energy; however, each one has unique properties.

THIAMIN (B_1): Thiamin supports the activity of nerves and muscles, including the heart. Inadequate thiamin levels can cause muscle weakness, pins-and-needles sensations, and numbness in the legs.

RIBOFLAVIN (B_2): This vitamin helps protect from oxidative damage and is needed for detoxification. A deficiency can cause itching and burning around the mouth, sensitivity to light, peripheral neuropathy, soreness of the tongue, migraine headaches, and seborrheic dermatitis (red, scaly patches of skin).

NIACIN (B₃): Niacin can help lower blood fats and stabilize your blood sugar. The collective group of symptoms that are a classic sign of a significant niacin deficiency is called pellagra and includes dermatitis, dementia, and dysentery (severe diarrhea).

PANTOTHENIC ACID (B₅): This vitamin helps your body respond to stress. If you are fatigued, weak, and/or depressed, or suffering from insomnia, you may have a B_5 deficiency.

PYRIDOXINE (B₆): Pyridoxine is important for the breakdown of starches and prevents the buildup of homocysteine (a compound linked to atherosclerosis and coronary artery disease) in the blood. B_6 is also important in the prevention of anemia.

FOLATE: Folate—not folic acid, which is synthetic and not found in nature—supports healthy red blood cells and proper nerve function, and, when taken during pregnancy, prevents the birth defect spina bifida. Low folate levels can cause elevated homocysteine and significant anemia.

BIOTIN: Biotin is needed for healthy hair and skin. Hair loss can result from a number of conditions, including alopecia (caused by multiple metabolic issues), male-pattern baldness from an excess of testosterone and dihydrotestosterone (DHT), and hypothyroidism. But if those reasons don't explain your thinning hair, think biotin deficiency.

COBALAMIN (B₁₂): Cobalamin allows nerves to develop properly and helps you metabolize protein, carbs, and fats. It is needed for red blood cell formation, and it reduces the buildup of homocysteine. Vitamin B_{12} is different from the other B vitamins; for proper absorption, it needs a ride into the small intestine from a protein called the intrinsic factor. While the other B vitamins are found in plant-based foods, B_{12} is found only in foods of animal origin, such as liver, meat, kidney, fish, shellfish, and eggs. B_{12} deficiency is often seen in strict vegetarians and vegans, the elderly, infants born to vegan mothers, and people suffering from autoimmune disorders in which the immune system targets the intrinsic factor. A B_{12} deficiency causes fatigue, anemia, nerve damage, numbness and tingling in the limbs, dementia, and memory loss. This collective list of symptoms is called pernicious anemia.

Now that you know more about the B vitamins and their functions, benefits, and signs of deficiency, you need to know where to find them. Asparagus, avocados, beans (legumes), bell peppers, broccoli, brown rice, dark green leafy vegetables, eggplant, green peas, lentils, mushrooms, squash, Swiss chard, tomatoes, wheat germ, and whole grains are all good sources of B vitamins, with the exception of B_{12}, which, again, is found only in animal-based foods.

Z NOTE: Risky procedures. If you have had or are considering gastric bypass surgery, it's important to keep in mind that gastric bypass causes significant malabsorption of vitamin B_{12}. If you are not familiar with the surgery, here is a quick overview: During normal digestion, food passes from the stomach into the small intestine, where nutrients are absorbed. As digestion continues, the broken-down food passes into the large intestine (colon), and waste is eventually eliminated. Gastric bypass surgery radically changes the way you digest your food and absorb nutrients.

The most common gastric bypass procedure is called the Roux-en-Y gastric bypass, in which the lower part of the stomach is "rearranged" surgically into a Y configuration: the stomach is divided into a large portion and a much smaller portion (the size of an egg). This smaller part is surgically stapled into a little pouch and connected directly to the middle of the small intestine, bypassing the upper portion. The larger portion of the stomach is then disconnected from the small intestine. The end result is a much smaller stomach, which forces you to eat less and feel less hungry.

According to the *Annals of Surgery*, after a Roux-en-Y gastric bypass, stomach acid secretion is virtually absent, and food-bound vitamin B_{12} is improperly digested and malabsorbed. The fact that stomach acid secretion virtually disappears following the procedure is a very serious issue. For one thing, protein digestion happens in the stomach; without stomach acid, protein is broken down and absorbed improperly, leading to protein deficiency. Without protein, the body and all of its intricate systems begin to fail. Stomach acid is also a disinfectant; without it, there is a higher risk of developing gut infections from pathogens ingested with food or water, for example *H. pylori*. An undetected and untreated *H. pylori* infection is associated with a high risk of developing lymphoma, a type of cancer, in the gut.

Moreover, if you don't stop eating processed foods, making your stomach smaller is a temporary Band-Aid. High-calorie foods will continue to flip the fat-storing switches regardless of how small your stomach is. Therefore, if you deprive yourself of nutrients by choice by eating a poor diet, or it is forced through invasive procedures, you increase your risk for chronic disease.

Having your stomach cut open and rearranged doesn't sound like a safe diet choice. Gastric bypass surgery is a major surgery with long-term health consequences. If you know someone considering this procedure, please show them this book and encourage them to read and apply the tools within. The only side effect of the food recommendations I make here is a lean and healthy body.

Jamie B. is a twenty-one-year-old cancer victor who struggled with her body composition for years. Following surgery to remove a brain tumor, she underwent radiation to ensure the cancer was destroyed. Unfortunately, the damage it caused created abnormal hormone levels, altered her metabolism, and resulted in extreme weight gain. For years she tried to control her weight through proper food choices and exercise, but the fight got to be too much. Jamie finally opted for gastric bypass surgery. Not long after the surgery, she began suffering from chronic headaches and fatigue, which became progressively worse with time. Two years following the surgery, she, accompanied by her mom, visited me to discuss possible treatment options for her current problems. In tears, Jamie said she was unable to have a social life, or go out and enjoy herself, because she had developed chronic diarrhea that occurred every time she took a bite of food. To add to her misery, she was also dealing with a viral infection, which was probably adding to her fatigue.

Upon reviewing her blood work, I saw clearly the long-term effects of the surgery. Jamie's body was not absorbing vitamin B_{12} and iron, which had resulted in severe anemia. Her blood work revealed a low red blood cell count, low hemoglobin and hematocrit levels, and extremely low iron levels. The unrelenting diarrhea was caused by abnormal stomach acid production and improper breakdown of the food she ate. Our immediate plan was to stop the diarrhea. I gave her digestive enzymes to take every time she had a bite of food. After the first time she used the enzymes, her diarrhea stopped. The next obstacle was to help her to digest and absorb vitamin B_{12} and iron. She started a scientifically formulated multivitamin with iron and a special B-vitamin complex. I encouraged her to continue to take the enzymes anytime she ate meat in order to break down the protein and facilitate B_{12} absorption. At her next visit, new blood work revealed improvements in her anemia, including a higher red blood cell count and improved hemoglobin, hematocrit, iron, and ferritin (iron storage) levels.

VITAMIN C

Of all the vitamins essential to health, vitamin C (ascorbic acid) is at the top of the list. Why? It is not made in the body, so it has to be taken in through the diet, thus making it essential. It is also a powerful antioxidant, important for building and maintaining healthy tissue through collagen synthesis. Vitamin C helps maintain healthy teeth and gums, promotes antibody production, and is needed for iron absorption. Last, vitamin C supports detoxification, increases HDL production, and is needed for the excretion or elimination of heavy metals.

Coronary artery disease is still the number one killer on the planet, despite the proliferation of cholesterol-lowering drugs, stents, and bypass surgeries. As I explained in chapter 1, current research states that coronary artery disease is *not* a consequence of cholesterol sticking to and clogging the arteries, but rather an inflammatory condition within the arterial walls. This inflammation allows the passage of LDL and white blood cells into the wall of the artery, where the LDL is oxidized, (damaged by free radicals). Eventually the damage within the arterial wall causes an eruption of material and debris within the lumen (opening of the artery), quickly shutting off the blood supply to the heart and leading to a sudden heart attack.

According to research published in the *Bratislava Medical Journal*, vitamin C protects LDL from oxidation. The researchers found that coronary artery disease is less pronounced in men with high blood levels of vitamin C. They also found that in parts of western Europe, deaths from cardiovascular causes fell rapidly following a movement to increase intake of vitamin C. Conversely, cardiovascular deaths are still growing in areas with known vitamin C deficiency.

In a research article published in the *New England Journal of Medicine*, subjects whose vitamin C intake exceeded 50 mg per day had a lower rate of death from all cardiovascular disease. Getting more than 50 mg per day is pretty easy; for instance, one kiwifruit provides 84 mg of vitamin C, while broccoli provides 81 mg per cup, chopped. If you have four or five servings of fruits and vegetables a day, that will provide enough vitamin C to prevent heart disease.

What about cancer? Since cancer was close to my heart, literally, I will point out the benefits of vitamin C in staving off cancer. It is a well-known fact that, under sustained environmental stress, free radicals are produced in the body. These free radicals can damage the DNA of the cells, which may cause the initial mutations within the cell that will eventually lead to cancer. Vitamin C is a powerful antioxidant that breaks down in the body, generating hydrogen peroxide, which is a reactive oxygen species (free radical) that can damage tissue. Normal cells produce enzymes that neutralize and eliminate the hydrogen peroxide, rendering it harmless. However, tumor cells lack these enzymes and are less capable of removing hydrogen peroxide, which ultimately leads to the cancer cells' death. Vitamin C can also inhibit cancer cell growth and blood vessel development to small tumors, a process called angiogenesis.

Regarding your dietary intake of vitamin C, the National Cancer Institute recommends five daily servings of plant-based foods—vegetables and fruits—to lower your risk for cancers of the mouth, throat, stomach, lung, colon, pancreas, and prostate. Vitamin C is readily available in citrus fruits (lemon, lime, grapefruit, orange, and tangerine, to name a few), as well as in broccoli, Brussels sprouts, cauliflower, kale, kiwifruit, red and green bell peppers, strawberries, and sweet potato. Other food sources include apples, black currants, cabbage, cantaloupe, guava, honeydew melon, mango, mustard greens, papaya, raspberries, red and green chiles, and spinach.

VITAMIN D: A POWERFUL HORMONE

You may be wondering why I didn't include vitamin D in the original list of nutrients found in plant-based foods. First, although it is called a vitamin, vitamin D is actually a hormone. Vitamins are obtained through diet, unlike hormones, which are made in the body. There are two forms of vitamin D: D_2 is found in fungi, like mushrooms, but not found in green leafy plants. D_3 is generated when your skin is exposed to UV radiation from sunlight (more on this on page 47). D_3 is also found in oily fish, cod-liver oil, herring, mackerel, salmon, sardines, tuna, and, to a lesser extent, egg yolks.

The classic manifestation of vitamin D deficiency in children is rickets, while in adults it causes osteomalacia; both conditions result in softening of the bones. However, low levels of vitamin D have been implicated in almost every major disease and many other disorders, including:

- Autoimmune disease
- Cancer
- Chronic pain
- Depression
- Heart disease
- High blood pressure
- Infertility
- Osteoporosis
- Psoriasis

How is vitamin D produced? When ultraviolet rays (specifically UVB) from the sun come in contact with the skin, it triggers the production of a chemical that travels to the liver, then to the kidneys to become the active form of vitamin D, called calcitriol. This helps the intestines absorb calcium and maintains the calcium and phosphate levels necessary for bone formation. It enhances muscle strength, has anti-inflammatory effects, and regulates the immune system. Calcitriol also helps control cell growth, which researchers have found can prevent cancer.

When patients come to see me about unresolved health issues, I often see common threads. One is a nutrient-deprived diet, and the other is a low level of vitamin D. One major cause of low vitamin D is fear of skin cancer, which has driven people to avoid the sun. Yet melanoma (a deadly form of skin cancer) is usually not located on parts of the body that get sun exposure. The *Journal of Skin Cancer* found that although outdoor workers get three to ten times the annual dose of UV radiation that indoor workers get, outdoor workers have similar or lower incidences of malignant melanoma. The human race has been out in the sun for millions of years, yet we are still around.

You may have heard that vitamin D is also important for bone health, and that's correct. Vitamin D is needed to absorb calcium from foods, which is used to build healthy bones and teeth. Not only is vitamin D responsible for the absorption of calcium, it's also important for bone mineralization, the process of adding calcium to the bone matrix (the structure within the bone) to make bones hard and durable. As mentioned earlier, severe vitamin D deficiency causes demineralized and deformed bones and the condition of softened bone known as rickets in children and osteomalacia in adults.

Since vitamin D is essential for bone health, a deficiency can contribute to osteoporosis, a common and often disabling bone disease usually diagnosed in postmenopausal women and the elderly. In patients with osteoporosis, bone-mineral density is reduced and the bone architecture breaks down, leaving empty, weak bones. Osteoporosis increases the risk of fractures of the long bones and hips, and spinal compression fractures, which lead to the stooped posture that appears as a hunchback. Spinal compression fractures are often very painful, and fractures of the hip are not only immobilizing, but can be life-threatening. The risk associated with hip fractures is deep-vein thrombosis, a condition in which a blood clot forms in the deep veins of the leg, which can then cause a pulmonary embolism, the blockage of a main artery in the lung—which, in turn, can cause sudden death. Need I say more?

What about the relationship between vitamin D and body composition? An article published in the *Nutrition Journal* showed evidence that taking a supplement with vitamin D and calcium helped get rid of body fat. The study was conducted with two groups. One group went on a calorie-restrictive diet of only 500 calories per day. The second group also reduced their calorie intake to 500 calories a day, but supplemented daily with vitamin D and calcium. Both groups followed the diet for twelve weeks. At the end of the study, the group taking the supplement of vitamin D and calcium showed a significant decrease in fat mass over the group who followed the calorie-restrictive diet alone.

In addition, population studies are revealing the relationship between grain/bread consumption and low levels of vitamin D. In "Cereal Grains: Humanity's Double-Edged Sword," an article in the *World Review of Nutrition and Dietetics*, it was noted that whole-grain products impair bone metabolism by limiting calcium intake and altering vitamin D metabolism. Population studies are also showing a widespread vitamin D deficiency in people who frequently consume whole-grain breads. And that's not taking into account the fact that most of the grain we're eating isn't "whole grain"—it's refined (even most "whole wheat" flour is refined), stripped of nutrients. If whole grains are depleting our vitamin D levels, then what's the processed stuff doing to us?

Z NOTE: The research on vitamin D is extraordinary. Facts found in the journal *Nature Reviews* found that calcitriol—the active form of vitamin D—had multiple effects on cancer. It was shown to inhibit abnormal cellular growth and decrease the spread of cancer. It also turned on a program in the cancer cells that caused them to commit suicide. Calcitriol was also shown to inhibit angiogenesis, thus starving cancer cells and tumors of their lifeline of nutrients.

Most of these studies have reported that higher blood levels of vitamin D are associated with lower rates of breast, colon, ovarian, kidney, pancreatic, prostate, and other cancers. Evidence published in the journal *Annals of Epidemiology* was surprising. It was projected that raising the year-round levels of vitamin D in the blood from 30 ng/ml to 40 to 60 ng/ml would prevent approximately 58,000 new cases of breast cancer and 49,000 new cases of colorectal cancer each year, in addition to preventing three-quarters of the deaths from those cancers. This is unheard of. By raising the levels of vitamin D beyond the "standard of care," thousands of people could be spared the emotional and physical devastation of cancer diagnosis and treatment, and their lives could be saved.

Among its countless benefits, vitamin D is also a powerful manipulator of the immune response. A deficiency of vitamin D—lower than 50ng/ml in the blood—is associated with increased susceptibility to infections and autoimmunity. Here's how that happens. Many tissues in the body, including the brain, intestine, breast, pancreas, bone marrow, skeletal muscle, and immune cells, express the vitamin D receptor (VDR)—a protein responsible for sensing vitamin D. The VDR, once activated by vitamin D, forms a complex that finds its way to the cell's nucleus and its DNA. Here, specific genes are turned on to produce proteins for different functions in the body. Vitamin D can boost your immune system while simultaneously regulating the arm of the immune system involved in autoimmunity. To prevent an autoimmune response, vitamin D suppresses T cells, the white blood cells that are programmed to attack the cells and tissues of your body, thus causing an autoimmune response. Low vitamin D is linked to autoimmune diseases, including Hashimoto's thyroiditis, multiple sclerosis, rheumatoid arthritis, diabetes mellitus, inflammatory bowel disease, Sjögren's disease, and systemic lupus erythematosus.

Finally, research is also discovering the relationship between cardiovascular disease and low vitamin D levels. The *Journal of Invasive Cardiology* reported that patients with lower vitamin D levels had a higher incidence of double- or triple-vessel coronary artery disease and diffuse coronary artery disease. Those with low vitamin D levels also exhibited dysfunction of the endothelium, the cells that line and protect the arterics, help regulate blood pressure, and protect against atherosclerosis and coronary artery disease.

> **CLINICAL NOTE:** A test to measure the amount of vitamin D in your blood is the only way to know whether you are getting enough vitamin D from the sun and/or supplements you are taking. The blood test you need is the 25(OH)D. The optimal range for vitamin D levels is 50 to 80 ng/ml, not 30 ng/ml—the current standard.

VITAMIN E

A fat-soluble vitamin abundant in vegetables, vitamin E is an antioxidant that helps prevent cell damage and plays a major role in protecting LDL from free radical damage. Vitamin E keeps the immune system in proper working order and helps reduce the proliferation of cells. It is considered the fertility vitamin, since studies have revealed its importance to reproductive health. A deficiency of vitamin E is characterized by muscle and nervous system disorders, cataracts, hemolytic anemia (the destruction of red blood cells), reproductive disorders (including a thin uterine lining), decreased sperm motility, and miscarriages.

Vitamin E is found in almonds, asparagus, avocado, beet greens, broccoli, collard greens, dandelion greens, dark green leafy vegetables, hazelnuts, pumpkin, sunflower seeds, sweet potato, turnips, and healthful vegetable oils, including olive and wheat germ oil.

VITAMIN K FOR K-OAGULATION

Vitamin K is another fat-soluble vitamin. There are two forms of vitamin K: K_1 from green plants, and K_2 from bacteria in the intestines. It is needed for healthy bones; however, the biggest role of vitamin K in the body is in blood clotting. The best food sources of vitamin K_1 are dark green leafy vegetables such as cabbage, lettuce, spinach, and turnip greens. Vitamin K_2, produced by gut bacteria and absorbed in the distal small intestine, has two crucial roles: it helps prevent atherosclerosis and osteoporosis.

> **Z NOTE:** Vitamin K deficiency is caused by a poor diet, and some pharmaceuticals, such as anti-clotting medications (Coumadin/warfarin) and broad-spectrum antibiotics (amoxicillin, streptomycin, and tetracycline).

Minerals to Rebuild

Minerals are essential nutrients that the body needs to carry out daily functions. Along with vitamins, they control and regulate a multitude of reactions in the body. The human body cannot create minerals; therefore, we must get them from foods—both plant- and animal-based. Plants absorb minerals from the soil, and we get most of our minerals from the plants we eat. Animals also eat mineral-rich plants, which we absorb in turn when we eat animal-based foods.

CALCIUM

Calcium is important for blood clotting and the passage of nutrients through cell walls, and it is essential for strong bones and teeth. As a dynamic "live" tissue, bone is constantly undergoing remodeling and turnover. Bone cells are constantly building and breaking down. This remodeling, essential to bone health, is dependent on calcium intake. Calcium is also needed for muscle contraction and to help nerves carry messages.

A calcium deficiency may result in muscle cramps, poor nerve firing, and bone demineralization or osteoporosis. Calcium-rich foods include beans, broccoli, Brussels sprouts, butternut squash, dark leafy greens, kale, spinach, Swiss chard, and turnips, but for the most part, any vegetable matter that can be eaten provides some measure of calcium. Fruits with calcium are blackberries, black currants, dates, grapefruit, orange, and pomegranate. Calcium is also found in eggs, perch, pollock, and sardines.

(Surprised that you're not seeing milk here? Turn to page 155 for more information on calcium and milk.)

COPPER

Copper, in small amounts, is essential for the absorption and storage of iron and the formation of red blood cells, among other functions. It also helps to regulate blood sugar and immune function. Copper deficiency may result in anemia, low white blood cell count, bone demineralization, poor wound healing, and weak muscles.

Copper-abundant foods include artichoke, avocado, beans, beef, blackberries, dates, kiwifruit, mango, nuts, parsnip, peas, potatoes, pumpkin, salmon, sardines, squash, sunflower seeds, sweet potato, Swiss chard, and turkey.

Z NOTE: A deficiency of copper may be a causative factor in congestive heart failure and an enlarged heart. A study published in the *European Heart Journal* found that those with chronic heart failure and ischemic heart disease had an improvement in heart function while taking a copper supplement. In addition to this study, multiple animal studies have shown that a copper deficiency in animals can induce cardiac enlargement and heart failure, which are then reversible with copper supplementation.

IODINE: THE TH-I-ROID NUTRIENT

Iodine is a mineral that is abundant in seaweed and other edible plants from the sea. It helps regulate energy production and promotes healthy skin, nails, and teeth. Its biggest role is to support normal function of the thyroid gland, which uses iodine to produce T3 and T4, hormones that are very important to a healthy body composition. Iodine deficiency can result in hypothyroidism. Lack of iodine also increases the risk of certain cancers, including thyroid, breast, and prostate cancers. Ironically, food companies know that processed foods have no nutritional value, so they add iodine to table salt. The problem is that most iodized salt has itself been processed and stripped of the more than eighty minerals found in natural salt.

Bromide, a compound in processed flours used in baked goods (bread, cakes, muffins, bagels, etc.), displaces iodine, so it's important to avoid those foods.

IRON

Iron is an essential mineral needed for the formation of hemoglobin, a protein in the blood that carries oxygen to tissues and organs throughout the body and brings carbon dioxide back to the lungs for elimination. Iron is also needed for the formation of myoglobin, which carries oxygen to the muscles, and for energy production, neurotransmitter production, and immune system health.

There are two forms of iron: heme iron and non-heme iron. Heme iron is found in clams, fish, meats, oysters, and poultry and is well absorbed by the body. Non-heme iron is found in fruits, vegetables, legumes, and cereals. Fortunately, plant-based foods also provide vitamin C, which promotes iron absorption from those foods.

Iron deficiency is the most common mineral deficiency, and according to the CDC is the leading cause of anemia in the United States. Iron deficiency is caused by either an increased need for iron, poor absorption of iron from foods, or a diet lacking in iron. Certain foods can decrease the absorption of iron: grains, certain beans, peanuts, tea, coffee, and fermented soy products all contain phytates, plant compounds that block the absorption of iron. Infants, pregnant women, and adolescent girls are at greatest risk of developing iron deficiency. Infants and the young need more iron because they are rapidly growing. Menstruation increases the demand for iron due to blood loss. Iron needs increase during pregnancy due to the requirements of the fetus. Vegans are at risk for iron deficiency because their diets do not include sources of heme iron. Those with internal bleeding disorders, including ulcers, colon cancer, and ulcerative colitis, are also at risk.

The effects of iron deficiency can include abnormal behavior, impaired mental cognition, impaired immune function, fatigue, weakness, problems regulating body temperature, and angular stomatitis (fissures or cracking of the skin at the corners of the mouth). Those with prolonged iron deficiency also develop brittle and spoon-shaped fingernails.

Iron loss can usually be treated with a balanced diet consisting of a variety of whole foods. Taking iron supplements if they are not needed can lead to oxidative stress and, for many, constipation, so try to address the deficiency with dietary changes before consulting with a qualified health care practitioner on whether you should supplement.

CLINICAL NOTE: Physicians are quick to recommend an iron supplement when someone feels fatigued or tired, but an iron supplement should be given only when evidence of an iron deficiency shows up in blood work. This will be seen as a low MCV and low MCHC. Other indications of iron-deficiency anemia include decreased hematocrit, hemoglobin, and ferritin levels.

MAGNESIUM

Magnesium is needed for many biochemical reactions in the body. It helps maintain and relax muscles and nerves, supports the immune system, and keeps bones strong. It is needed to produce energy from the foods we eat, help regulate blood sugar, promote normal blood pressure, and keep the heart rhythm steady. Magnesium can also act as a mild sedative, which helps ensure a good night's sleep.

Magnesium-rich foods include almonds, artichoke, avocado, bananas, beans, beef, beets, blackberries, Brazil nuts, butternut squash,
cashews, fish, hazelnuts, kiwifruit, peas, pecans, pistachios, pumpkin
seeds, quinoa, raspberries, shrimp, spinach, spirulina, walnuts, and
wheat germ.

Like other mineral deficiencies, the main reason for a magnesium
deficiency is a nutrient-deprived diet. However, gastrointestinal disorders such as Crohn's disease can limit the body's ability to absorb
magnesium, and chronic diarrhea can also result in a magnesium deficiency.

This may come as a shock, but alcohol—yes, alcohol—can deplete
magnesium. According to a study published in the *Journal of the American College of Nutrition*, alcohol consumption acts as a magnesium
diuretic, causing a "vigorous" increase in magnesium loss through the
urine. Chronic intake of alcohol also depletes the body's stores of magnesium and the rate at which magnesium is absorbed. Additionally,
alcohol contributes to vitamin D deficiency, which can also lower magnesium levels. Chemotherapy, diuretics, antibiotics, physical stress,
and excessive exercising can cause a loss of magnesium as well.

When magnesium levels get low enough, symptoms occur. You may
have heard of cardiac arrhythmias, muscle cramping, and restless leg
syndrome as symptoms of low magnesium, but how about anxiety,
hyperactivity, and difficulty falling asleep? Adequate magnesium is
needed for the normal functioning of the brain and nervous system.
It is also needed for electrolyte balance, which also affects the nervous
system.

RON'S STORY

Ron came to me complaining of restless leg syndrome—a set of symptoms characterized by uncomfortable sensations in the legs and an
urgency to move the legs. The symptoms always occur at night while

resting or trying to sleep. I quickly learned that Ron enjoyed alcohol at night, and was consuming too many nutrient-deprived foods. Following an assessment of his blood work, along with bioelectrical-impedance testing to evaluate his body fat and metabolism, we implemented a food plan. To help him with the restless legs, I prescribed magnesium glycinate to be taken a few hours before bed. Ron also agreed to reduce his drinking at night. Within a few days, the symptoms in his legs disappeared, and he reported sleeping better than he could remember.

CLINICAL NOTE: I prescribe magnesium only once I fully understand a patient's condition and know of any medications he or she is taking. When considering whether you should supplement with magnesium, or any other nutrient, it's important to know what condition or health issue you are trying to resolve and to determine if that supplement will be of benefit.

Second, there are endless possibilities for interactions between prescription drugs and nutraceuticals (dietary supplements). Before you take concentrated single nutrient supplements or supplements with multiple nutrient ingredients, I suggest you consult with a health care professional seasoned in nutrition and nutritional biochemistry, to make sure you are not risking any adverse drug/nutrient interactions.

MANGANESE

Manganese is needed for enzyme reactions controlling metabolism, energy, and thyroid-hormone function. It is also important in the regulation of blood sugar during periods of fasting (anytime you're not eating). A deficiency of manganese is rare. It is abundant in anchovies, asparagus, avocado, bananas, beans, blackberries, blueberries, cranberries, eggs, grapefruit, herring, kale, nuts, pineapple, raspberries, brown rice, sardines, spirulina, squash, strawberries, sweet potatoes, and Swiss chard.

PHOSPHOROUS

After calcium, phosphorous is the second most abundant mineral in the body. The skeleton contains roughly 85 percent of total body phosphorous. Besides its role in the structural component of teeth and bones, it is important in maintaining healthy cell membranes, as well as high-energy compounds that are needed for metabolism.

Phosphorous is abundant in many foods, and is well absorbed; therefore, deficiency is highly unlikely. However, people at risk for deficiency are alcoholics and those who abuse antacids containing magnesium and aluminum, which can cause phosphorous malabsorption and increased urinary loss of phosphorous.

Phosphorous is found in artichoke, avocado, most beans, black currants, Brussels sprouts, eggs, fish, kiwifruit, meat, nuts (including Brazil nuts and cashews), parsnips, peas, poultry, pumpkin seeds, sunflower seeds, and sweet potato.

POTASSIUM

Potassium is the third most abundant mineral in the body. It is needed for nerve firing, muscle contraction, and, more important, proper heart function. Potassium interacts with sodium and chloride to control fluid, pH, and electrolyte balance.

Potassium-rich foods include almonds, avocado, bamboo shoots, bananas, most beans, beef, bok choy, Brussels sprouts, carrots, cherries, chicken, clams, coconut, dates, fish (especially salmon), grapefruit, kiwifruit, steel-cut oats, papaya, parsnips, pumpkin seeds, sardines, spinach, sunflower seeds, sweet potatoes, Swiss chard, tomatoes, and turkey.

Clinically, I see many endurance athletes who succumb to a loss of potassium, or hypokalemia, due to excessive sweating. They commonly complain of muscle cramping, heart irregularities, fatigue, and weakness. This is due not only to direct loss of potassium but also to depletion of potassium in the muscles. Potassium is stored with muscle sugar (glycogen) and is lost when muscles use up that glycogen to get through a workout.

High levels of stress hormones, diuretic use, and malnutrition can also cause hypokalemia. When potassium is deficient, it results in heart failure, muscle weakness, paralysis (in extreme situations), kidney dysfunction, and problems with elevated blood sugar.

If you exercise daily, you should drink water not only all day, but during and right after exercising in order to replenish electrolytes lost in the workout. I have included a tasty, homemade electrolyte recipe on page 433 for creating your own sports drink. I suggest you use it to replenish fluids and electrolytes instead of wasting money on crappy sports drinks loaded with high-fructose corn syrup.

SELENIUM

Selenium has two important functions. It is needed to produce powerful antioxidants called selenoproteins, which have the ability to render free radicals harmless. More important, it gobbles up the free radicals that damage LDL. Also, due to its role in regulating thyroid hormones, selenium is needed for normal growth and metabolism.

The major food sources of selenium are seafood and organ meats. Other sources include eggs, grains, meat, and poultry; smaller amounts are found in asparagus, bananas, beans, Brazil nuts (highest selenium content), Brussels sprouts, cashews, coconut, parsnips, black-eyed peas, long-grain brown rice, and spinach.

CLINICAL NOTE: The function of the thyroid is to take iodine and the amino acid tyrosine and make the thyroid hormones thyroxine (T4) and triiodothyronine (T3). T4 and T3 are released into the blood and transported throughout the body, where they act on nearly every cell. Their job is to increase metabolism, help control the proper development of all cells, and regulate the metabolism of macronutrients. Circulating T4 is converted into T3 in the liver by enzymes that are dependent on zinc, selenium, magnesium, vitamin B_6, vitamin B_{12}, as well as the amino acids cysteine, glutamine, and glycine. If you have symptoms of thyroid dysfunction but your blood work "looks fine," focus on the levels of free T4 and free T3. If free T4 is normal and free T3 is low, it may be a conversion issue due to a lack of the nutrients listed above.

SODIUM

Sodium has gotten a bad rap. In small amounts, sodium is an essential mineral needed to balance fluids and electrolytes, and regulate blood volume and pH. Along with potassium, sodium is needed to transmit nerve impulses and regulate muscle function. However, as we know, Americans eat far too much sodium chloride (salt).

As a daily requirement, the magic number for salt is 2,400 mg, or roughly 1 teaspoon. The American Heart Association recommends no more than 1,500 mg of sodium per day. The concern is that high amounts of dietary sodium can lead to increased blood volume and high blood pressure, which can cause heart disease.

If you are salt-sensitive, lowering your sodium intake involves more than just leaving the salt shaker in the spice rack. Unless you are paying attention to food labels or eating mostly home-cooked meals, you are probably consuming too much salt, as most of the salt we ingest is found in processed and fast foods. Let's look at the sodium content of some of these items.

At McDonald's, a Big Mac has a "whopping" 970 mg of sodium, a double cheeseburger 1,050 mg, and Premium Crispy Chicken Club Sandwich tops the list at 1,410 mg.

At the grocery deli counter, a 2-ounce serving (about four thin slices) of deli-style smoked ham has about 660 mg of sodium; 2 ounces of regular ham has 590 mg; and four thin slices (roughly 4 ounces) of deli turkey breast has 600 mg. While we're on the topic of lunch, let's look at the sodium content of a popular packaged "food-like" product fed to children: Lunchables. Manufactured by Oscar Mayer, the plastic-wrapped Turkey & Cheddar Lunchable contains 1,100 mg of sodium per serving. The recommended daily allowance of sodium for children four to eight years old is 1,200 mg.

And don't even get me started on hot dogs—a plain hot dog on a white-flour bun contains 717 mg of sodium; add chili and cheese, and you reach 1,264 mg.

What better way to spend a rainy Saturday afternoon than at the movies with a bag of popcorn? Air-popped popcorn can be a relatively harmless snack, but movie popcorn is a wolf in sheep's clothing. A large bag of popcorn has 1,500 mg of sodium—and that doesn't include the yellow "butter" they squirt all over it.

Sodium is also hidden in cured meats (such as sausage and bacon), breads and other baked goods, microwaveable foods, and many foods from Chinese and other takeout restaurants, where sodium is added to dishes in various forms, such as sodium nitrite, sodium saccharin, sodium benzoate, and monosodium glutamate (MSG, or free glutamic acid).

What about salt for seasoning foods and cooking? Salt is a crystalline mineral made up of sodium (Na) and chloride (Cl)—both essential for human life. These elements serve to help the brain and nerves send electrical impulses, absorb and transport nutrients, maintain blood pressure, and maintain the balance of our fluids. The majority of sodium from salts in the Western diet is found in processed and fast foods. The amount of sodium in processed foods can encourage many health problems, including high blood pressure. This said, if you eat nutrient-dense whole foods, you don't need to worry about adding a little natural salt to your meals to bring out and enhance the taste.

There are different varieties of salt to choose from, including kosher, pink Himalayan, sea salt, iodized sea salt, and regular iodized table salt—each with a unique texture and flavor. In the recipes in this book, I recommend using sea salt and pink Himalayan salt for their naturally occurring minerals (and because they lend a briny flavor to different foods). Use whichever salt you like the taste of in your recipes.

Z NOTE: MSG is a white powder made from the amino acid glutamate, which occurs naturally in seaweed, sugar beets, vegetables, and grains containing gluten. The sodium component of MSG turns it into a salt. MSG enhances the flavors of food, and it is added to canned vegetables and soups, processed meats, Chinese food and other takeout options, dressings, junk-food snacks (Doritos, Cheetos, and any other snacks made with cheese powder), hot dogs, smoked meats, grated Parmesan cheese from a can, and soy sauce. MSG is also found in powdered spice mixes, instant soup packets, and dry dressing mixes.

Even though MSG is used in many foods, it can cause a wide range of side effects, including migraine headaches, asthma, rashes, hives, vomiting, heart irregularities, depression, skin flushing, numbness and tingling, nausea, and weakness. To figure out why, I picked up a book called *Excitotoxins: The Taste That Kills,* by Dr. Russell L. Blaylock. In the book, Dr. Blaylock explores the dangers of artificial flavor enhancers like MSG, as well as zero-calorie sweeteners like aspartame. Citing hundreds of scientific studies, he uncovers the harmful effects of MSG on the brain and nervous system.

Basically, glutamate is a naturally occurring amino acid, and its role is to stimulate the brain and nervous system as a neurotransmitter. At normal levels, it is important for memory, learning, and muscle tone. However, an excess of glutamate can overstimulate the nervous system, causing nerve cell death. MSG is known as an excitotoxin due to its potential role in nervous system damage. (Excitotoxins are compounds that can overstimulate neurons until the point of exhaustion and eventual nerve cell death.)

If MSG can potentially damage the nervous system, can it affect body composition? A study published in the journal *Obesity* linked MSG to excess weight and obesity. More than 750 Chinese men and women, ages forty to fifty-nine, were studied. Of those who cooked at home, roughly 82 percent used MSG in their food. That group was further divided into three groups.

Adjusted for calorie intake and physical activity, those who used the most MSG were three times more likely to be overweight. The study mentioned that MSG can damage appetite control mechanisms in the brain, as well as affect how we metabolize fat.

ZINC

This metallic ion is important in many key functions in the body, including carbohydrate and protein metabolism, alcohol detoxification, wound healing, vision, growth, balancing blood sugar, smell and taste perception, DNA repair, immune function, and defense against free radicals.

Zinc is important during pregnancy for the growth and development of the fetus, due to the rapid division of cells. It is also needed for growth in infants, children, and teens, and can help alleviate the symptoms of premenstrual syndrome. Zinc also plays a vital role in both male and female fertility. It is needed to maintain sperm count, motility, prostate health, and testosterone levels in men. A study published in the *Asian Journal of Andrology* found zinc levels to be directly related to sperm development and sperm count. A deficiency of zinc was also found to cause a dysfunction of the gonads, as well as decreased testosterone levels. In women, zinc plays a role in sexual development, the menstrual cycle, and the production of healthy eggs and ovulation. A deficiency of zinc during pregnancy can lead to miscarriages and abnormal fetal development.

The immune system is dependent on zinc. When zinc is deficient, lymphocytes (one type of white blood cell) are less able to fight off infection and tumor cells. Zinc-rich foods include asparagus, avocado, most beans, beef, blackberries, Brussels sprouts, cashews, chicken, eggs, fish, oats, peas, pomegranate, pumpkin seeds, raspberries, brown rice, seafood (especially oysters), spirulina, sunflower seeds, Swiss chard, turkey, and wheat germ.

Phytonutrients: Rebuild with Color

Fruits and vegetables are the most nutrient-dense foods you can eat. They are low in calories but high in water content and fiber, which satisfies the appetite and improves blood sugar and bowel health. In addition to the abundance of vitamins and minerals found in fruits and vegetables, they also contain phytochemicals. Phytochemicals are a broad category of plant compounds that do not fall under the classification of vitamin or mineral. Some phytochemicals give fruits and vegetables their color, while others provide distinctive tastes and smells. You may be familiar with lycopene, which is found in deep-red tomatoes, or the anthocyanins that give blueberries their dark purple color. A compound called allicin, which contains sulfur, is responsible for the pungent smell of garlic, just as catechins in tea cause its slightly bitter taste.

Plants contain thousands of compounds that protect them in their environment. Scientific research shows how, when we consume those plants, the phytochemicals work synergistically with vitamins, minerals, and fiber to protect us from disease and, in some cases, prevent it.

RED FRUITS AND VEGETABLES

The phytochemicals found in red fruits and vegetables comprise a group of valuable compounds: quercetin, ellagic acid, hesperidin, lycopene, and anthocyanins. Lycopene and anthocyanins are powerful red-pigmented antioxidants. These nutrients reduce the risk of cancer, reduce tumor growth, lower blood pressure, scavenge free radicals, reduce LDL levels, and reduce arthritic inflammation.

Lycopene, found in tomatoes and many other plant-based foods, helps to prevent atherosclerosis and coronary artery disease. In fact, data published in the *American Journal of Clinical Nutrition* showed that lycopene protects low density lipoprotein (LDL) from the damaging effects of free radicals, rendering it less harmful to the arteries. The study also found that people with low blood-serum concentrations of lycopene had thicker coronary arteries, a condition associated with atherosclerosis and coronary artery disease.

The phytochemical quercitin inhibits the growth of colon cancer. A study published in the *International Journal of Cancer* showed that using a very small amount of quercetin, colon cancer cell growth was halted. According to a study published in *Cancer Research*, quercetin was also effective in causing apoptosis (cell suicide) in leukemia and lymphoma cells.

The anthocyanins in fruits and vegetables help prevent hardening of the arteries, lower blood pressure, reduce inflammation, and prevent cancer, while ellagic acid helps prevent cancer by neutralizing toxins found in processed meats and tobacco smoke.

All these compounds are found in red apples, beets, cherries, currants, red grapes, guava, kidney beans, red onion, red bell peppers, radicchio, radishes, raspberries, rhubarb, strawberries, tomatoes, and watermelon.

BLUE AND PURPLE FRUITS AND VEGETABLES

Blue and purple fruits and vegetables contain anthocyanins, ellagic acid, resveratrol, flavonoids, quercetin, lutein, tannins, and zeaxanthin, giving them the highest antioxidant action of all plant-based foods. These nutrients lower LDL levels, improve immune function, support digestion, improve mineral absorption, and reduce inflammation, tumor growth, and risk of developing coronary artery disease.

Anthocyanin-rich berries are particularly powerful. During the past few decades, research has shown the therapeutic effects of anthocyanins on diseases, including cancer. In one study, an extract made up of six berries—wild blueberry, bilberry, cranberry, elderberry, raspberry, and strawberry—was used to determine their antioxidant efficacy and anti-angiogenic properties. (Angiogenesis, as mentioned earlier, is the process by which cancer cells create new blood vessels to supply tumors with blood and nutrients.) The six-berry extract was found to inhibit angiogenesis in tumors.

Additionally, anthocyanins protect cells from oxidative stress, improve memory, and lower risk for developing cancer. These compounds are abundant in blue, purple, and black fruits and vegetables, including black beans, blackberries, black currants, blueberries, purple cabbage, eggplant, elderberries, figs, purple grapes, plums, purple potatoes, prunes, and raisins.

Z NOTE: Research on the health benefits of anthocyanins against chronic disease is ongoing. Many studies are coming to the same conclusion regarding the effect of anthocyanins found in dark blue and purple fruits and berries on the mechanisms involved in the development of cardiovascular disease, and two of these studies are worth mentioning here. Nitric oxide is a signaling molecule produced by the endothelium (the lining of the arteries). Nitric oxide relaxes the muscles within the arteries, causing arterial dilation, improved blood flow, and reduced blood pressure. Collective data published in *Advances in Nutrition* revealed that anthocyanins found in berries improve the release of nitric oxide and protect the endothelium from damage. It also noted that anthocyanins shut down the inflammation responsible for the development of coronary artery disease.

In another study, published in the journal *Angiology*, researchers found that anthocyanins contained in the nutritional supplement OPC-3 improved circulation and reduced cardiovascular risk factors. A randomized, double-blind, placebo-controlled, parallel group study was conducted. The control group received a two-month supply of OPC-3, which contains extracts from grape seed, bilberry, citrus, pine bark, and red wine. The placebo group received a mixture of fructose, apple fiber, and food dyes. The study showed that those who took the OPC-3 had an improvement in blood pressure and, more impressive, a significant decrease in levels of the inflammatory marker C-reactive protein, a major predictor of cardiovascular disease risk.

ORANGE AND YELLOW FRUITS AND VEGETABLES

Orange and yellow plant-based foods contain beta-carotene, flavonoids, lycopene, zeaxanthin, and lutein. Beta-carotene is a strong, red-orange-pigmented antioxidant that can be converted into vitamin A. It also helps to protect the skin, maintain the immune system, and reduce the risk of blindness and strokes.

Along with protecting your skin and eyes, beta-carotene and lycopene greatly reduce the risk for cancer and heart disease, while lutein and zeaxanthin reduce the risk of disorders of the eye. A study published in the *Archives of Ophthalmology* measured demographic, lifestyle, and medical characteristics for 4,519 participants aged sixty to eighty. Those with a high dietary intake of lutein and zeaxanthin were less likely to develop age-related macular degeneration. Research shows that these carotenoids can also help to detoxify drugs and foreign chemicals. Omitting carotenoid-rich vegetables from your diet may weaken your immune system.

Orange and yellow foods include apricots, butternut squash, cantaloupe, carrots, grapefruit, pumpkins, lemon, mango, nectarines, orange, pineapple, yellow bell peppers, orange bell peppers, peaches, winter squash, sweet potatoes, and tangerines.

WARNING: Grapefruit contains furanocoumarins, compounds that can prevent the breakdown of certain medications—including heart drugs, cholesterol-lowering medications, and chemo drugs—in the body. This can lead to fatal toxicity. If you take medications of any kind, ask your doctor if any drug interactions may occur if you eat grapefruit or especially if you drink grapefruit juice.

GREEN FRUITS AND VEGETABLES

Green leafy vegetables are an excellent source of folate (a B vitamin), potassium, vitamin K, vitamin C, and omega-3 fatty acids. Green vegetables get their different hues from a phytochemical called chlorophyll.

In addition to chlorophyll, green foods—specifically cruciferous vegetables—contain a class of phytochemicals called glucosinolates, which are sulfur-containing compounds that are responsible for the pungent aroma and bitter taste of some vegetables.

Crucifers such as broccoli, Brussels sprouts, cabbage, cauliflower, and kale are believed to help prevent macular degeneration of the eyes and the formation of cataracts. More important is the protection they provide against cancer. There is now evidence showing that compounds in cruciferous vegetables can stop the growth of breast cancer by making estrogen less potent. Cruciferous vegetables also contain a chemical known as indole-3-carbinol (I3C), which can alter estrogen metabolism and subsequently protect women from breast cancer. Studies published in *Cancer Research* and the *Journal of Biological Chemistry* found that I3C suppressed the growth of estrogen-dependent and estrogen-independent breast cancer cell lines by favoring 2-hydroxyestrone, which prevents breast cancer cells from growing. It was also found that I3C shut down breast cancer tumor growth and the spread of breast cancer by deactivating 16-alpha-hydroxyestrone, which causes breast cells to grow. (For more on 2- and 16-alpha-hydroxyestrone, see page 56.)

Crucifers are also strong detoxifiers, capable of combating and neutralizing carcinogens. These powerful vegetables help clear toxic compounds from the body, whether those compounds come from junk food or the environment.

Green fruits and vegetables include green apples, artichokes, arugula, asparagus, avocados, bok choy, broccoli, Brussels sprouts, green cabbage, celery, chives, cucumbers, fresh herbs, grapes, green bell peppers, green chiles, leafy greens, honeydew melon, kale, kiwifruit, leeks, lettuce, limes, parsley, peas, spinach, Swiss chard, and zucchini.

WHITE AND TAN FRUITS AND VEGETABLES

White fruits and vegetables are colored by anthoxanthins. They also contain important phytochemicals, such as allicin (found in garlic), organosulfur compounds, fructan, flavonoids, quercetin (found in onions), and beta-glucans (found in mushrooms). These nutrients stimulate the immune system and reduce the risk of certain cancers.

Garlic and onion belong to the genus *Allium*, which also includes leeks, chives, shallots, and scallions. Besides warding off vampires, garlic has been used in cooking and medicine for centuries, all over the world. Garlic contains a mixture of phytochemicals, and it also supplies vitamins C and B$_6$. The sulfur compounds in garlic not only give it its distinctive smell but are thought to protect against heart disease and cancer. In addition, garlic contains saponins, which have been shown to act as anti-inflammatory and antimicrobial agents against bacteria, yeast, parasites, fungi, and viruses.

Have you ever wondered why you cry when chopping onions? When you cut into an onion, it releases enzymes that produce sulfenic (not sulfuric) acid, which further converts into syn-Propanethial S-oxide, the compound responsible for your tears. Onions also contain sulfur compounds, saponins, fructans, and two major flavonoids, quercetin and kaempferol. Both are powerful antioxidants and are important for immune function and healthy gene expression. Fructans are indigestible parts of the onion, which help maintain beneficial bacteria in the gut.

What about ginger? Ginger is a rhizome (an underground stem) known for its spicy and sharp taste, as well as its medicinal properties. Its most common use is to soothe the stomach. The phenols and oils in ginger can relieve stomach symptoms from acid reflux to motion sickness. The nutrients found in this white rhizome can provide pain relief from arthritis, muscle soreness, and menstrual cramps.

Mushrooms, such as reishi, maitake, shiitake, and white button, are among the many functional foods known to inhibit tumor growth by enhancing immune function. A clinical study reported that beta-glucans—long carbohydrates found in mushrooms—stimulate the cancer-killing white blood cells called natural killer cells. How long did the killing response last? They found the activity of natural killer cells in lung, breast, and liver cancer to exceed one year. That is *amazing*.

The phytochemicals in white button mushrooms were also found to inhibit the growth of breast cancer cells by blocking an enzyme needed for the cellular growth. In addition to the powerhouse phytochemicals they contain, mushrooms are an excellent source of non-heme iron, phosphorus, potassium, B vitamins, copper, and zinc. Mushrooms also provide immunotherapy for anyone with a compromised immune system or cancer, especially hormone-sensitive cancers.

White and tan fruits and vegetables include bananas, cauliflower, chickpeas, cucumbers, figs, garlic, ginger, great northern beans, Jerusalem artichoke, leeks, lentils, mushrooms, onions, parsnips, pinto beans, shallots, turnips, white corn, white peaches, and white potatoes.

Z NOTE: Breast cancer cells produce an enzyme called aromatase, which raises estrogen levels, subsequently allowing cancer cells to proliferate and spread. A study published in the *Journal of Nutrition* showed that the phytochemicals in white button mushrooms blocked the production of aromatase, thus decreasing cancer cell growth.

As you can see, fruits and vegetables are among the most nutritious foods that you can eat. They are packed with vitamins, minerals, antioxidants, phytochemicals, and other unique compounds that promote optimal health. By eating a variety of fruits and vegetables of different colors, you are guaranteed a diverse range of plant-based nutrients. If you are rebuilding from a health crisis and/or taking steps to prevent recurrence, prevent chronic disease, and get lean, I recommend eating five or six servings of vegetables and low-sugar fruits every day. When designing your diet, be sure to include plenty of vegetables and fruits in your meals and certainly as snacks.

Three "Z Rules" for a
Healthy Body Composition

This is not a complicated regimen—rules are made to be broken, and that's especially true for people who have tried a dozen different diets and found that none of them work. In this book, I'm going to keep it simple.

I think there are three main reasons people become overfat or struggle to shed fat. First, they eat high-calorie, nutrient-deficient, crappy foods. Second, they eat their biggest meal at night. Third, they are not performing the right fat-burning exercises. So I have three rules. That's right: just three. But though there are only a few of them, these guidelines will make all the difference in your body composition.

1. Eat high-nutrient, low-calorie foods roughly five or six times throughout the day each day.
2. Eat little to no carbs (especially refined white carbs) or excessive animal protein meals after 6 or 7 p.m.
3. Do high-intensity interval training (HIIT).

That's not so hard, is it? You don't have to count calories; I've already done it for you in the recipe section. You don't have to cut back on the amount of food you're eating. The tools in this plan will help you eat according to the way your body works best. That's what really cuts the weight. Let's look at the first two rules and see exactly what they mean for you. (Rule #3 will be covered in chapter 4.)

Z RULE #1: EAT HIGH-NUTRIENT, LOW-CALORIE FOODS ROUGHLY FIVE OR SIX TIMES THROUGHOUT THE DAY EACH DAY.
Okay, how is processed, empty-calorie food bad for you? Let me count the ways. Do you suffer from heart disease, cancer, diabetes, obesity,

autoimmune disease, digestive issues, mood disorders, fatigue, insomnia, sleep apnea, poor healing, hormone imbalances, low libido, skin issues, or arthritis? Are you afflicted with dementia, Alzheimer's disease, ADHD, osteoporosis, suppressed immune function, or chronic colds and allergies?

If so, you are suffering from PFD—Processed-Food Disorder. This is a condition caused by eating too many highly processed, refined, high-calorie, low-nutrient foods.

You may remember the war the government waged against Big Tobacco in the name of health for American citizens. That same war is going on today—only the fight is over the foods we can buy at any supermarket in the country. As a person who understands nutrition so well, I am discouraged that the processed- and junk-food industries are given a free pass to manufacture, advertise, and distribute synthetic non-foods. More and more clinical studies are showing that these foods are the root causes of most, if not all, chronic diseases, from diabetes to heart disease to cancer. Meanwhile, small farms producing whole foods are unable to compete in a market where the cost to run a farm is more than the money it can earn. Huge agribusinesses like Monsanto and Perdue Farms use their power in the market and their huge profits to ensure their top position, squashing small farmers. If we continue to buy processed foods, we are collectively handing over billions of dollars to an industry that could not care less about us.

So processed, sugar- and fat-laden non-food is out. By the same token, "going on a diet" and restricting calories in order to lose weight will also not make you healthier. Why? When you overly restrict calories, your appetite increases and your ability to sense when you're full decreases. This not only creates food cravings but also triggers frequent overeating of high-calorie, low-nutrient foods. That happens because the body goes into starvation mode. Instead of using the fat you have stored up, the body reacts to what it perceives as famine conditions by breaking down muscle for energy and hanging on to body fat as an emergency energy source. That is an unhealthy cycle that only gets worse the longer you restrict your calorie intake.

According to research published in the journal *Nutrition & Metabolism*, calorie restriction alone (i.e., without exercise) is not a sustainable long-term solution for improving body composition. More than half of the people who lose weight (fat) as a result of restricting calories will gain it back. They can also make themselves sick, because major calorie restriction also means nutrient restriction. A three-year study of the dietary habits of 16,000 Americans found that many people are deficient in nutrients including vitamin B_6, folate, and thiamin, as well as calcium and magnesium. In a scientific review published in the *Journal of the American Medical Association*, researchers found that "inadequate intake of several vitamins has been linked to chronic diseases, including coronary artery disease, cancer, and osteoporosis." The specific vitamins they are referring to are vitamins B_6, B_{12}, and folate, as well as vitamins A, C, D, E, and K.

In contrast, researchers have found that a diet high in nutrients and low in calories, with lower carbs, higher protein, and some fat, showed improvements in body fat percentage and lean muscle mass—a better body composition, and reduced risk of developing chronic disease. Realize that food is information for your body. Healthful foods regulate your body functions, cellular functions, and genes. By eating a nonprocessed, highly nutritious diet, you stop making fat and also prevent and reverse disease. Your fork, not your genes, determines your fate.

Z RULE #2. EAT LITTLE TO NO CARBS OR EXCESSIVE ANIMAL PROTEIN MEALS AFTER 6 OR 7 P.M.

I can hear the complaints now. "Huh? I can't do that. That's impossible. I don't get home until seven. What am I supposed to eat?" Or "That's when my family eats dinner." Or "I work late, so I eat late." Okay, I know it sounds rough, but this rule is probably the single most powerful factor in losing fat—ever.

In our fast-paced society, the concept of eating small amounts of nutrient-dense foods throughout the day has been abandoned. Although humans are programmed to eat three meals a day, most people skip breakfast and eat their biggest meal at dinner. Here's the deal. While our bodies require a certain amount of food and calories to function properly, timing is everything. If you require 1,500 calories to sustain you through the day, what happens if you eat most of those calories at night? Those unused calories are stored as fat. Evolutionally speaking, we are meant to graze—eat small meals frequently throughout the day. This includes breakfast, so don't skip it! According to research published in the *American Journal of Clinical Nutrition*, omitting breakfast impairs blood fats (triglycerides, HDL, and LDL) and causes you to gain weight. Skipping breakfast because of "dieting" or being too busy to eat will send signals to your body that will make you fat. Eat when you get up in the morning. Quick tip here: Eat high-protein, not high-carb, breakfasts.

The key to fat loss is not only to burn it or get rid of it, but to stop making it. Food is the control switch: it provides us with energy and helps regulate our hormones. To improve your body composition, you need to understand how to control these hormones. Certain hormones store fat, and others burn it. Your fat-storing hormones include insulin, estrogen, and cortisol. Your fat-burning hormones include glucagon, human growth hormone (HGH), testosterone, the thyroid hormone T3, and norepinephrine. The release of these hormones is triggered by the type of foods you eat, the exercise you get, and the stress you endure. Let's examine three key hormones involved with storing or burning fat: insulin, glucagon, and cortisol. Then we will discuss the relationship between estrogen and body fat.

RICH'S STORY

Rich works in construction, mainly in stone and masonry. He's up at the crack of dawn and works till dusk. During his daily operations, he has to manage the job and oversee his crew, making sure they are doing a good job. He came to me because he was having a hard time managing his weight. With his long work hours and driving from job to job daily, he found it difficult to eat healthful foods at the most favorable times of the day. He sometimes skipped breakfast, ate bags of nuts—not a handful here and there, but *bags*—during the day, ate high-calorie foods for lunch, and then consumed far too much food at night before going to bed. Eating large amounts of protein and carbs late at night caused a surge of insulin that was released during his sleep. This resulted in a lot of excessive body fat.

After I gave him a plan, he was excited to make some changes. He began eating a healthful breakfast consisting of eggs mixed with vegetables, with sweet potato and fruit on the side. He took food to work to eat throughout the day. The biggest change was at night; he ate fewer carbs and less protein at the end of his long days. In a few weeks, his belly fat came off. He had more energy to meet the demands of his job, as well as enough energy to get back to the gym.

INSULIN: Insulin is released into the blood in response to blood glucose levels. When you eat carbs, your blood sugar goes up; this signals the pancreas to make insulin. Insulin takes sugar out of the blood and stores it in the liver and muscles as a substance called glycogen, which is a source of energy for the body. Once the liver and muscles are filled with glycogen, the rest of the blood sugar is stored as fat. Therefore, a rise in blood sugar produces a rise in insulin, which creates the potential for storing fat. Insulin is the fat-storage hormone.

The following are some functions of insulin:

- Insulin lowers blood sugar.
- Insulin shuttles sugar to the liver, muscles, and fat for energy.
- Insulin converts sugar and protein into fat.

GLUCAGON: Conversely to insulin, glucagon is released when your blood sugar is low, as well as after you've eaten protein. Eating protein stimulates the release of glucagon, which causes fat cells to release fat to be used for energy. By eating adequate amounts of protein, you can control your glucagon levels during the day and night to help you get rid of fat. Even better, when you are not digesting food—for example, when you are sleeping—you shut off insulin and release glucagon, allowing you to burn fat while you sleep. This causes the fat stores around your belly to be used for fuel. Glucagon is the fat-burning hormone.

Some functions of glucagon are:

- Glucagon raises blood sugar when it's low.
- Glucagon stimulates the release of fat to be burned for energy.

FRANK'S STORY

Frank O. was fed up with his high cholesterol and LDL levels. He was frustrated with his weight and low energy. After I reviewed his blood work and lifestyle, it was clear that his current diet was making him sick and overfat. We had to make some changes.

First, we removed refined carbs—white breads, pastas, and white rice—which produced higher-than-normal blood sugar and insulin. With too many of the wrong calories, insulin was storing his excess blood sugar as fat. Second, we added three to four daily servings of protein from lean meat and fish to his diet. At each meal, he replaced the simple, refined carbs he was used to eating with sweet potato, wild rice, carrots, and beets. He also included dark leafy greens and vegetables with each meal. By eliminating the simple carbs and increasing his lean protein intake, he reduced his blood sugar and insulin levels and increased his glucagon levels.

To further stimulate the production of glucagon, Frank started high-intensity exercises three to four times a week. After implementing these simple steps, he proudly told me, "I have lost thirty pounds, cut my body fat percentage in half, and lowered my cholesterol and blood pressure. I have more energy to do the things I enjoy outside of work."

Individual foods, and foods in combination, affect insulin and glucagon levels. If you require 1,500 calories a day and you eat those calories during the day and not at night, you will turn on the fat-burning switch (glucagon) and burn fat while you sleep. If you eat lots of calories at night, insulin will store those unused calories as fat while you sleep. Which do you want happening?

Have you ever heard of the sumo-wrestler diet? (This is no joke.) In order for sumo wrestlers to get as big and fat as they can, they consume roughly 20,000 calories a day. These calories are divided between two meals, both followed by a period of sleep. They skip breakfast and drink lots of beer (for added calories) with their monster meals. The sleep period causes the body to store this enormous caloric load as fat . . . lots of fat. Sadly, these wrestlers have a short life expectancy of sixty to sixty-five years due to their unhealthful lifestyle and the diseases (heart disease, high blood pressure, and diabetes) that develop from it.

The standard American diet (SAD) is not too different, although I don't know anyone who eats 10,000-calorie meals. However, many people skip breakfast and then eat a couple of big meals later—the biggest one at dinner, fairly close to bedtime. Dinner is usually a combination of high-carb, low-protein foods. That combination sets you up for major fat storage while you sleep—just like a sumo wrestler, even though that's not what you're trying to do.

To lose weight, you need to eat most of your food while the sun is out, and little to no food while the moon is out. If you eat dinner in the evening, choose foods that don't raise insulin, such as greens and nonstarchy vegetables (check the list at the end of this chapter for examples). Dinner should consist of plenty of low-calorie greens with perhaps a tiny piece of protein (3 ounces), along with a drop of olive oil and vinegar. Try a nondairy vegetable soup, a tiny piece of flounder or cod, and a mixed-greens salad. You will find an endless number of foods you can use to create low-calorie, non-insulin-raising meals. Later in this chapter, you will learn how to create a food plan specific to you, based on your caloric needs.

Before we turn away from insulin, I want to include a word to the wise for diabetics. When managing insulin resistance and diabetes, always combine a small amount of complex carbohydrates with a protein at meals. This will produce a slow rise in blood sugar and, thus, a slow rise in insulin. The key to reversing blood sugar spikes is to stop eating simple carbohydrates that flood your body with blood sugar. Eating mainly greens with lean protein and a small amount of slow-burning carbs, like sweet potato, squash, and beets, is the best way to regulate blood sugar.

CORTISOL: Cortisol is the stress hormone. In times of stress, the brain tells the adrenal glands (located above the kidneys) to secrete cortisol. This hormone blocks inflammation and helps regulate the allergic reaction. So what does this have to do with weight loss? When we restrict calories too much (such as by skipping breakfast and/or eating our largest meal at dinner), blood sugar levels drop. Cortisol is released into the body to help manage this blood sugar loss. When blood sugar gets too low, cortisol breaks down muscle to create sugar for the brain and nervous system to use as energy. When you turn on this hormone, you are producing exactly the opposite of what you want for fat loss.

In stressful moments, cortisol helps the body deal with the stressors; this is a normal response. However, when stress is chronic, the prolonged release of cortisol can cause sleep issues, anxiety, muscle wasting, immune suppression, and an increase in belly fat. According to *Obesity Reviews*, chronic stress "inhibits the secretion of growth hormone, testosterone, and 17 beta-estradiol (estrogen), all of which counteract cortisol's effects. The net result is an accumulation of visceral fat." In another article, from the journal *Psychosomatic Medicine*, researchers found that high cortisol levels cause circulating fat to be deposited deep in the abdomen as visceral fat, the dangerous fat linked to diabetes, heart disease, and cancers.

ESTROGEN AND BODY FAT: Estrogen, a fat-storing hormone, is the main female sex hormone; it gives women their secondary sex characteristics and development of the reproductive organs. During and after menopause, estrogen levels drop. This causes fat to be stored in and around the belly, thighs, and buttocks. However, the relationship between estrogen and body fat is a double-edged sword. If estrogen levels plummet after menopause, fat may be stored around the lower body. When there is excess body fat—in both women and men—estrogen levels can rise. Fat tissue contains an enzyme called aromatase, which converts other hormones like testosterone into estrogen. When your body fat increases, so does aromatase activity, and thus your levels of circulating estrogen. The consequences of high estrogen in women include uterine fibroids, breast cancer, and infertility; in men, impotence, prostatic enlargement, and prostate cancer may result; in both men and women, excess estrogen may lead to thyroid dysfunction, high blood pressure, and more body fat. The good news is that eating a variety of whole foods and doing high-intensity exercise help combat the effects of fat storage, and thus maintain normal aromatase and estrogen levels.

Three Foods That Kill

If nutrient-dense foods prevent disease and help you get rid of fat, then are there foods that can make you ill and increase fat? Yes, indeed. Let's examine a few food sources that we consume every day—foods that many of us have been eating since childhood and don't really think about—but that scientific evidence is showing can make us both fat and sick. Which foods these are might surprise you. But you know what they say: the truth will set you free—free to make you feel a whole lot better about yourself.

Through years of scientific research, I have learned some alarming facts about three basic food sources in our diet: refined flours and grains that make up bread and baked goods; dairy; and refined processed sugars. That's right, the three worst sources of food are refined grains, dairy, and sugar—what I call the "Three Foods That Kill." That sounds outrageous, doesn't it? Let's take a closer look at what clinical tests have to show us.

REFINED GRAINS

We've been led to believe that grains (including wheat, maize, rice, barley, sorghum, oats, rye, and millet) are a healthful food source that provides vitamins, minerals, and especially fiber. Let's not forget that grains are also low in fat. Digging through the scientific and historical research reveals that humans did not always consume grains, and certainly not grains that were refined.

Before the agricultural revolution (roughly ten thousand years ago), humans were hunter-gatherers. Our forebears' food sources consisted of wild meats, fruits, and vegetables. They rarely ate any grains because most grains had to be cultivated through farming. For the last two million years, our genetic makeup was shaped by the food sources that were commonly consumed; grains were not. According to Loren Cordain, PhD, in an article titled "Cereal Grains: Humanity's Double-Edged Sword," the addition of grains to the human diet roughly ten thousand years ago "represents a dramatic departure from those foods to which we are genetically adapted." He also states that the addition of grains to our modern diet is responsible for many of the most common chronic diseases today. You may be saying, "So what?" Grains are mentioned in the Bible, so how bad can they be?

To begin with, unprocessed whole grains do not contain such vital nutrients as vitamin A, beta-carotene, vitamin B_{12}, vitamin C, and vitamin D. Furthermore, in order to be used to make bread and other baked goods, grains must be processed, which depletes the naturally occurring nutrients in the grain. This means breads and processed flours have to be fortified; some of the nutrients stripped out during processing are added back to increase the grain product's nutritional value. Finally, when people eat breads and refined grains, they tend to eat less meat, fruits, and vegetables. That causes even more nutrient deficiencies, which is dangerous to your health.

The reality is, refined grains—and even whole grains—contain phytic acid, an anti-nutrient that prevents the absorption of nutrients including zinc, iron, copper, calcium, magnesium, and phosphorous. According to the World Health Organization, phytates in grains have been identified as a major cause of iron-deficiency anemia. Besides preventing the absorption of nutrients, refined grains—such as those used to make breads and pastas—are broken down into glucose, which will trigger a surge of insulin. Insulin works to help the body use that glucose as fuel, but any excess glucose will be stored as fat.

SUSAN'S STORY

Susan Q. came to see me with fatigue, major stomach pain after eating, and aches and pains, as well as a general sense of not feeling well. She also suffered from chronic neck pain. As with most patients I see, I tried to get to the root of her health issues in order to find the most effective treatment. My tentative diagnosis for Susan was that she had either food allergies, an infection in her gut, or a sensitivity to gluten. Because blood testing was the most logical place to start, I had her tested for sensitivity to gluten. The tests came back positive. Because this is a serious issue, I recommended that Susan eliminate any grains containing gluten, including wheat, barley, rye, spelt, and triticale, from her diet, as well as any products made with those grains. Within days, Susan's stomach started to feel better, and her fatigue had diminished. Now, gluten-free and more aware of the factors affecting her health, she can make food choices that won't be hazardous to her health.

Grains also contain gluten. Gluten makes pizza and bread dough pliable and elastic and gives other baked goods a pleasing texture, but in the body, its effect is less benign. In genetically susceptible individuals, gluten can trigger a severe immune reaction in the intestine, whereby the white blood cells surrounding the gut destroy the villi lining the intestine; this is the condition known as celiac disease. The *World Gastroenterology Organisation Practice Guidelines* state that the prevalence of celiac disease in a healthy population is 1 in 100. Most people don't know they have an immune reaction to gluten until symptoms appear, at which point the damage to the intestines has been done.

For celiac suffers, the hidden danger is not the intestinal damage but the potentially life-threatening diseases that can be triggered by a reaction to gluten. These include autoimmune diseases such as dermatitis, type 1 diabetes, Hashimoto's thyroiditis, rheumatoid arthritis, kidney disease, and possibly multiple sclerosis. Reaction to gluten has also been shown to cause different types of cancer, including malignant lymphomas (non-Hodgkin's lymphoma and T-cell lymphomas), small-bowel cancer, large intestine cancer, and oropharyngeal tumors. The mechanism for this disease was covered in chapter 1, in the section The Leaky Gut Connection. For more on celiac disease, see chapter 1, page 66.

CLINICAL NOTE: The only definitive indicators of celiac disease are elevated IgA tissue transglutaminase or IgA endomysial antibodies and a small bowel biopsy to confirm damage to the villi. For more information, see chapter 8, Testing the Disease Terrain.

THE GLUTEN-FREE TRAP

The gluten hazard is now so well known that many cookbooks have come out loaded with recipes for gluten-free this and gluten-free that. Researchers and consumers are realizing that many foods contain gluten and, thus, can cause health problems. Due to this awareness, food companies are jumping on the gluten-free bandwagon.

Companies prey on us using slick and emotionally touching marketing to get us to buy their products; they take advantage of the newest food fads and exploit our health issues. "Gluten-free" is currently the big marketing ploy. Yes, if you are sensitive to gluten, you have to avoid it. But beware of agenda-driven marketing ploys. Don't buy packaged foods just because they say "gluten-free"; read the labels. Food companies incorporate additives, including soy lecithin and other emulsifying agents that make foods chewy and gooey, to mimic the textural effects created by gluten. These companies also add lots of refined sugar and fats that have health implications when eaten too much.

Grains can be categorized as refined or whole. When grains are refined, each seed has been mechanically stripped of its bran and germ by sifting or grinding, leaving only the endosperm. The **bran**, in its natural state, is a seed's protective outer layer that contains fiber. The **germ** is the part of the seed that sprouts; it contains vitamins and minerals. The **endosperm** is the starchy portion of the seed that can be ground to make flour.

The ground grain is then bleached, and the chemical bromine is added; this strengthens doughs made with the bromated flour. Finally, B vitamins and iron are added to the flour in an attempt to restore nutrients stripped out by the refinement process. Even so, refined flours and grain are still devoid of nutrients and fiber. Examples of refined flours and grains include white (all-purpose) flour, white rice, whole wheat flour, cornmeal, Cream of Wheat, Cream of Rice.

Refined grains are hazardous for several reasons:

- They have no fiber.
- They are too starchy and cause rapid blood sugar spikes.
- They contain added chemicals as a result of the refining processes they undergo.
- They have to be enriched because they are nutritionally naked.
- They have been bleached to lighten their color, or have had artificial flavorings and colors added to make them pretty and tasty.

Whole grains, by comparison, are intact seeds that still contain their bran and germ. Because whole grains have not been destroyed by refining processes, it makes sense that whole grains are a more healthful choice than refined grains and flours.

I realize it would be hard to eliminate all grains from your diet, and I won't ask you to. Based on my reading and observations, I've found brown, wild, and black rices; gluten-free steel-cut oats; millet; and quinoa to be the least problematic. The preparation of these grains involves soaking and boiling, which helps break down phytates and other chemicals that can prevent the absorption of nutrients. Even so, *eat grains sparingly*. In Part III, I have included some super-tasty recipes that contain brown rice, brown rice pasta, brown rice crackers, quinoa, and steel-cut oats.

However, based on the current research, I recommend eating no refined flours or refined grains or products that contain them. (Okay, perhaps a cookie once in a while, or a piece of birthday cake on *your* birthday—eating junk very occasionally is different from making it a part of your daily or weekly diet.) And of course, if you have an autoimmune problem, or you have digestive trouble when eating grains, absolutely stay away from both refined and whole grains that contain gluten.

Z NOTE: Gluten has wreaked havoc on the health of millions of people and is currently the most researched protein known to cause autoimmunity. However, it's not the *only* protein linked to autoimmune disease. If you have gone gluten-free and your autoimmune condition has not improved or has only marginally improved, you should know that other proteins can provoke the same immune reaction as gluten, a phenomenon known as cross-reactivity. Data published in *Food and Nutrition Sciences* show that proteins found in cow's milk (including butyrophilin, whey proteins, and casein), milk chocolate, yeast, oats, corn, millet, instant coffee, and rice are all cross-reactive with gluten. If you are dealing with an autoimmune dysfunction or some other immune issue, it's best to eliminate these cross-reactive foods.

DAIRY

Milk has long been heralded as the ultimate source of calcium for our bones. An advertisement used to say, "It does a body good." We got it in school lunches. We dipped cookies in it, and even added sugar and food dyes to it to create new flavors. It has become a staple in American culture, like Superman. This iconic food source is *milk*.

Milk has some very good properties. Breast milk is the primary food source for a developing newborn before the introduction of solid foods. In addition to essential nutrients, breast milk contains growth factors, antimicrobials (virus and bacteria fighters), cytokines, and hormones. But after infancy, the milk we drink is not human breast milk. We drink the milk of other species, and that is abnormal. We are the only mammals that drink milk after weaning, and it's not even our own milk.

Here are a few reasons why we should not drink milk. Cow's milk has roughly three times the amount of protein as human breast milk. The protein component in cow's milk is suited for the development of calves, which grow up to weigh 1,320 pounds. I don't know of any 1,320-pound humans. Both cow's milk and human breast milk contain casein and whey proteins, but cow's milk has a higher ratio of casein to whey—typically 80:20 versus roughly 40:60 in breast milk. The high proportion of casein in cow's milk has been linked to many health issues in humans, specifically allergies and type 1 diabetes.

More and more research is coming to the same conclusion: milk does a body bad. According to research published in the journals *Medical Hypothesis*, *American Journal of Clinical Nutrition*, and *Cancer Epidemiology, Biomarkers & Prevention*, dairy products have been linked to breast cancer, colorectal cancer, and prostate cancer. The American Academy of Pediatrics now recommends that infants not be given cow's milk during their first year of life. Research is finding that giving infants cow's milk may cause the immune system to attack the body, thus creating conditions like type 1 diabetes.

If you still aren't convinced, think about it this way: Most milks contain traces of hormones and antibiotics. And did you know that cow's milk—even organic milk—contains white blood cells (pus)? When a cow's udder becomes infected from exposure to milking machines and human hands, white blood cells rush in to fight the infection. These white blood cells are passed into the milk that you drink . . . gross! The dairy industry monitors the amount of white blood cells in milk, calling it the "somatic cell count"—a measure of the level of infection in the cows.

BRETT'S STORY

Brett H., a young businessman, suffered from an inflammatory condition in his colon called colitis. He often had debilitating pain, blood in his stool, and fatigue. He was afraid to leave the house, and always had to be near a restroom in case of an emergency. His biggest heartbreak was not being able to sit in a stadium to watch his favorite baseball or football teams play. General practitioners offered him no solutions, only symptom relief via steroids and super-strong anti-inflammatories that made him feel tired. After our first consultation, he immediately eliminated grains containing gluten from his diet, as well as all dairy products, including milk and cheese. He wasn't a big vegetable eater, but he agreed to eat four to five servings of greens a day. To cool the inflammation in his gut, I recommended the powdered amino acid glutamine, a fish oil supplement, and an anti-inflammatory probiotic. We communicated every couple of weeks to discuss his health and any changes in his colitis. Within two months, Brett returned to my office elated to tell me that he had stopped taking the powerful drugs and had few, if any, symptoms of the colitis. Play ball!

A FAMILY'S STORY

I was treating a family for a host of physical ailments resulting mainly from physical activity and sports. The youngest son, Sam, was in high school and having a hard time getting through soccer season because of chronic hip and leg pain. After a thorough examination, I found the cause of his hip and leg pain to be a weak hip flexor (psoas). I treated him with spinal manipulation and prescribed exercises to be done daily at home. In only half a dozen visits, his pain was gone and life was good again. His mother, Lia, pleased with his results, wondered if I could help her younger daughter, Nina, who was struggling with eczema on her arms and legs. I suggested she eliminate dairy from her diet and substitute rice milk or almond milk. After several months, Lia ecstatically reported that Nina's eczema had cleared up, and Sam was still pain-free.

Dairy products are produced from or contain the milk of mammals, including cows, buffalo, goats, and sheep. Food items that fall into the dairy category include:

- Milk
- Cream
- Cheese

- Butter
  - Cultured dairy—yogurt, cottage cheese, sour cream, and dips
  - Frozen desserts—ice cream
  - Custard
  - Pudding

The dairy industry wants us to drink milk and eat cheese because that's their business, the same way fast-food companies want us to eat their deep-fried foods and the tobacco companies would like us to keep smoking. Oddly, if I handed you a glass of human breast milk to add to your coffee, I'm sure you'd be grossed out. But to millions of people, drinking the milk from a pregnant cow is normal.

Wait! What about calcium? For years, the dairy industry has brainwashed us into thinking we have to drink milk to get calcium. However, current research is showing little evidence to support this propaganda... I mean, claim. The authors of a paper in the journal *Pediatrics* reviewed collective studies on dairy consumption, high calcium intake, and bone mineral density. They found that high calcium intake from milk and dairy products had no impact on bone mineralization in children. Additional research shows that although the United States is one of the highest consumers of dairy products, its rate of osteoporosis and bone fractures is also very high. According to the Nurses' Health Study, which followed 77,761 women ages thirty-four to fifty-nine for twelve years, women who consumed dairy products had significantly *more* bone fractures than those who drank little to no milk.

Milk does a body bad. Dark green vegetables and healthful protein are better sources of calcium. Are there any dairy products you can have? No, not even regular ice cream, cheeses, or regular yogurt. Read the previous paragraphs again. I know this goes against all we've been told, but it's true. The good news is that the food industry has seized the opportunity and is providing more nutritious and better-tasting substitutes for cow and goat milk, including rice milk, almond milk, and coconut milk. Rice milk and almond milk are delicious in steel-cut oats, protein shakes, and smoothies. Coconut milk and almond milk are excellent in coffee, and make super-delicious ice cream and yogurt. (But that doesn't mean you should polish off an entire container of it.)

SUGARS—NOT SO SWEET

Earlier in this chapter, you learned how different sugars are metabolized differently. Refined sugars (sucrose) and synthetic sugars (high-fructose corn syrup) are very common ingredients in processed foods. Sucrose has different aliases: table sugar, white sugar, and cane sugar. Table sugar is completely devoid of nutrients and loaded with calories. If used in high amounts, sucrose can act as a preservative; therefore, it is found in just about all baked goods, desserts, and junk foods. In other words, you're getting fat so that food-industry products can have a longer shelf life. It should go without saying that artificial sweeteners, such as saccharine, sucralose, and aspartame, are not acceptable substitutes.

Like sucrose, high-fructose corn syrup (HFCS) has no fiber, which causes the body to process it faster. The consumption of sucrose and high-fructose corn syrup has been proven to help cause heart disease, diabetes, and obesity, among many other serious health issues. These sugars also cause the development of visceral fat, which in both men and women can cause abnormally high estrogen levels and elevated C-reactive protein, a protein that indicates that your fat has become toxic. Visceral fat also increases your risk for diabetes, heart disease, and certain cancers.

Let's not forget about the ill effects of sugar on your blood vessels. A diet including refined white carbohydrates (sugars) can lead to the onset of type 2 diabetes. Eating refined sugar over the long term causes the cells to reject signals from insulin—the hormone that helps glucose (blood sugar) enter your cells to be used for energy. You may be familiar with insulin resistance, which occurs when you have frequent high blood glucose levels; eventually, the cells ignore the signal from insulin. Poor insulin signaling leads to chronic high blood sugar, the condition called type 2 diabetes.

Diabetes is associated with atherosclerosis, coronary artery disease, and other causes of cardiovascular dysfunction. Data published in the *American Journal of Clinical Nutrition* show that a diet high in refined carbohydrates increases the risk for coronary artery disease. Research published in the *Journal of Medical Biochemistry* found that insulin reduced the production of nitric oxide, while high blood sugar (hyperglycemia) injured the endothelium, further lowering nitric-oxide production. Reduced nitric-oxide production and function are crucial steps in the development of atherosclerosis.

Atherosclerosis accounts for 80 percent of all deaths among people diagnosed with diabetes—more specifically, type 2 diabetes. Data published in *Cardiovascular Diabetology* and the *Journal of Lipid Research* show that high blood sugar causes changes in the blood vessel itself that promote atherosclerosis. These alterations include damage to fats and proteins (glycation), oxidation of LDL, inflammation, and tissue damage. Last, diabetes was shown to reduce HDL's ability to remove unwanted cholesterol from the atherosclerotic lesion—a local or focal area of the arterial wall where a plaque develops. That's why the biggest cause of atherosclerosis and coronary artery disease is a processed-food diet. Processed meats, hydrogenated trans fats, and refined sugar appear to do the most damage to the cardiovascular system. Sugar goes by many different names. Read labels, and avoid foods containing the following: barley malt, blackstrap molasses, brown sugar, cane sugar, confectioners' sugar, corn sweetener, corn syrup, date sugar, dextrin, dextrose, d-mannose, evaporated cane juice, fruit juice concentrate, glucose, high-fructose corn syrup (HFCS), honey, lactose, malt syrup, maltodextrin, maltose, maple syrup, molasses, raw sugar, sucrose, syrup, table sugar, turbinado sugar. (Fructose, naturally occurring in fruit or added in small quantities to foods, is acceptable.)

KAREN'S STORY

Karen M. originally came to see me for treatment for dizziness, high cholesterol, and high LDL levels. After I put her on a lifestyle-change program, Karen's blood fats returned to normal levels, and she was very pleased. But several months later, she returned in a panic. "Dr. Z, my cholesterol and LDL levels are high again. Now what?"

After questioning her about changes in her lifestyle, she said, "I fell off the wagon and am eating sugar again—cookies, cakes, pies, and ice cream." I asked her why she went to the dark side, and her response was, "I was getting away with it. I know it's unhealthy, but I continued to binge anyway. I wasn't feeling bad, so I continued to eat junk, even though I know it's bad for me." She made an interesting point. This sums up the mind-set many people have when they are eating just for taste. Maybe we feel immortal, so we push our health limits until we're sick and dying. Is this not like a child pushing boundaries until there is some consequence that sets the boundary?

Knowing that high-sugar, refined junk caused her blood fats to elevate, Karen eagerly got back to healthful eating, including protein, healthful fats, and green and other vibrantly colored vegetables. While she craved processed simple sugars, we substituted healthful low-sugar fruits and starchy vegetables. Over the next couple of months, Karen's sugar cravings disappeared, and her cholesterol and LDL levels went back to normal.

The Glycemic Index

The glycemic index (GI) is a very useful guide to how your body's sugar levels will respond when you eat certain foods. The GI is an estimate of how much each gram of carbohydrate in a food will raise a person's blood sugar (glucose) after that food is eaten. In this rating system, pure glucose has a value of 100. Carbohydrates that break down quickly during digestion are given a high glycemic index, while carbs that break down more slowly have a low glycemic index. Here are the major differences between the two:

- Low GI means a smaller rise in blood glucose levels after meals.
- Low GI diets can help you lose weight.
- Low GI diets can improve the body's sensitivity to insulin.
- Low GI diets can improve control of diabetes.
- Low GI foods keep you feeling fuller for longer.
- Low GI diets can prolong physical endurance.
- High GI foods help refuel carbohydrate stores after exercise.

GLYCEMIC INDEX RANGE

Low GI = 55 or less

Medium GI = 55 to 69

High GI = 70 or more

If you eat foods with a high glycemic index, you will digest them quickly, which will raise your blood sugar quickly. High and fast blood sugar means high insulin levels, and insulin drives chronic disease and will make you fat.

The higher the number given to a food source, the higher the blood sugar response. For example: watermelon has a glycemic index of 70, which is a high value. Eating watermelon will cause a high blood sugar response. Mushrooms have a low glycemic index of 10, so they don't raise blood sugar too much or too fast.

As mentioned before, foods that raise blood sugar also raise insulin levels. The problem with high-glycemic foods is that they cause a quick rise in insulin with a subsequent quick drop in blood sugar, known as hypoglycemia, the typical crash you experience after eating refined carbs and high-sugar foods.

Some foods have a high glycemic index, but they don't provoke the same blood sugar response. For example, carrots have a high glycemic index, but they don't raise blood sugar like pasta made from refined flour does. Why is that? Since we tend to eat only a small amount of carrots, the blood sugar response is minor. Also, eating foods containing fiber will help slow the absorption of sugars, preventing a fast rise in blood sugar—unlike refined white flours and sugars, which have no fiber, and thus cause a rapid rise in blood sugar.

If you have a health issue like diabetes or hypoglycemia, or you are trying to lose fat, eat healthful foods and be mindful of the glycemic index. Check the lists of foods on page 189 of this chapter and in Part III on page 356. If you have a problem managing your blood sugar in conditions like insulin resistance or type 2 diabetes, try to stay away from high-glycemic fruits: banana, mango, papaya, pineapple, and watermelon. This recommendation is not forever, just until you get your blood sugar under control.

WARNING: Whatever you do, stay away from the high-sugar meal-replacement drinks like the classic ones, Ensure and Boost, given to hospital patients with advanced disease. Why? An 8-ounce bottle of Ensure has 22 grams of sucrose (table sugar); Boost has 20 grams of sugar; both contain almost as much as an 8-ounce bottle of Coca-Cola, which has 27 grams of sucrose. Also avoid energy drinks, "diet" sodas, and any beverage containing more than 10 calories.

Z NOTE: I am surprised by the number of patients I see trying to recover from illness by replacing whole fruits and vegetables with juicing. Whether you are rebuilding from a disease or trying to get rid of your excessive body fat, I'm all for juicing vegetables periodically in small amounts, but not as a substitute for eating the whole food source. Mother Nature created fruits and vegetables in their packaged whole-food form with just the right amount of fructose and fiber. The fructose is bound to the fiber that breaks down slowly during digestion. The slow digestion prevents a rapid influx of the fructose, which ends up in the liver and is turned into stored energy (glycogen). The liver can metabolize small amounts of fructose, roughly 20 to 25 grams, without being overloaded. We run into issues when the amount of fructose exceeds 20 to 25 grams taken in through the juicing of fruits and vegetables, or through processed high-fructose corn syrup found in junk foods and soft drinks. When we take in too much fructose—as Dr. Jeff Bland puts it, "fructose in a pharmaceutical dose"—the liver gets overwhelmed, in turn causing abnormal levels of triglycerides (fats), and insulin. This can lead to major metabolic issues and hinder your rebuild. In nutrition guidelines, eating four or five servings of fruit and vegetables means eating the whole food form and not juicing four or five times a day. If you do decide to juice, do it infrequently and in small amounts.

Other Problematic Foods

Grains, dairy, and sugar aren't the only foods you should avoid. Other problematic foods include soy, partially hydrogenated vegetable oils, and alcohol.

SOY

Another food often touted as a health food is soy. But, like grains, soybeans contain phytates, the compounds that prevent the absorption of nutrients. Soy also contains enzyme inhibitors that block the action of enzymes needed for proper protein digestion. Consuming soy-based foods can lead to reduced protein digestion, bloating, and gastrointestinal discomfort.

You should also be aware that there are two forms of soy: fermented and unfermented. You may be familiar with fermented soy products like miso, natto, and tempeh. The fermenting process involves cooking or soaking the soybeans, then treating them with magnesium chloride. Fermentation makes the nutrients in the soy available for the body. In its natural state, unfermented soy is loaded with antinutrients, which have been linked to digestive disorders, allergies, malnutrition, and immuno-suppression. Examples of unfermented soy foods include tofu, soy milk, soy burgers, soy cheese, soy ice cream, edamame (soybeans), and soy protein isolate (found in many protein powders and protein bars).

Last, 90 percent of all soybeans grown in the United States are genetically modified to resist the herbicide Roundup. Yes, the giant chemical company Monsanto has somehow been allowed to engineer the Roundup Ready gene that makes soybeans impervious to the poison Roundup. Supposedly, soybeans resistant to Roundup make farming easier and soybeans less expensive. Here's the caveat: GMOs have been linked to infertility, low-birth-weight babies, birth defects, allergies, and a plethora of other health problems. If you decide to eat fermented soy-based foods, eat them sparingly.

PARTIALLY HYDROGENATED VEGETABLE OIL

What is partially hydrogenated vegetable oil? Simply put, you take refined vegetable oil, add nickel, heat it to a high temperature, blow hydrogen through it, and you have hydrogenated vegetable oil—a.k.a. synthetic trans fat. What's the purpose of doing that? The processed-food industry puts that toxic stuff into foods to improve the shelf life. They are concerned about their profits, not human health.

When hydrogenated trans fats were invented in 1902, they were the first man-made fat to join the American food chain. According to the American Heart Association, in 1911, Crisco vegetable shortening was introduced. During World War II, the use of margarine rapidly rose because butter was rationed. A study published in 1974 in the *Journal of the American Oil Chemists' Society* estimated that the annual consumption of trans fats went up 81 percent from 1937 to 1972. Data from the Departments of Nutrition and Epidemiology at the Harvard School of Public Health indicate that the use of partially hydrogenated vegetable oils increased steadily until about 1960, displacing animal fats in the American diet.

The CDC reports that deaths due to coronary artery disease peaked in the mid-1960s. That statistic correlates with the highest rates of consumption of hydrogenated vegetable oil. Looking over the data, is it a coincidence that death from coronary artery disease peaked around 1960 when use of hydrogenated trans fats was at its highest? Similarly, data published in the journal *Atherosclerosis* show that when the use of hydrogenated fats goes up, death rates rise; likewise, when trans fat use goes down, death rates decline.

What is the connection between partially hydrogenated fats and coronary artery disease? Data found in the journal *Atherosclerosis*, the *Journal of Lipid Research*, and the *Annual Review of Nutrition* show that hydrogenated vegetable oils raise plasma LDL, triglycerides, and lipoprotein(a) at the same time that they lower plasma HDL. The research shows that hydrogenated fats increase systemic inflammation within the arteries, damage the arterial endothelium, and inhibit cyclooxygenase, an enzyme needed for proper blood flow. This creates an arterial nightmare.

Not surprisingly, hydrogenated fats have been shown to increase the number of sudden cardiac arrests. Researchers published data in the journal *Circulation* and the *American Journal of Clinical Nutrition* showing that synthetic trans fats become incorporated into the cell membrane of red blood cells. This creates inflammation, which ultimately increases the incidence of sudden death from heart disease.

The harmful effects of hydrogenated trans fats are now well documented. In a statement found on the FDA's website dated November 7, 2013, the FDA announced its preliminary determination that hydrogenated oils are not safe for human consumption. Here's the kicker: if the FDA "finalizes its preliminary determination" that hydrogenated oils/ fats be considered "food additives" and unsafe for use in food, it would require the processed-food industry to find a suitable alternative. If the ruling goes through, the industry will still have a grace period during which foods containing hydrogenated fats will be available on grocery store shelves.

Whatever the FDA decides, the first step in rebuilding from disease is making the decision to eliminate these toxic and inflammatory compounds from *your* diet. This can be hard, because trans fats are ubiquitous and hide in places we might not think of, including:

- Bread, cakes, doughnuts, cookies, muffins, pies, and other baked goods; cake mixes, pancake mixes, and other powdered food mixes
- Sugary frostings on cakes, muffins, and doughnuts
- Crackers made from refined flour
- Peanut butter (except freshly ground)
- Frozen meals, including frozen baked products
- Most frozen meat- and fish-based processed foods
- French fries
- Whipped toppings
- Margarines and vegetable shortening (Crisco)
- Powdered mashed potatoes
- Taco shells
- Cocoa mix
- Most breakfast cereals
- Microwave popcorn
- Many snack chips (potato, corn)
- Frozen pizza, burritos, frozen snack foods
- Low-fat ice cream
- Instant noodle cups
- Pasta and sauce mixes
- Pet food—it's no wonder that pets are suffering and dying from the same diseases humans do.

Note that foods labeled "0 trans fats" may, by law, contain small amounts of trans fats. Look for foods labeled "no trans fats" or "trans fat free." Here's the interesting part: there are naturally occurring trans fats in meat and dairy. Unlike harmful partially hydrogenated trans fats, however, the fats found in meat and dairy products are not a concern. In fact, several studies, including one out of *Advances in Nutrition*, have concluded that a moderate intake of trans fats from ruminant animals does not appear to be harmful.

> While we're on the subject of processed food, you should also avoid canned foods unless they are unsweetened, low-sodium/no-salt-added, and organic. Try to find products in cans labeled "BPA-free," as BPA is used to coat the inside of most cans and can leach into foods. Processed foods containing trans fats often contain artificial flavors, food dyes, and coloring as well— avoid these like the plague.

MEAT, EGGS, AND FISH

Avoid beef, poultry, and eggs raised on factory farms, which use grain feed, antibiotics, and hormones. Instead look for grass-fed beef raised without antibiotics or hormones, free-range poultry, and organic cage-free eggs. Farm-raised fish may contain petroleum dyes used for coloring, so look for sustainable, wild-caught seafood. Finally, cured meats (deli, sausages, bacon) can contain nitrates, so look for types that are organic with no preservatives or sugar.

READ IT BEFORE YOU EAT IT

In order to rebuild yourself from a disease, prevent recurrence, and get rid of body fat, you must stay away from highly processed, nutrient-naked, "food-like" substances that can and will interfere with your efforts to rebuild.

The processing of foods and food-like substances strips the fiber, vitamins, and minerals out of the food source, making it an empty shell lacking nutrition. Companies have to fortify (add back certain vitamins) to make those foods consumer-ready. These same companies also add hidden toxic fats, salts, and sugars in order to increase shelf life and improve palatability. We have been trained to read the top section of a food label (calories, fat, salt, sugar, and protein) but not the important part—the ingredients. Many packaged foods are loaded with junk hidden among the ingredients.

Do you know what you are about to eat? Could you identify or even pronounce all the ingredients on the label? Are the ingredients natural or synthetic? Do you know what all of them are? The only way to know what you are eating is to read the whole label, including the ingredients, not just the top of the label, and look them up if you're unfamiliar with them (or better yet, avoid foods with ingredients you can't readily identify).

On the label, look at:

SUGAR. In the top portion of the label, see how many grams of sugar are listed. Check the ingredients to see if any sugars are among the first three ingredients (see page 160 for a list of aliases for sugar on nutrition labels). Note: Four grams of sugar equals 1 teaspoon.

FAT. The top portion of the label indicates the total fat grams, followed by a breakdown of the amounts of different types of fat. Monounsaturated and polyunsaturated fats are healthful. Saturated fats—those found in animal foods like grass-fed beef and plant-based foods like coconut—are also healthful. However, steer clear of trans fats (refer back to page 165 if you need a refresher on why). Look at the list of ingredients. If you see the words *hydrogenated or partially hydrogenated*, do not buy. Those are both types of trans fats. Beware of the ingredient listed as just "vegetable oil," which is easily oxidized, making it hazardous to your health.

SALT. Salt is a mineral substance made of sodium and chloride; both are essential to good health. However, the salt found in many processed foods is processed salt. Many times the sodium content in packaged foods is MSG, which can be hazardous to your health (see page 132). In order to determine if the sodium content of a food is too high, here is my formula: in one serving, the amount of sodium in milligrams should not exceed the number of calories.

ARTIFICIAL FLAVORS AND COLORINGS. Stay away from toxic, unnatural food dyes and flavors. Many synthetic food dyes are made from petrochemicals (petroleum-based). Why would you eat anything labeled artificial?

Does this mean you can't eat something from a package? No. When choosing packaged or processed foods, look for ones that have few ingredients (five or fewer is a good guideline) that you recognize and can pronounce. Remember, when shopping, stay around the perimeter of the grocery store, where you will find whole, unprocessed, real foods, and bypass the dairy section. Also remember that whole foods have no labels or multisyllabic ingredients. What are the ingredients in an apple? Apple.

ALCOHOL AND NUTRIENT DEFICIENCY

When counseling people on nutrition, the most common question I hear is "What about alcohol?" I realize that telling you you shouldn't drink alcohol creates resistance. However, if you are rebuilding from a serious health issue, I would say give it up. I'm not saying you can't have a drink once in a while—but if you're having a glass of wine or a couple of beers every night, you should try to cut them out. Ultimately, it's your decision. To help you, I will give you the facts on alcohol consumption—then you can decide.

Besides being the number one recreational drug and the number one cause of liver cirrhosis, alcohol—ethanol in the form of wine, beer, or spirits—is one of the main causes of nutrient malabsorption and malnutrition in the United States. Alcohol causes malabsorption of vitamins A, B_1, B_6, folate, magnesium, potassium, and zinc. It is also a diuretic, causing a loss of water and electrolytes. The health issues that can arise from alcohol consumption include pancreatitis, liver cirrhosis, fatty liver, hemorrhagic stroke, gastrointestinal issues, muscle wasting in the limbs, and an increased risk for cancers of the esophagus, stomach, small intestine, colon, and bladder, as well as estrogen-sensitive breast cancer. Lung cancer is also a major risk because of the synergistic effects of drinking and smoking. Drinking alcohol also increases susceptibility to gout.

When you drink alcohol, enzymes in the body turn the ethanol it contains into acetaldehyde, a compound more toxic than the ethanol itself. Acetaldehyde can damage the liver and cause free radical damage, and is responsible for the hangover effect. Acetaldehyde also causes flushing of the face and a blotchy appearance on the skin, including the reddish/purple tone commonly seen on the noses of alcoholics.

Ethanol also disrupts multiple metabolic pathways in the body that can affect your body composition. It can cause muscle wasting and increased body fat. You may be familiar with a connection between drinking alcohol and unhealthful eating. Sipping wine or a cocktail often also involves eating cheese and crackers, bread, and/or fried foods. As you become more intoxicated, you start to care less about what and how much you're eating. Both of these scenarios increase your intake of calories and sugars, which causes your body to make fat. Second, having more than one drink introduces more calories than you are likely to burn before bed, causing you to store those calories as fat.

Drinking alcohol also has a dramatic effect on how you burn fat. Inside your body, acetaldehyde is rapidly converted into acetate—a short-chain fatty acid that the body uses for energy. But because you are burning that acetate for energy, your body holds on to the fat it would otherwise be converting into fuel.

What time of day you drink is also an important factor. Most people drink at night, and drinking before, during, or after dinner turns on the fat-making process. If you are in the habit of drinking alcohol at night and you can't seem to get rid of belly bulge, you may want to reconsider that cocktail.

WARNING: Taking acetaminophen (Tylenol) after drinking creates a toxin called NAPQI (pronounced *NAP-key*), which is extremely harmful to the liver.

The second and third most-asked questions are "What about chocolate?" and "What about caffeine?" There are health benefits to consuming both chocolate and caffeine.

Dark chocolate is a good source of antioxidants, polyphenols, flavanols, and catechins. Flavanols can stimulate the endothelium lining of the arteries to produce nitric oxide, a gas that regulates blood pressure. The cacao in dark chocolate can protect LDL from getting oxidized by free radicals, which provides some protection from atherosclerosis and heart disease. The cacao in dark chocolate may also improve cognitive function in those with mental impairment. Eating small amounts of dark chocolate—a couple of squares, or about 1 ounce—provides nutritional fiber and minerals, including iron, magnesium, manganese, and copper.

When shopping for chocolate, be aware that a lot of the chocolate sold is crap. Choose quality organic dark chocolate—not milk chocolate—with 70 percent or higher cacao content. Remember, eating a couple of squares has health benefits. That doesn't mean eating an entire chocolate bar.

If you enjoy a cup or two of coffee a day, you are not alone. Besides a tasty and satisfying everyday ritual, a cup of coffee and the caffeine it contains also have health benefits. Caffeine can decrease fatigue, improve memory and cognitive function, help burn body fat for fuel, and protect against type 2 diabetes and depression. Coffee is a good source of antioxidants and B vitamins. However, too much caffeine—more than three cups of coffee in a six-hour span—can cause increased blood pressure, nervousness, insomnia, stomach upset, increased heart rate, and jitters. When going for that cup of joe, you'll want to avoid adding nasty and unhealthful flavoring syrups and sugars, creams and artificial creamers, and flavors to it. I suggest using a little unsweetened almond milk or coconut milk, or just drinking it black.

Food Substitutions

Instead of this . . .	Use this . . .
DAIRY from cows, goats, sheep	
Milk	Rice milk, almond milk, coconut milk, or hemp milk
Yogurt	Yogurt made with coconut milk, almond milk, or rice milk
Cream	Coconut-milk creamer (unsweetened) Coconut cream Almond milk thickened with rice flour
Cheese	Daiya dairy-free cheese *(see Resources)*
Butter	Avocado oil and grape-seed oil for high-heat cooking; olive oil and others for flavor *(see OILS & FATS in this chart)*
Ice cream	Ice cream made with coconut milk, almond milk, or rice milk
SWEETENERS	
Natural sweeteners including: Sugar (cane, brown, raw) Evaporated cane sugar Dextrose Glucose Sucrose Corn syrup High-fructose corn syrup Maple syrup Maltodextrin Sugar alcohols (erythritol, maltitol, mannitol)	In *very* small amounts: Agave syrup Coconut palm sugar Fructose (from whole fresh or dried fruits) Honey (organic only)

Instead of this . . .	Use this . . .
Artificial sweeteners including: Aspartame (Equal, NutraSweet) Saccharine (Sweet'N Low) Sucralose (Splenda)	Rebaudioside or reb A (Rebiana) Stevia (Stevia, Sweet Leaf)
GRAINS	
Wheat Rye Barley Oats (rolled, instant) Corn Products made from these grains, including pasta and baked goods	Brown rice Brown rice pasta Wild rice Quinoa Oats (steel-cut) Almond flour or meal Coconut flour
OILS & FATS	
Hydrogenated and partially hydrogenated oils Corn oil Soybean oil Cottonseed oil Sunflower oil Processed vegetable oils Shortening Lard Butter	Avocado oil (for high-heat cooking and flavor) Olive oil (for salads and flavor) Coconut oil (for baking) Nut oils (such as almond and walnut, for flavor) Grape-seed oil (for high-heat cooking)
SALT	
Refined salt	Sea salt Pink Himalayan salt Kosher salt (without additives)
CONDIMENTS	
Any condiment containing sugars, preservatives, high-fructose corn syrup, or artificial color	Ketchup (sweetened with agave) Tomato paste (made with only tomato and salt) Umeboshi vinegar *(see Note, page 416)* Tamari Gluten-free soy sauce

Your Caloric Needs

Now that you have a basic understanding of *what* to eat, let's talk about *how much* you should eat. In order for you to lose the fat, you have to know how many daily calories you need. In the following paragraph, I've given you a formula to determine the amount of food you should eat based on your specific metabolism and activity level. Just like getting a custom suit, dress, or shoes made, the formula gives you a way to find out how much food—really nutrients—you require in order to rebuild from disease and prevent recurrence. The formula and your calculation will also let you know how many calories you need to consume to get rid of fat and maintain or increase your lean muscle. The process allows you to create a custom-tailored food plan.

To figure out how many calories you should eat per day to lose weight, you need to calculate your basal metabolic rate (BMR), the number of calories you would burn in a 24-hour period if your body were completely at rest.

BASAL METABOLIC RATE (BMR)
CALCULATION (FROM THE HARRIS-BENEDICT EQUATION)

For women:
655 + (4.35 x weight in pounds) + (4.7 x height in inches) − (4.7 x age in years)

For men:
66 + (6.23 x weight in pounds) + (12.7 x height in inches) − (6.76 x age in years)

I'll use myself as an example. I'm 50 years old, 6 feet tall, and weigh 195 pounds. Before we start, let's convert that height into inches: 6 feet = 6 x 12 inches = 72 inches. Using the formula above, my BMR is:

66 + (6.23 x **195**) + (12.7 x **72**) − (6.76 x **50**) or 66 + 1,214.85 + 914.4 − 338 = 1,857.25

So my body would burn 1,857.25 calories in a 24-hour period, even if I just lay in bed all day. Try it for yourself—plug in your numbers and see what you get.

ACTIVITY FACTOR CALCULATION

Once you figure out your BMR, you must determine how active you are, which we will call the activity factor. Why is this necessary? Whether you are sedentary or very physically active, you are burning calories—just at different rates. The following chart gives some examples of what activities define each activity level. If you are active in some way but don't see it listed, just look for a similar activity and figure out where you fall.

ACTIVITY ADJUSTMENT

Sedentary or very light activity: Seated activities (computer work, reading, telephone work, driving), about 2 hours of walking/standing daily	**Use BMR**
Mild activity: Some walking throughout the day, standing activities (teaching, retail work), golf, light housework	1.2
Moderate activity: Fast walking, housework, gardening, carrying light loads, cycling, weight-lifting	1.3
Strenuous activity: Dancing, skiing, physical labor (construction, moving cargo, road work), some running; very little sitting throughout the day	1.5
Extreme activity: Endurance training, tennis, swimming, long-distance cycling/running, team sports (football, soccer, basketball)	1.7

Let's continue with myself as the example: I'm on my feet six to eight hours a day at my practice, and I work out four or five days a week, weight training for 40 minutes every other day and doing 20 minutes of HIIT on the other days; due to my busy work week, I sometimes miss a day or two. I would classify my activity level at strenuous (1.5).

Your total metabolic rate (TMR) is your BMR multiplied by your activity factor. This is the number of calories that serves as your baseline. In my case, it looks like this:

1,857.25 [my BMR] x 1.5 [my activity factor] = 2,785 [total calories my body will burn in a day]

From this number, you need to decide how many calories to subtract to start getting rid of the fat. In order to do this, you need to calculate your body fat percentage.

BODY FAT PERCENTAGE CALCULATION

There are different methods for measuring body fat. The most accurate and cost-effective way is to be tested via bioelectrical impedance. However, to give you a general sense of your body fat percentage, researchers have created another formula. It will not calculate the exact percentage, but it will give you a guideline as you go forward to determine if you are losing body fat and/or muscle. This equation is called the Jackson-Pollock formula.

Adult Body Fat % = (1.61 x BMI) + (0.13 x age) − (12.1 x your gender value) − 13.9

Gender values: men = 1, women = 0

You can also buy body fat calipers that use skin-fold testing to determine body fat. This method involves pinching the skin and fat over different parts of your body and putting roughly seven measurements into a formula to calculate your fat percentage.

Once you have calculated your body fat percentage, look at the charts on the next page to see where you fall. One chart is for men and the other for women. Your percentage will indicate whether you are at a healthy fat level. For a forty-five-year-old woman, a body fat percentage between 23 and 28 is ideal, and 29 to 34 percent is average.

As you can see on the charts, average body fat percentages go up with age. As we age, physical and metabolic changes take place that increase body fat. This increased fat is sometimes seen around the organs (visceral fat), under the skin (subcutaneous fat), and even inside the muscles (intramuscular fat). The greatest reason for the deposition of fat within the muscles—technically called intermuscular adipose tissue (IMAT)—is inactivity. It is safe to say that as many people age, their physical activity diminishes. Research out of the *American Journal of Clinical Nutrition* states low physical activity prevents the burning of fat within the muscle, which creates an environment for fat accumulation.

BODY FAT % MEASUREMENT CHART FOR MEN

AGE																	
18-20	2.0	3.9	6.2	8.5	10.5	12.5	14.3	16.0	17.5	18.9	20.2	21.3	22.3	23.1	23.8	24.3	24.9
21-25	2.5	4.9	7.3	9.5	11.6	13.6	15.4	17.0	18.6	20.0	21.2	22.3	23.3	24.2	24.9	25.4	25.8
26-30	3.5	6.0	8.4	10.6	12.7	14.6	16.4	18.1	19.6	21.0	22.3	23.4	24.4	25.2	25.9	26.5	26.9
31-35	4.5	7.1	9.4	11.7	13.7	15.7	17.5	19.2	20.7	22.1	23.4	24.5	25.5	26.3	27.0	27.5	28.0
36-40	5.6	8.1	10.5	12.7	14.8	16.8	18.6	20.2	21.8	23.2	24.4	25.6	26.5	27.4	28.1	28.6	29.0
41-45	6.7	9.2	11.5	13.8	15.9	17.8	19.6	21.3	22.8	24.7	25.5	26.6	27.6	28.4	29.1	29.7	30.1
46-50	7.7	10.2	12.6	14.8	16.9	18.9	20.7	22.4	23.9	25.3	26.6	27.7	28.7	29.5	30.2	30.7	31.2
51-55	8.8	11.3	13.7	15.9	18.0	20.0	21.8	23.4	25.0	26.4	27.6	28.7	29.7	30.6	31.2	31.8	32.2
56 & up	9.9	12.4	14.7	17.0	19.1	21.0	22.8	24.5	26.0	27.4	28.7	29.8	30.8	31.6	32.3	32.9	33.3

LEAN · IDEAL · AVERAGE · ABOVE AVERAGE

BODY FAT % MEASUREMENT CHART FOR WOMEN

AGE																	
18-20	11.3	13.5	15.7	17.7	19.7	21.5	23.2	24.8	26.3	27.7	29.0	30.2	31.3	32.3	33.1	33.9	34.6
21-25	11.9	14.2	16.3	18.4	20.3	22.1	23.8	25.5	27.0	28.4	29.6	30.8	31.9	32.9	33.8	34.5	35.2
26-30	12.5	14.8	16.9	19.0	20.9	22.7	24.5	26.1	27.6	29.0	30.3	31.5	32.5	33.5	34.4	35.2	35.8
31-35	13.2	15.4	17.6	19.6	21.5	23.4	25.1	26.7	28.2	29.6	30.9	32.1	33.2	34.1	35.0	35.8	36.4
36-40	13.8	16.0	18.2	20.2	22.2	24.0	25.7	27.3	28.8	30.2	31.5	32.7	33.8	34.8	35.6	36.4	37.0
41-45	14.4	16.7	18.8	20.8	22.8	24.6	26.3	27.9	29.4	30.8	32.1	33.3	34.4	35.4	36.3	37.0	37.7
46-50	15.0	17.3	19.4	21.5	23.4	25.2	26.9	28.6	30.1	31.5	32.8	34.0	35.0	36.0	36.9	37.6	38.3
51-55	15.6	17.9	20.0	22.1	24.0	25.9	27.6	29.2	30.7	32.1	33.4	34.6	35.6	36.6	37.5	38.3	38.9
56 & up	16.3	18.5	20.7	22.7	24.6	26.5	28.2	29.8	31.3	32.7	34.0	35.2	36.3	37.1	38.1	38.9	39.5

LEAN · IDEAL · AVERAGE · ABOVE AVERAGE

FAT LOSS ADJUSTMENT CALCULATION

Once you have calculated your TMR and your body fat percentage, you can determine how many calories to cut from your diet in order to start losing fat. Use the chart on page 179 to determine how many calories to subtract from your TMR. The key here is to not severely restrict calories. You want to take away only a small number of calories, so your body doesn't release cortisol and hold on to fat. Fat loss is a process, not an event.

Each person's fat loss needs are different. For example, if person A had a body fat percentage of more than 30, subtracting 300 to 600 calories would be appropriate. If person B had a slight increased body fat percentage, subtracting the same 300 to 600 calories would be too drastic. Modify your caloric intake based on *your* metabolic rate and body fat percentage. This makes your diet customized and tailored to you.

FAT LOSS ADJUSTMENT

Men:

If you have a healthy body fat percentage:	No subtraction of calories
If you have an increased body fat percentage:	Subtract 200 to 500 calories
If your body fat percentage is more than 30%:	Subtract 300 to 600 calories

Women:

If you have a healthy body fat percentage:	No subtraction of calories
If you have an increased body fat percentage:	Subtract 100 to 300 calories
If your body fat percentage is more than 30%:	Subtract 300 to 500 calories

DAILY CALORIC INTAKE CALCULATION

Now calculate how many calories you need to eat daily by subtracting the calories from the fat loss adjustment table from your TMR. This is your daily caloric intake.

CALCULATE YOUR DAILY CALORIC INTAKE	
Basal Metabolic Rate (BMR):	
Activity Adjustment:	x
Total Metabolic Rate (TMR):	
Fat Loss Adjustment:	–
Your Daily Caloric Intake*	=

*This is the amount of food you eat each day.

DR. Z'S EAT RIGHT RECOMMENDATIONS

1. Whatever you do, don't skip breakfast. According to research published in the *American Journal of Clinical Nutrition*, skipping breakfast can make you fat. Skipping breakfast alters the way insulin talks to the cells. This increases blood sugar, which is then stored as fat. So start the day with protein and a complex carb. Check out the breakfast ideas starting on page 360.

2. Remember to eat frequently, five or six times a day. This allows better blood sugar control, increases your metabolism, feeds the muscles, and gets rid of fat.

3. Spice it up. Adding healthful spices to pop the flavors of food makes eating enjoyable and tasty. Examples of healthful spices include curry powder, dry mustard, ginger, oregano, basil, parsley, cayenne pepper, cumin, and garlic. See the list of spices that go well with specific foods, including poultry, beef, fish, eggs, vegetables, soups, and stews, on page 183.

4. Drink six to eight glasses of water per day. Water transports oxygen and nutrients to the cells, detoxifies them, helps to regulate body temperature, boosts metabolism, and moisturizes joints, as well as a thousand other benefits. Most of us are "dry"—walking

around dehydrated. We lose water constantly throughout the day, especially during the warmer months due to sweating. You can't replace water by downing coffee or a beer. Alcoholic and caffeinated drinks are diuretics, which cause you to lose water. Research published in the journal *Metabolism* found that hydrating the body increases fat burning. In another study, published in the journal *Lancet*, researchers suggested that increased hydration actually increases the number of enzymes that cause fat burning. Last, a study found in the *European Journal of Clinical Nutrition* reaffirms the effects of water on fat burning. The researchers found when the body is hydrated, fat is burned and muscle is preserved. Drinking water is definitely a must for sustainable fat loss and a healthy body composition.

5. Legumes are an excellent source of carbs and protein, but unfortunately, some people lack the enzyme alpha-galactosidase, which is needed to break down beans and cruciferous vegetables (such as broccoli, cauliflower, Brussels sprouts, and cabbage). After eating these food sources, bacteria in the gut help to break them down and produce large amounts of carbon dioxide and hydrogen. This causes bloating, gas, and pain. The solution to this discomfort is to take a supplement containing the missing enzyme. The supplement I use personally is Digest from Transformation Enzymes. It contains alpha-galactosidase, as well as other enzymes to help you break down beans and cruciferous vegetables, thus preventing unpleasant symptoms.

6. Be careful with peanuts. Even if you don't have a peanut allergy, eat them sparingly, or better yet, eat tree nuts (peanuts are actually a legume) and seeds, including walnuts, macadamia nuts, pecans, pine nuts, pistachios, cashews, almonds, Brazil nuts, and pumpkin seeds. People with peanut allergies may be allergic for one of two reasons. First, peanuts contain an insect-protective protein called lectin. Unlike other proteins, which are broken

down during digestion, lectins aren't digested at all. They can attach to the intestine where immune cells are parked, waiting to attack invaders and unwanted proteins in our food. For many people, eating peanuts triggers the immune system to attack the lectins, causing an internal war, which can lead to conditions like leaky gut syndrome, autoimmune conditions, and allergies. Second, peanuts can be contaminated during storage. Either from the soil or a poor storage environment, peanuts can be infected with a mold called *Aspergillus flavus*. *Aspergillus* releases aflatoxin, which not only is carcinogenic but also causes the nasty allergies associated with peanuts.

Your Custom-Made Diet

What's new about this plan compared to other diet programs? You will work smarter, not harder. You will choose the diet that fits your needs. Whatever diet you pick, you will not starve. You will not give up in frustration. You are going to see how these changes will affect your palate—and your health—for the better, and for the long run.

I provide sample diets to show you what a 1,300- and 1,500-calorie food plan looks like. Take a look at those samples, then fill in the worksheet on page 194 with your own food choices. Each meal should have protein, some carbs, some fat, and lots of nonstarchy vegetables. You can plug the calorie counts from the recipes in Part III right into your daily food plans, or you can choose foods you like from the lists I have provided to create your own meals and snacks. Serving sizes and their respective calories are already calculated for you. You just need to decide what you like to eat. Depending on your lifestyle, you pick the foods and recipes convenient for you. If you like to make super-tasty meals loaded with nutrients, turn to Part III. While some of these recipes take a few minutes to prepare, others take very little time. Many of the foods on the optimal-foods lists and in the recipes are "grab and go" food items. If you choose a recipe that requires preparation time, save time by making enough for leftovers. See Dr. Z's Fast Food on page 192 for other ideas for quick meals.

SPICE UP YOUR DIET

Food	Herbs, Spices & Other Seasonings
Poultry	Aniseed, black pepper, cardamom, cayenne pepper, celery seed, coriander, curry, fennel, garlic, ginger, lemon, marjoram, mustard, onion powder, oregano, paprika, red pepper flakes, sage, salt, savory, thyme
Beef	Black pepper, cayenne pepper, chili powder, chipotle, curry powder, fenugreek, garlic, horseradish, mustard, onion, oregano, sage, salt, savory
Fish/Shellfish	Bay leaf, capers, dill, garlic, horseradish, lemon, marjoram, mustard, onion, parsley, rosemary, saffron, salt, tarragon, thyme
Stews & Soups	Bay leaf, celery seed, chervil, chili powder, cilantro, cumin, curry powder, garlic, ginger, horseradish, marjoram, mustard, nutmeg, onion, oregano, paprika, parsley, saffron, salt, soy sauce (organic gluten-free), thyme
Eggs	Basil, chervil, curry powder, dill, onion, paprika, pepper, rosemary, salt, tarragon, thyme
Vegetables	Basil, black pepper, cardamom, celery seed, chives, coriander, cumin, fennel, garlic, ginger, lemon, mint, onion, oregano, parsley, salt, sesame seed, thyme
Oatmeal	Allspice, aniseed, cinnamon, clove, cocoa (unsweetened), coconut, nutmeg, salt, vanilla

You can use your own recipes or recipes from other sources; just make sure you take the time to calculate their calorie content. Use a site like Nutrition Data (www.nutritiondata.self.com) to find the calorie counts for the individual ingredients in the recipe, add them up, then divide the total calories by the number of servings to get the calories per serving and plug that number into your meal planning worksheet. This approach requires a little bit of work at first, but it makes your dieting adventure easy and enjoyable. Be sure to replace unhealthful ingredients with healthful ones so you are not eating too many or the wrong kind of calories. For example, if you are used to eating regular white or wheat pasta, replace it with brown rice pasta; if a recipe calls for cow's milk, substitute nondairy milk from the optimal foods lists on page 189.

Don't drive yourself crazy when putting your meals together—just try to get as close to your daily calorie requirements as possible. (For example, in the 1,300-calorie sample plan, the calories add up to roughly 1,361.) But if your total metabolic rate requires you to eat 1,300 calories, then eat 1,300 calories—don't try to lose more fat by cutting more calories. It may seem like a lot of food, but don't forget that the foods you are eating are high in nutrients and low in calories, so while you may be eating *more* than you were in the past, you're also eating *better*.

Eat most of your meals during the day, and eat less at night. If you eat dinner late, I suggest having just a small piece of protein and a hearty portion of greens. If you are hungry at night, eat vegetables with few calories and lots of nutrients. Remember, you don't want to store fat while you sleep, so at night, don't eat foods that raise insulin. Stick to nonstarchy vegetables, like Brussels sprouts, bell peppers, or cucumber to satisfy your hunger.

MEAL PLANNING WORKSHEET (SAMPLE 1)

1,300 CALORIES	
MORNING MEAL Protein: 2 whole eggs Carb: ½ sweet potato Fat: 1 teaspoon avocado oil Additional foods: 1 serving nonstarchy vegetables 1 cup blueberries	Start your day with protein: eggs, veggie burger, chicken. Add a complex carb, some fat, and a nonstarchy vegetable. Include a fruit.
SNACK 10 almonds 1 medium apple ½ cup carrots	8 to 10 almonds is the limit. No need to overeat at snack time.
MIDDAY MEAL Protein: 3 to 4 ounces chicken Carb: ½ cup brown rice with black beans Fat: ¼ avocado Additional foods: 1 serving nonstarchy vegetables	Pick another protein: turkey burger, chicken salad, or chicken with green salad and ¼ avocado (2 servings). Have another nonstarchy vegetable and legumes on the side.
SNACK 6 to 8 brown rice crackers ¼ cup hummus	Remember: Eat most of your calories before dark.
EVENING MEAL Protein: 3 to 4 ounces fish Carb: ½ cup lentil soup Fat: 1 teaspoon olive oil Additional foods: 1 serving nonstarchy vegetables	Low calories now that it's getting later in the day.
SNACK Nonstarchy vegetable Herbal tea	If you're hungry after dinner, eat half a cucumber or red bell pepper.

MEAL PLANNING WORKSHEET (SAMPLE 2)

1,300 CALORIES	
MORNING MEAL Scrambled Eggs & Sun-Dried Tomatoes (page 367) ½ cup strawberries and ½ cup blueberries ½ cup Roasted Brussels Sprouts (page 424)	Eggs with sun-dried tomatoes provide 318 calories. Berries have about 75 calories. Sun-dried tomatoes and the oil used to cook the eggs provide some fat.
SNACK 1 medium apple 6 to 8 ounces fresh-brewed unsweetened green tea	An apple has 70 calories, and the tea has no calories. Green tea is a great fat burner!
MIDDAY MEAL Turkey Bolognese (page 417) Mixed green salad with 1 teaspoon vinaigrette	This meal includes protein, fat, and carbs (brown rice pasta) with about 392 calories. The oil in the salad dressing has 40 calories.
SNACK 1 cup broccoli ¼ cup Hummus (page 436)	Broccoli with hummus provides about 120 calories.
EVENING MEAL Salmon Salad (page 385) with sliced cucumbers and tomatoes Pantry Salad (page 380)	This meal includes protein, fat, and carbs. Salmon Salad has 186 calories. The Pantry Salad and dressing are 110 calories.
SNACK Tomato with fresh basil and a few drops of olive oil Herbal tea	This has about 50 calories.

MEAL PLANNING WORKSHEET (SAMPLE 3)

1,500 CALORIES	
MORNING MEAL Protein: 3 egg whites & 1 large egg Carb: ½ sweet potato Fat: 2 teaspoons avocado oil Additional foods: 1 serving nonstarchy vegetables 1 cup mixed berries	Egg whites plus a whole egg provide 150 calories. Add chopped spinach or collard greens. Sweet potato and oil for frying provide 205 calories. Berries have 75 calories.
SNACK 10 almonds 1 medium apple ½ cup carrots	Almonds, apple, and ½ cup carrots provide 225 calories.
MIDDAY MEAL Protein: 3 to 4 ounces chicken Carb: 1 medium carrot Fat: 1 tablespoon oil Additional foods: 1 serving nonstarchy vegetables	Grilled chicken over green salad with a carrot and olive oil provide a total of 300 calories.
SNACK 1 brown rice cake 1 tablespoon almond butter	This combination provides 135 calories.
EVENING MEAL Protein: 3 to 4 ounces fish Carb: ½ cup lentil soup Fat: 1 tablespoon olive oil Additional foods: 1 serving nonstarchy vegetables	3 to 4 ounces wild salmon baked or broiled with lemon and dill, soup, and a green salad with vinaigrette provide a total of 385 calories.
SNACK Red and yellow bell peppers Herbal tea	Depending on the amount you eat, this has 25 to 50 calories.

MEAL PLANNING WORKSHEET (SAMPLE 4)

1,500 CALORIES	
MORNING MEAL Scrambled Eggs & Sun-Dried Tomatoes (page 367) Fresh-brewed green tea	This medley provides protein, carb, and fat in one dish for 318 calories.
SNACK Ambrosia Fruit Salad (page 440)	The fruit and coconut in this salad will satisfy your sweet tooth for 188 calories.
MIDDAY MEAL Curried Chicken Salad (page 374) Spiced Sweet Potato Cubes (page 427)	Chicken salad provides 367 calories. The sweet potatoes add 123 calories.
SNACK Broccoli and Hummus	One cup provides 139 calories.
EVENING MEAL Summer Poached Salmon (page 411) Pantry Salad (page 380)	One serving of salmon provides 359 calories. Use the salad recipe or what you have on hand. Calories should be about 110.
SNACK Nonstarchy vegetable	Tomatoes and cucumbers have about 50 calories.

OPTIMAL FOODS

Dairy Alternatives

Almond milk, unsweetened (1 cup = 50 calories)

Coconut milk beverage, unsweetened (1 cup = 50 calories)

Coconut milk yogurt, unsweetened (1 ounce = 80 calories)

Hemp milk, unsweetened (1 cup = 130 calories)

Rice milk, unsweetened (1 cup = 70 calories)

Fruits

Choose whole fruit rather than juice. Juice has a much higher glycemic index because the fiber has been removed.

Low Glycemic Index:

A serving of berries is 1 cup.

Blackberry (62 calories)

Blueberry (84 calories)

Boysenberry (166 calories)

Cranberry (46 calories)

Elderberry (106 calories)

Gooseberry (66 calories)

Loganberry (81 calories)

Raspberry (64 calories)

Strawberry (50 calories)

Medium Glycemic Index:

Apple (1 = 95 calories)

Apricot (1 = 17 calories)

Cherry (15 = 75 calories)

Grapefruit (1 = 82 calories)

Kiwifruit (1 = 50 calories)

Lemon/lime (1 = 17 calories)

Melon (1 slice = 50 calories)

Nectarine (1 = 62 calories)

Orange (1 = 62 calories)

Passion fruit (1 = 17 calories)

Peach (1 = 38 calories)

Pear (1 = 96 calories)

Persimmon (1 = 118 calories)

Prune (4 = 80 calories)

Tangerine (1 = 47 calories)

High Glycemic Index:
_____

Eat sparingly or after a workout.

Banana (1 small = 90 calories)

Grape (15 = 30 calories)

Mango (1 = 135 calories)

Papaya (1 small = 59 calories)

Pineapple (1 cup = 83 calories

Raisin (1.5-ounce box = 129 calories)

Watermelon (2 cups cubed = 92 calories)

Protein
_____

Eat 3 to 4 servings per day.

Animal Sources
_____

Choose free-range, cage-free, grass-fed, with no hormones or antibiotics added. Avoid farm-raised fish. One serving is 150 calories.

Poultry (lean, 3 to 4 ounces): chicken, turkey

Cold-water fish (3 ounces or ¾ cup canned in water): cod, halibut, mackerel, salmon, tuna

Shellfish (3 ounces or ¾ cup canned in water): crab, lobster, shrimp

Red meat (lean, 3 to 4 ounces): beef, lamb

Game (3 to 4 ounces): buffalo, ostrich, venison

Eggs (2 large, or 3 whites plus 1 large)

Plant Sources
_____

Calories per serving vary.

"Veggie" burger, gluten-free (4 ounces = 100 calories)

Tempeh (½ cup = 165 calories)

Nonstarchy Vegetables
_____

Unlimited raw or cooked; juiced (use sparingly). One serving is 10 to 25 calories; eat a minimum of 3 to 4 servings per day.

Arugula

Asparagus

Bamboo shoots

Bean sprouts

Beet greens

Bell pepper

Nonstarchy Vegetables (cont.)

Bok choy	Kale
Broccoli	Leek
Broccoflower	Lettuce (all types)
Brussels sprouts	Mushroom (all types)
Cabbage (all types)	Mustard greens
Cauliflower	Okra
Celery	Onion
Chicory	Radicchio
Chive	Radish
Collard greens	Romaine
Cucumber	Scallion
Dandelion greens	Shallot
Eggplant	Snow pea
Endive	Spinach
Escarole	Swiss chard
Fennel	Spaghetti squash
Garlic	Summer squash
Green beans	Tomato
Hearts of palm	Water chestnut
Jalapeño	Watercress
	Zucchini

High-Fiber Starchy Vegetables

Up to 3 servings per day. Serving size is ½ cup.

Acorn squash (56 calories)	Pumpkin (142 calories)
Artichoke heart (42 calories)	Sweet potato (125 calories)
Beet (37 calories)	Turnip (17 calories)
Butternut squash (40 calories)	Winter squash (40 calories)
Carrot (27 calories; 2 raw medium = 50 calories; ½ cup baby = 30 calories)	Yam (79 calories)

DR. Z'S FAST FOOD

Protein
- Rotisserie chicken (hot for one meal, cold for chicken salad)
- Applegate deli meats (turkey, chicken)
- Applegate chicken and turkey sausages (only those with no sugar added)
- Canned tuna (American Tuna is low in mercury)
- Sautéed ground meats and vegetables for a quick stew
- Grilled chicken, kebabs, burgers
- Omelets with mushrooms and other vegetables

Produce
- Salad mixes, romaine hearts, lettuce, spinach
- Baby carrots, celery sticks, broccoli florets in bags
- Trader Joe's steamed beets (serve hot, or cold in salads)
- Frozen vegetables and fruits are often as good as fresh, since they are frozen shortly after picking. Frozen peas, lima beans, green beans, spinach, and berries are available almost everywhere.

Lentils and Grains
- Trader Joe's cooked lentils and rice (basmati, jasmine)
- Eden Organics canned beans (cans are BPA-free)
- Gluten-free steel-cut oats (cook in quantity and freeze for use later)

Snacks (foods to pack in a cooler and bring to work)
- Nuts (raw walnuts, almonds, cashews)
- Seeds (pumpkin, sunflower)
- Nut butters (unsweetened)
- Brown rice crackers (with nut butter, hummus, avocado)
- Celery or cucumber with nut butter
- Cut carrots, broccoli, cauliflower, apples, sugar snap peas
- Hummus

- Hard-boiled eggs
- Berries (especially strawberries and blueberries)
- Healthful low-sugar protein bars. (Be careful on this one. Many protein bars are very high in sugar. Even with low-sugar bars, eat half and save the other half for later.)

Your Optimal Diet

In conversation, you frequently hear things like, "My grandfather ate crap and drank his whole life and never got sick," "He never smoked a cigarette in his life and developed lung cancer," and "Why does she get to eat whatever she wants and not gain a pound?" How can this be? The old saying "No two people are alike" is the truth. Each person, including you, has a unique genetic blueprint. What you look like, how fast you heal, how you respond to stress, and how well your body manages the calories you take in from food—all are unique to you. So how could we all follow the same diet? A diet that works for someone else may not work for you.

The key is to fill your plate with nutrient-dense foods, including colorful vegetables and protein, without loading up on calories. Each meal should consist of roughly 30 to 40 percent protein, 20 percent fat, and 40 percent carbohydrates. This provides you with not only a variety of food sources, but also the nutrients needed to rebuild from disease and get rid of fat. Your snacks should include nuts/seeds, legumes, vegetables, a limited selection of grains, and fruits.

It's also important to remember portion control. When eating protein, common sense tells us not to eat a 12- to 16-ounce steak, just as eating an entire pound of nuts is too extreme. One simple way to remember portion sizes is by tying them to everyday objects: A 3- to 4-ounce piece of meat, for example, is about the size of a deck of cards. A 3- to 4-ounce piece of fish is about the size of a checkbook. One cup equals a baseball, ½ cup equals a lightbulb, and 1 tablespoon is about the size of a poker chip. Here's another way to think about portion size: the right amount of protein for you is the size of your palm; a serving of carbs should be roughly the size of your clenched fist. While portion sizes don't have to be exact, you should have at least a rough idea of how much you're eating so you don't consume too many calories.

MEAL PLANNING WORKSHEET

_____ CALORIES
MORNING MEAL   Protein: Carb: Fat: Additional foods:
SNACK
MIDDAY MEAL   Protein: Carb: Fat: Additional foods:
SNACK
EVENING MEAL   Protein: Carb: Fat: Additional foods:
SNACK

To recap, the options for creating your own food plan are:

- Pick from the optimal-foods lists and put those foods and their calorie counts into your meal plan.
- Use the recipes provided to make meals and plug their calorie counts into your meal plan.
- Use your own recipes or recipes from other sources, replacing unhealthful ingredients with healthful alternatives, then calculating the calories per serving.

Supplement Your Diet

Modern agricultural practices and the depletion of nutrients in the soil, coupled with diets heavy in nutrient-deficient processed foods, the onslaught of environmental pollutants, and increasing use of pharmaceuticals, have created widespread chronic nutrient deprivation. For example, it's a well-known fact that cholesterol-lowering drugs cause the depletion of coenzyme Q10—a vitamin-like substance needed to produce energy—while smoking causes a rapid depletion of vitamin C. Sadly, without vital vitamins, minerals, and other plant-based compounds, over time we slowly develop tissue and organ dysfunctions and, eventually, chronic disease. Nutritional supplements, or "nutraceuticals," such as vitamins, minerals, probiotics, herbs, and enzymes, can provide a portion of our daily nutritional needs, filling in the potholes for people who could become ill due to lack of proper nutrition and toxic or stressful lifestyles.

It is well established that nutraceuticals are also important for anyone recovering and rebuilding from disease and/or a medical procedure. For example, research in the journal *Cancer Research* showed that the compounds indole-3-carbinol (I3C), curcumin, and epigallocatechin-3-gallate (EGCG, found in green tea) not only prevented cancer but also, in combination with cancer therapies, enhanced the antitumor activity of the therapies. The same dietary compounds were also shown to decrease the toxicity caused by chemotherapy and radiation. Regarding heart disease, a study in the *New England Journal of Medicine* found vitamin E to be a powerful antioxidant that prevented the oxidation of LDL—a crucial step in the development of atherosclerosis and coronary artery disease. Last, studies published in *Diabetes Care* and *Diabetology & Metabolic Syndrome* reported that zinc and magnesium were found to help reduce the risk of diabetes as well as regulate the high blood sugar associated with diabetes.

While rebuilding myself from toxic chemotherapy, radiation, and surgery, I ate a whole-food diet consisting of plant-based foods, healthful protein, fats, and carbs. To supplement that diet, I took probiotics and digestive enzymes, vitamin C, vitamin D, B vitamins, anti-inflammatory nutrients, a multivitamin, essential fats, and specific herbs shown to improve bone-marrow suppression and anemia. Following this diet and supplement protocol, I was able to reverse the side effects of my cancer treatments and recover quickly.

Taking supplements to recover, rebuild, and heal is essential; however, what worked for me may not work for you, so talk to your health care provider and do your research before establishing a supplement regimen. And remember that supplements are not meant to, and cannot, replace a healthful diet. They are intended to fill in any gaps and add therapeutically to a diet of whole, nutrient-dense foods, to help offset excess stress and facilitate healing and repair.

WILLIAM'S STORY

William is a highly successful seventy-six-year-old entrepreneur and businessman. At thirty-eight years old, he was told by his family doctor that he wouldn't live past the young age of fifty if he didn't get his blood pressure down and lose 50 pounds. From that point on, he began working out, and decided to change to a more plant-based diet. Around the same time, at his annual physical exam at the Cooper Clinic in Texas, a faulty mitral valve—the valve between the left atrium and left ventricle of the heart—was found. It was successfully repaired at the Cleveland Clinic in Ohio. Fast-forward to years later: Back at the Cooper Clinic, a faulty tricuspid valve—a muscular valve separating the right atrium from the right ventricle—was found in William's heart, and he was instructed to get yearly evaluations to monitor his heart for issues associated with it.

In his pursuit of better health, William attended a talk I gave in the Florida Keys on the causes of chronic disease. After the talk, we discussed some of his health issues and decided it was best to do a full health workup. He and his wife flew to my clinic a few weeks later. A review of his health history revealed atrial fibrillation (AFib), mild hypertension, increased urinary frequency, and "mild" coronary atherosclerosis. Following a thorough evaluation, we also found high blood sugar, elevated inflammatory markers, anemia, low vitamin D, low testosterone, and low thyroid hormone T3 (interestingly, his thyroid was producing enough T4, but his T3 was very low). William has exercised practically every day for years, combining weights with cardio, and has maintained excellent body composition, with only 13 percent body fat.

An assessment of his internal terrain showed abnormal blood sugar (dysglycemia) due to his protein-deficient and high-fructose diet; a lack of amino acids from infrequent protein consumption and high blood sugar; and elevated blood pressure caused by an inability of the blood vessels to produce enough nitric oxide. The atherosclerosis most likely had begun years ago, when he wasn't taking care of himself. Eating poorly damaged the lining of the arteries, which allowed inflammation to occur. The imbalance of his thyroid hormones—normal T4 but very low T3—was due to a conversion problem in the liver, where specific enzymes were unable to convert T4 into T3, the active thyroid hormone. Last, his low testosterone was not just an "age-related" reaction. Factors including high blood sugar, stress levels, and low protein intake can all decrease levels of circulating testosterone.

I worked with William on his nutrient intake by increasing protein, plant-based foods, and healthful fats in his diet. I recommended more weight training and shorter periods of cardio to shift his body composition toward more lean muscle. I also recommended specific nutrients to regulate his blood sugar, improve testosterone production, regulate levels of thyroid hormones, and reduce his blood pressure. Roughly six months later, we retested his biomarkers and the affected systems. He was excited to find his testosterone and T3 levels had returned to normal; his blood sugar was at a healthy level; the inflammatory marker C-reactive protein had cooled off; and he had gained 10 pounds of lean muscle—at seventy-six years old—while maintaining his 13 percent body fat. He eliminated all but one of his blood pressure meds.

However, he was still dealing with the AFib. With concerns about this heart condition, he was off to the Cooper Clinic for a consult and evaluation of this electrical misfire. From advanced diagnostic testing, it was determined that his AFib was due to his faulty tricuspid valve. The purpose of this valve is to prevent a backflow of blood into the right atrium of the heart. Consequently, his faulty valve also caused an enlarged right ventricle, which is associated with an increased risk of heart failure and cardiovascular death. Weeks later, William was admitted to the hospital to have the faulty valve repaired.

Knowing this would be major surgery, William and I discussed a protocol to implement after the surgery to quickly get him on his feet, back to working out, and certainly back to a normal life. While waiting to have the drains removed after surgery, he blew into a plastic tube daily to reinflate his lungs. Soon he was discharged from the hospital with a prescription medication to prevent a dangerous blood clot, but with no other instructions but to "take it easy."

When he was settled at home, he was back on his food plan and determined to quickly get back to normal. With the AFib resolved and the faulty tricuspid valve repaired, I designed a nutraceutical plan to help heal his sternum, as well as the soft-tissue trauma associated with the procedure. Coupled with his excellent health going into the surgery and his post-surgical nutrient protocol, he was exercising again in four weeks, and ten weeks later he was back to his full work-out routine, his life, boating, and all the things he enjoys.

There is a perception among the general public and in the health care community that nutraceuticals have a more gentle biological response in the body than pharmaceuticals. The reality is that natural products possess powerful biological activity that often parallels the strength of pharmaceutical compounds. For example, niacin is a B vitamin that, when taken in higher doses, can trigger the blood vessels at the surface of the skin to dilate, causing a tingling sensation and red appearance called "niacin flush." People who have a rough time with insomnia often have elevated nighttime cortisol levels. The supplement phosphatidylserine has been known to reduce cortisol, allowing those a sound night's sleep.

When considering nutritional support, there are some things you should keep in mind before you run off to some vitamin store to buy the next miracle supplement as seen on TV:

- Be aware that some medications and/or medical conditions do not pair well with certain supplements. For example, St. John's Wort (an herbal supplement) should not be taken with antidepressant medication. Consult with a health professional who is well versed in nutrition before you start taking any supplements, to find out if they can affect the intended function of the medication you take and to make sure there are no contraindications.
- Consider your specific needs. Are you looking for a multivitamin, a specialty product, or help with a specific health condition? Are you

currently being treated for a health condition or rebuilding from one? Medications can cause depletion of some vitamins and minerals, so it's important to know what nutrient(s) may be lost from taking a specific drug.

· Choose a company that uses good manufacturing practices (GMP), pharmaceutical-grade production and ingredients, and strict quality-control measures. Look for supplements that are tested and analyzed for quality and purity, and have been shown to be effective for their intended use.

There is no one-size-fits-all supplement plan that will work for everyone. Be sure to consult with a qualified health professional who can assist you in developing a plan based on your specific needs. As part of your program to rebuild, you may want to consider the following:

· A probiotic to re-inoculate the gut. Pharmaceuticals, including chemotherapy, antibiotics, and steroids, can wipe out normal gut flora, causing a host of problems.

· Digestive enzymes taken with each meal will help you break down your food so you can digest and absorb nutrients more efficiently. Enzymes will also help to reduce the inflammation produced by certain foods.

· Glutamine, deglycyrrhizinated licorice (DGL), and aloe vera are nutrients that support and help to heal the intestinal lining, which is critical for digestion and immune function. This is very important for anyone with leaky gut syndrome (for more on leaky gut, see page 64).

· Vitamin D is mandatory for good health. Extensive research has repeatedly shown that a deficiency of vitamin D has been linked to most of the major chronic diseases (see the section on vitamin D starting on page 116).

· Antioxidants, including vitamin C, vitamin E, beta-carotene, and grape-seed extract, are important for neutralizing free radicals and preventing them from causing damage. Vitamin E and vitamin C are important in reducing free radical damage to circulating LDL—and preventing DNA damage in cells that can lead to the development of cancer.

- Detoxifying nutrients, such as indole-3-carbinol (I3C), selenium, and N-acetylcysteine are all important in improving liver detoxification while reducing inflammation. I3C is found in cruciferous vegetables, and its benefits are discussed on page 138.

- Omega-3 essential fatty acids, such as those in fish oil supplements. Chemotherapy, specifically the drug vincristine, can cause peripheral neuropathy (tingling) in the hands and feet due to nerve damage. The DHA and EPA components of fish oil can assist in healing damaged nerves. DHA and EPA are also important to reduce inflammation seen in atherosclerosis and other inflammatory diseases.

- A multivitamin/mineral formula will provide an array of vitamins and minerals that can be lost due to pharmaceutical use and/or trauma from surgery. A powdered multivitamin in an isotonic formula is warranted after gastric bypass surgery, as this type of surgery causes malabsorption and severe nutrient deficiency (see page 112 for more information).

- If you suffer from gastroesophageal reflux disease (GERD, commonly referred to as acid reflux) or a peptic ulcer, you may have an *H. pylori* bacterial infection. The best way to test for this is stool testing. I use and recommend the testing from Genova Diagnostics (www .gdx.net) and BioHealth Laboratory (www.biohealthlab.com). I have had the greatest success treating *H. pylori* infections with two nutraceutical products: Bio-HPF and Neutrophil Plus from Biotics Research Corporation (www.bioticsresearch.com).

CHRISTINA'S STORY

Christina is a schoolteacher who came to see me suffering with stomach pain, bloating, and symptoms of gastritis (inflammation of the stomach lining). Her family doctor recommended the usual antacids, in addition to a wait-and-see approach. If her symptoms didn't clear up, she was instructed to return for a follow-up visit. After consulting with her, I decided to order stool testing to evaluate her gut symptoms. The tests results revealed an *H. pylori* infection. Because the standard pharmaceutical approach to treating this infection is often ineffective, I ordered two nutraceutical products to assist in eliminating the *H. pylori*. Following roughly six weeks of treatment, then a retest, the infection was gone, and so were her symptoms.

Z NOTE: *Helicobacter pylori* is a hardy, corkscrew-shaped bacterium that can cause gastritis, stomach ulcers, abdominal pain, bad breath, bloating, belching, nausea, black stool, and fatigue. According to the *Danish Medical Bulletin,* 85 percent of all people infected with it will never develop symptoms, but roughly 15 percent will get sick or even die due to the infection. Why? *H. pylori* causes peptic ulcers, duodenal ulcers, gastric (stomach) cancer, and a type of cancer called mucosa-associated lymphoid tissue (MALT) lymphoma in the gut. The most accurate and noninvasive testing for *H. pylori* is fecal antigen testing (stool testing). The use of antibiotics or proton pump inhibitors prior to diagnosis can lead to false negative results, so these drugs should be paused up to a month prior to testing.

Supplements to Rebuild from Disease

The association between diet and disease highlights a primary role of nutritional therapy in the form of concentrated nutrients found in nutraceuticals. There are many single- and multi-nutrient supplements that can be used to rebuild from and prevent chronic health conditions and disease. Let's review what the research community is saying about the use of supplements and their benefits for specific conditions.

NUTRACEUTICALS TO REBUILD FROM HEART DISEASE

The most important actions to take when rebuilding the blood vessels that supply your heart with blood include eliminating smoking, processed foods, and stressors. To rebuild and prevent vessel disease, you must eat a whole-food diet loaded with nutrients, antioxidants, and natural anti-inflammatories. For those who have lived a stressful, toxic, and nutrient-deprived lifestyle, taking nutraceuticals is strongly recommended.

To assist in rebuilding from vessel disease, the goal is to use concentrated nutrients to:

* Protect and preserve the function of the endothelium (the cells lining the arteries)
* Prevent and reduce LDL oxidation
* Reduce inflammation and prevent plaque formation

There is significant evidence in the literature that oxidative stress (free radical damage) is a major contributing factor in the development and progression of atherosclerosis and coronary artery disease. To neutralize the damaging effects of free radicals or reactive oxygen species (ROS), the body has a built-in antioxidant system. However, that system can be overwhelmed by a damaging lifestyle: poor diet, physical inactivity, and a toxic burden of smoking, as well as air- and food-borne pollutants. When your body has been "abused," the antioxidant system fails to get rid of free radicals, which leads to the oxidation of protein and fats, including the LDL particle.

If you are looking to prevent and rebuild from coronary artery disease, consider restoring your antioxidant system and reducing inflammation with the following nutraceuticals.

Vitamin C (Ascorbic Acid)

Vitamin C is an essential nutrient and powerful antioxidant that is protective in several different stages of atherosclerosis. Vitamin C enhances nitric oxide function, thus improving the endothelium and blood vessel function. In fact, a study published in the *Journal of the American College of Cardiology* found that a low blood level of vitamin C is a predictor of an unstable coronary syndrome. Vitamin C was also found to have a profound effect on protecting LDL from the oxidizing effects of homocysteine and other circulating free radicals.

Not only did Vitamin C protect LDL from free radical damage; it protected HDL from the same fate. HDL is the sanitation worker that gets rid of unwanted cholesterol that has accumulated in the artery as a consequence of oxidized LDL. HDL also acts as a powerful antioxidant. By preventing free radical damage, vitamin C thus preserves HDL's powerful function.

N-Acetylcysteine (NAC)

NAC provides the nutrient cysteine, which is responsible for producing glutathione—the most powerful intracellular antioxidant. Studies found in the *Journal of Atherosclerosis and Thrombosis* and the *Journal of the American College of Cardiology* showed that NAC reduced levels of the inflammatory marker C-reactive protein and reduced inflammation by shutting down NF-kB, the orchestrator of inflammation.

R-Alpha-Lipoic Acid

Researchers from the Emory University School of Medicine published data in the journal *Circulation* showing that 300 milligrams of lipoic acid was significant in reducing inflammation and improving endothelial function by 50 percent in those taking it for only four weeks. Alpha-lipoic acid has also been shown to reduce LDL oxidation and improve blood sugar levels that could adversely affect the artery and promote atherosclerosis. Alpha-lipoic acid is also needed to recycle vitamin C and vitamin E, both powerful antioxidants needed to rebuild and prevent inflammation and artery disease.

Fish Oils (Omega-3 Fatty Acids)

Omega-3 fatty acids that contain EPA and DHA have been shown to reduce the inflammation associated with atherosclerosis. One of the components of the inflammatory process seen with atherosclerosis is overproduction of inflammatory cytokines (messengers), including interleukins 1, 2, and 6, and tumor necrosis factor. These messengers recruit the immune system to join in the war of inflammation developing in the wall of the arteries.

The EPA and DHA in marine omega-3 fatty acids were found to reduce inflammation by reducing the function of NF-kB and the production of these inflammatory compounds. The DHA found in marine omega-3 fatty acids was shown to increase release of nitric oxide from the endothelium, reduce constriction of the artery, and reduce white blood cells sticking to the endothelium and vessel wall. Last, data published in the journal *Circulation* indicate that the dietary intake of omega-3 fatty acids reduce overall mortality and sudden death due to coronary heart disease.

Coenzyme Q10 (CoQ10)

CoQ10 is a powerful antioxidant that helps provide us with energy and has been shown to regenerate the vitamins E, C, A and beta-carotene in the body; increase HDL; and prevent the oxidation of LDL. If you are taking a statin, you must take a CoQ10 supplement. Cholesterol-lowering drugs not only prevent the production of cholesterol in the liver but also stop the formation of CoQ10. Why is this a big deal? The heart, liver, and kidneys rely on CoQ10 to help provide their energy. And according to the *Proceedings of the National Academy of Sciences*, CoQ10 protects LDL from oxidation even more than vitamin E does.

Flavonoids

Dietary flavonoids are a group of compounds found in various yellow, red, blue, and purple plant-based foods. Flavonoids have been shown to have beneficial effects in the prevention of cardiovascular disease. One such flavonoid—Pycnogenol (pine bark extract) from the French maritime pine—was found to inhibit LDL oxidation and increase nitric oxide activity. Pycnogenol was also found to improve endothelial function. Flavonoids found in the skin of red grapes and grape seeds were shown to reduce oxidized LDL and dramatically reduce inflammation. In a study published in the journal *Angiology*, researchers found that the nutritional supplement OPC-3 improved circulation and reduced cardiovascular risk factors. In a randomized, double-blind, placebo-controlled, parallel group study, the control group received a two-month supply of OPC-3, which contains extracts from grape seed, bilberry, citrus, pine bark (Pycnogenol), and red wine. The placebo group received a mixture of fruit sugar, apple fiber, and food dyes. The study showed that those who took the OPC-3 had an improvement in blood pressure and, more impressive, a significant decrease in the inflammatory marker C-reactive protein.

Z NOTE: The plant-based compounds in OPC-3 can interfere with the drug Coumadin (warfarin). Coumadin is an anticoagulant drug that prevents the liver from making clotting factors, and thus prevents the blood from clotting. If you are taking Coumadin or another anticoagulant, consult with a qualified health care professional seasoned in nutrient-drug interactions for advice before supplementing with OPC-3.

Niacin

If you are currently taking a cholesterol-lowering drug, you may want to also take niacin to reduce the vessel-wall inflammation associated with atherosclerosis. Niacin with a statin appears to be a powerful combination therapy at reducing atherosclerotic progression. In studies published in the *New England Journal of Medicine* and the *Journal of Cardiovascular Nursing*, niacin, in combination with a cholesterol-lowering drug, was extremely effective at not only reducing LDL but also increasing HDL levels. The niacin-statin combination caused a significant regression of the inflammation in the walls of arteries.

Niacin also has a reputation of causing the warm, tingling, and itchy, prickly skin symptoms known as "niacin flush." If you are concerned about niacin flush, the symptoms associated with it can be managed in several ways:

- Take niacin before bed.
- Avoid spicy foods, alcohol, and hot beverages at the time you take niacin.
- Avoid hot showers at the time you take niacin, as the hot water can increase flushing.
- Take 325 mg of aspirin with niacin, which has been shown to reduce the flushing symptoms.

You may consider working with a health care provider who can help you regulate the potential symptoms of taking niacin, so you can continue the therapy and its exceptional benefits.

Vitamin D

Let's not forget vitamin D. We talked about it in detail starting on page 116, but regarding vitamin D and heart disease, the *Journal of Invasive Cardiology* reported that patients with lower vitamin D levels had multiple coronary artery disease with atherosclerosis and endothelial dysfunction. Data published in the *Journal of Clinical Endocrinology and Metabolism* showed that a lack of vitamin D was also associated with endothelial dysfunction and increased LDL oxidation.

CLINICAL NOTE: How much vitamin D_3 should you take? This depends on what your blood levels look like. The Vitamin D Council and the Endocrine Society recommend up to 10,000 IU/day, while the Food and Nutrition Board recommends 4,000 IU/day. To make it less confusing, if your blood work shows that your serum vitamin D level 25(OH)D is below 50 ng/ml, start with 5,000 IU a day for a couple of months, then retest your blood levels. If you are between 50 and 80 ng/ml, continue on that dose. If you are above 80 ng/ml, reduce by 2,000 IU and wait another couple of months. If the 25(OH)D has improved but is not quite in the therapeutic range, take another 2,000 IU a day and test again in two months.

When testing your blood for vitamin D levels, the therapeutic range is between 50 and 80 ng/ml; the old standard of 30 ng/ml is inadequate. Having objective testing to reveal what you need is the most accurate way to determine your vitamin D needs.

My recommendations are based on studies that have shown these specific nutraceuticals to be beneficial in controlling, preventing, and reversing the oxidation and inflammation involved in the development of atherosclerosis and coronary artery disease. But remember, as with all supplementation, there is no one-size-fits-all supplement protocol for those with known atherosclerosis and coronary artery disease.

NUTRACEUTICALS TO REBUILD DURING CANCER CARE

People dealing with cancer can become deficient in nutrients as a result of their disease, as well as the treatment of the disease. Some become malnourished to the point of causing severe changes in body composition, including muscle wasting (cachexia). While cancer, as a major metabolic disease, can cause malnutrition, chemotherapy and radiation (radiotherapy) are often the direct cause of malnutrition.

Chemotherapy destroys cancer cells that are rapidly dividing. Unfortunately, chemo also destroys other cells that rapidly divide in the body, including cells in the mouth, stomach, small and large intestine, hair follicles, blood cells, sperm, and eggs. This can cause side effects that can be unbearable. Major chemo side effects that cause malnutrition are nausea, vomiting, diarrhea, mouth sores, and poor appetite. All of these can result in weight loss and muscle wasting, and even organ damage.

Radiotherapy is another cause of nutrient deficiency and malnutrition. According to the *Journal of Nutrition*, radiation therapy damages normal cells by depleting the cellular antioxidants vitamins E, A, and C and selenium. Data found in the journal *Integrative Cancer Therapies* show that radiation therapy can have long-lasting effects on antioxidant levels, which sometimes don't come back to baseline.

The first action many people take when diagnosed with cancer is a major overhaul of their diet. In their search for the best anticancer nutrition, most people get confusing and conflicting dietary advice from family, friends, and coworkers; the news media; the supplement industry; trade magazines; and personal stories that circulate through social media. What's one to believe?

Before my second round of chemo, I was elbows-deep in the research not only to understand the mechanisms of my disease but also to gain a greater understanding of what nutraceuticals I could take to rebuild myself back to excellent health. I was also interested in knowing more about using targeted nutrition and concentrated supplements to enhance my chemo while reducing its toxicity and awful side effects.

Like everyone else, I was told to refrain from taking supplements and antioxidants during chemotherapy because, supposedly, concentrated nutrients and antioxidants would negate the effects of certain chemotherapeutic agents and radiation. Rather than take that at face value, I reviewed the data myself. The results of some 280 peer-reviewed studies since the 1970s, spanning 8,521 patients (5,081 of whom were given nutritional supplements), suggested that nutrients and antioxidants do not interfere with the cell-killing functions of chemotherapy. Furthermore, antioxidants and other nutrients were shown to enhance the therapeutic activity of cancer therapies, reduce toxicity, protect healthy tissues, and reduce side effects. Of the 5,081 patients who took supplements, 3,738 had increased survival.

Personally, I chose to take targeted nutrients during my second round of chemo, as well as after my surgery. I had very few side effects through chemotherapy, and eight weeks following major surgery, I was working out again to rebuild my health and body.

Another bit of irresponsible and dangerous advice doctors give people during their chemo, or any other medical care, is to "eat whatever you want" or "calories in, calories out" or to eat plenty of calories to keep one's weight up. But calories are not just calories, and there are three reasons to ignore this advice:

1. Typically, nutrient-deficient, high-calorie foods contain too much sugar, which causes not only large spikes in blood sugar but also a surge of the hormone insulin to deal with high blood sugar. Both high sugar and insulin have been shown to promote cancer growth and make cancer cells resistant to chemotherapy.
2. High-calorie foods raise blood sugar and insulin, which can and will increase body fat. Body fat is a hormone-producing organ that spits out cancer-promoting hormones and inflammation. Body fat also produces an enzyme called aromatase, which turns testosterone and other hormones into estrogen. High estro-

gen can be dangerous for those with cancer of the breast, ovary, uterus, and endometrium.

3. Nutrient deficiency is one of the major causes of cancer. If you recall from chapter 1, nutrient deficiency has the same damaging effects on DNA as radiation. Deficiencies of folate, vitamin B_6, B_{12}, niacin, vitamin C, vitamin E, iron, and zinc cause DNA damage that will contribute to the formation of cancer. Most high-calorie foods are void of these important nutrients.

To stress this important point again: people going through cancer care suffer from malnutrition, nutrient malabsorption, and often changes in body composition varying from cachexia to increased body fat. Cancer patients often have low antioxidant levels prior to chemotherapy treatment, perhaps because of poor appetite, or because cancer cells may use more antioxidants than normal cells. Chemotherapy and radiation "use up" antioxidants due to interactions of those therapies with the different metabolic processes of the body. The B vitamins, including folate, pyroxidine (B_6), riboflavin (B_2), as well as vitamins C, E, and other nutrients, also become deficient during cancer care. This sets the stage for secondary cancers to develop due to DNA damage and the inability of damaged cells to heal themselves.

The goal of incorporating a targeted nutraceutical protocol into a standard chemotherapy regimen is to help restore nutrients lost during cancer care and to mitigate the often debilitating side effects of toxic anticancer agents, enhancing the therapeutic effects of chemo, while at the same time preserving the integrity of healthy tissues. By doing so, you will have a better quality of life during your cancer care. It is my experience working with cancer patients that those who follow a guided nutrient protocol are able to tolerate full doses of anticancer agents without interruptions in their treatment schedules. They are able to tolerate the treatments to the end. Ultimately, as a result, they have better outcomes and much higher survival rates.

Whether you are in the throes of cancer care or just about to start treatment, I strongly suggest you incorporate nutraceuticals into your cancer treatment as a parallel set of steps. Here are five reasons to use nutraceuticals to support your cancer treatment:

- To begin your personal rebuild even during cancer care
- To reduce side effects
- To enhance the function of chemotherapy
- To reduce chemo resistance to the anticancer agents
- To replenish lost nutrients and antioxidants from anticancer drugs or radiation

It is difficult to provide specifics regarding which nutraceuticals you should take, because your cancer is genetically unique to you. However, even without knowing all aspects of your disease, individual pathology, and diagnosis, there are guidelines you can follow to have a much better outcome, and certainly fewer side effects from the treatment.

If you or your oncology team have any concerns regarding the use of nutraceuticals co-administered with your chemo regimen, consider using supplements the day or two after an infusion of chemo. In between the infusions, the concentrated nutrients will help clean up the internal damage from the drugs; that will help reduce the side effects and maintain your blood counts as they drop from the effects of the chemo.

Supplements to Aid Digestion and the Gastrointestinal Tract

DIGESTIVE ENZYMES: Enzymes taken with each meal will help break down the food you eat, so you can get the most nutritional value from that food. Enzymes may also help in the fight against cancer. Data from *Planta Medica* showed that bromelain, a proteolytic enzyme (one that breaks down protein), reduced the amount of metastasis seen with lung cancer.

ALOE VERA JUICE: Aloe vera has been known to help with digestion; regulate bowel movements; normalize pH and acid/alkaline balance; and encourage normal gut flora (bacteria). It is best to take aloe on an empty stomach before meals. Aloe vera is also an excellent natural anti-inflammatory.

ALOE VERA PILL: Constipation is a very common and uncomfortable side effect of chemotherapy. Commercial laxatives often use chemical ingredients that can be harsh on the gut. Similar to aloe juice, concentrated aloe leaf in a pill form can be taken to relieve chemo-induced constipation. It works by drawing water into the colon to allow for better movement of waste through the bowel and elimination.

L-GLUTAMINE: Glutamine is the most abundant amino acid in muscle. Besides stimulating the production of growth hormone, glutamine is a metabolic fuel for the brain, liver, kidneys, skeletal muscles, and cells of the immune system. L-glutamine acts as an anti-inflammatory and is needed for the growth and repair of the intestinal lining. Cancer creates a state of glutamine deficiency, which is aggravated by the toxic effects of anticancer agents. According to the *Indian Journal of Medical and Paediatric Oncology*, glutamine supplementation was found to reduce mucositis (painful inflammation of the mucous membranes lining the digestive tract), as well as the painful mouth sores caused by chemotherapy. It was also shown to reduce chemo-induced peripheral neuropathies (burning and tingling) in the hands and feet.

Antioxidants to Protect Healthy Cells and Tissues

VITAMIN C: Vitamin C (ascorbate) is an essential vitamin; it is not made in the body, so it must come from the diet. For years, it has been proven to be a powerful antioxidant and anticancer agent. In the latter capacity, vitamin C has a profound effect on tumor metabolism. Tumors contain regions of low oxygen, a state called hypoxia. To survive a low-oxygen environment, cancer cells spit out a protein called hypoxia-inducible factor 1 (HIF1). This protein causes the production of new blood vessels to feed the tumor with nutrients and oxygen for its survival. Not a good situation. Good news from *Biochemical Pharmacology*: Vitamin C was found to block the production of HIF1, thus preventing blood-vessel growth to tumors and causing their eventual starvation. It was also found that vitamin C, in combination with other antioxidants (vitamin A, vitamin E, and selenium), did not protect cancer cells from the cytotoxic effects of chemotherapy. Regarding antioxidant functions, a study in the *Journal of Pharmaceutical and Biomedical Sciences* showed vitamin C reduced the toxicity associated with the chemotherapy drug Adriamycin (a.k.a. Red Death) by neutralizing the free radical damage caused by the drug.

Vitamin C was also found to weaken cancer cells, thus making them vulnerable to the functions of chemotherapy. Research found in the *Journal of Chemotherapy* demonstrates that vitamin C enhanced the antitumor activity of different anticancer agents by sensitizing cancer cells to the chemo, thus causing those cancer cells to die. Vitamin C was also found to shut down the orchestrator of inflammation NF-kB, a crucial player in the development and progression of all cancers. Studies found in both *In Vivo* and *Biochemical Journal* demonstrated that vitamin C enhanced chemo-responsiveness and served as a potent sensitizer in chemo-resistant lymphoma and lung-cancer cell lines.

Free radical damage (oxidative stress) caused by chemotherapy, combined with low vitamin C levels and poor antioxidant systems, is a major reason behind the toxicity and side effects associated with chemotherapy and radiotherapy. Results from a six-month observational study conducted on children being treated for acute lymphoblastic leukemia were published in the *American Journal of Clinical Nutrition*. Those children with low dietary antioxidants had more side effects, greater toxicity, and delays in their cancer care. Those with greater vitamin C intakes had fewer therapy delays and less toxicity, and spent fewer days in the hospital.

OLIGOMERIC PROANTHOCYANIDIN COMPLEXES (OPCS): OPCs are powerful antioxidants extracted from grape seeds and maritime pine bark. OPCs consist of compounds called polyphenols and bioflavonoids. Bioflavonoids are plant chemicals that give fruits and vegetables their beautiful bright colors. Polyphenols are super antioxidants found in grapes, red wine, blueberries, green tea, and other plant-based foods. Why is this important? OPCs have powerful effects against cancer, and they have been shown to mitigate the side effects associated with chemo toxicity. A study in the journal *Prostate* demonstrated that OPCs were able to suppress the growth of prostate-cancer cells, while turning on genes that caused the cancer cells to kill themselves (apoptosis).

The *Journal of Cancer Prevention* and the *International Journal of Oncology* published additional studies that showed the OPC Pycnogenol (pine bark extract) and the OPCs found in cranberries also turned on genes to cause apoptosis, thus preventing blood vessel development to feed cancer cells and reducing cancer cell proliferation.

Anticancer Nutrients

VITAMIN D$_3$: The active form of vitamin D, calcitriol, has a large spectrum of anticancer properties. From the *Journal of Cancer*, calcitriol enhanced the cancer-killing effects of most chemotherapeutic agents and radiation. Calcitriol was also shown to prevent cancer cell proliferation; prevent cell invasiveness and metastasis; induce cancer cell suicide (apoptosis); and prevent the development of blood vessels by developing tumors. In order for calcitriol to have these anticancer effects, it has to be at sufficient levels. The levels of vitamin D in the blood measured as 25 hydroxyvitamin D (25[OH]D) have to be above 50 ng/ml to have any cancer-fighting function.

Data presented in a report from *Cancer Research* demonstrated that pretreating breast cancer cells with vitamin D sensitized those cells to the effects of two heavy-hitting breast cancer drugs: Adriamycin (Red Death) and paclitaxel.

Low vitamin D levels correlate with increased incidences of most cancers, notably colon and breast cancers. Research on vitamin D and cancer out of the *Journal of Clinical Oncology* states that women with early-stage breast cancer whose vitamin D levels were below 20 ng/ml had poor prognoses. Not only were the initial levels of vitamin D dangerously low in the individuals in the study, but it was also shown that levels of 25-(OH)D decreased from 9.03 ng/ml at baseline to 6.75 ng/ml after just four cycles of chemotherapy.

Information from *Nutrition and Cancer* reveals that vitamin D deficiency was also found in 83 percent of those diagnosed with colorectal cancer. Those with low vitamin D (below 30 ng/ml) correlated with poorer overall survival odds. It was also stated that higher levels of vitamin D after a diagnosis of colorectal cancer improved survival. The *Journal of Clinical Oncology* presented similar findings in those with lymphoma. Vitamin D deficiency (less than 25 ng/ml) was associated with inferior overall survival, while those with higher levels of vitamin D had greater long-term survival.

How much vitamin D should you take? See the Clinical Note on page 208. You should strive to get your level of vitamin D between 50 and 80 ng/ml and keep it there in order for it to have therapeutic effects against cancer and to enhance the function of chemotherapy.

GREEN TEA (EGCG): Tea is the most consumed beverage in the world; 20 percent of the 2.5 million tons of tea leaves produced are sold as green tea, which is also one of the most healthful beverages on the planet. It is loaded with antioxidants and other phytochemicals that have robust effects in the body. One of the most powerful disease-fighting compounds found in green tea is epigallocatechin-3-gallate (EGCG). EGCG has gained much attention in medical research due to its impressive effects on cancer prevention and as a chemotherapeutic agent. Multiple studies published in *Carcinogenesis,* the *American Journal of Epidemiology,* and *Cancer Epidemiology, Biomarkers & Prevention* show that green tea reduced the risk of developing breast, prostate, and colorectal cancer.

Green tea, with the EGCG it contains, will not only reduce the risk of developing cancer; it has a profound effect on several mechanisms of carcinogenesis and can enhance the function of chemotherapy. The journals *Cancer and Metastasis Reviews* and *Carcinogenesis* report that EGCG can reactivate genes that suppress cancer growth and proliferation and shut down several mechanisms involved in cancer metastasis. EGCG has also been shown to reduce inflammation, extinguish free radicals, and induce apoptosis in cancer cells of the lung, colon, pancreas, skin, and breast.

Supplements That Enhance Chemotherapy

The greatest obstacle in the successful therapeutic effects of chemotherapy is chemo resistance. What is chemo resistance? Basically, cancer cells become resistant to the cell-killing effects of the drugs. Attempts by the oncology community to overcome resistance involve combining different types of drugs with the hope of minimizing toxicity and bone marrow damage.

There is a reason for this problem. Typically, tumors consist of a mixed population of cells, some of which are chemo-sensitive and some of which are chemo-resistant. Chemotherapy kills the chemo-sensitive cells, leaving behind the resistant cells. Chemo-resistant cells have "pumps" in their cell membranes that actively expel or spit out chemotherapy drugs. Researchers have identified two pumps: P-glycoprotein and multidrug resistance-associated protein (MRP). Pharmaceutical companies are scrambling to create the next anticancer drug in hopes of unplugging these pumps and taking down drug resistance, thereby creating a better therapeutic response to chemotherapy.

While this is costly and time consuming, the quest for chemo-sensitizing drugs has also uncovered natural compounds that can reverse drug resistance by inhibiting the chemo-resistant pumps. Recently, studies have documented the ability of phytochemicals to "sensitize" cancer cells to anticancer drugs. Natural compounds, including vitamin C, vitamin D, epigallocatechin-3-gallate (EGCG), and curcumin, can reverse drug resistance by inhibiting the pumps.

The following are some natural chemo sensitizers that overcome chemo resistance:

VITAMIN D: Known to regulate calcium and phosphorous metabolism, vitamin D is also a potent anticancer agent, playing important roles in antitumor pathways. Vitamin D shuts down cancer cell growth and proliferation; it induces apoptosis (programmed cell suicide), prevents blood vessel growth to tumors, and can reverse drug-resistance in cancer cells. Data from *Genetics and Molecular Research, Cell,* and *Cancer Discovery* demonstrate that vitamin D sensitized cancer cells to anticancer drugs by shutting down the P-glycoprotein and MPR pumps, and it reduced inflammation—another cause of chemo resistance. Research published in *Nature Reviews* states that administering vitamin D before or simultaneously with chemotherapy treatment was optimal to chemo-sensitize cancer cells to the killing effects of chemotherapy. Vitamin D after treatment did not have the same effect.

EPIGALLOCATECHIN-3-GALLATE (EGCG): Epigallocatechin-3-gallate (EGCG), the miracle compound found in green tea, continues to be a promising and proven anticancer agent. It has been shown to halt cancer cell growth and proliferation, activate apoptosis, prevent angiogenesis, and reduce inflammation. EGCG also increases the accumulation of anticancer drugs in cancer cells by blocking the P-glycoprotein pump. A study out of the *Journal of Pharmacology & Clinical Toxicology* showed that EGCG was extremely effective at shutting down P-glycoprotein activity and dramatically reducing chemo-resistance in breast cancer cells by up to 90 percent. In another study found in *Breast Cancer Research* involving the use of EGCG, researchers demonstrated that EGCG sensitized breast cancer cells to the anticancer agent Taxol.

EGCG was found not only to reduce chemo-resistance in different types of cancer but also to sensitize these different cancers to many of the common chemotherapy drugs, including Taxol, doxorubicin (Adriamycin, Rubex), cisplatin (Platinol), and 5-fluorouracil (Efudex, Fluoroplex). EGCG has also been shown to protect against toxicity that comes with the use of chemotherapy.

Besides being one of the most popular beverages on the planet, green tea should be heralded as one of the most potent natural anticancer compounds that should be part of mainstream chemotherapy regimens.

NOTE: EGCG was found to interfere with the therapeutic effects of the anticancer drug bortezomib (Velcade).

CURCUMIN: Curcumin, the yellow pigment in turmeric, is far more than just a coloring agent. Extensive research on this potent compound has revealed that curcumin is an effective chemo-sensitizer and radio-sensitizer (making cells sensitive to radiation). Research in *Nutrition and Cancer* reveals that curcumin sensitizes cancers of the breast, colon, pancreas, stomach, blood, liver, lung, prostate, bladder, ovary, head and neck, and brain, and in multiple myeloma, leukemia, and lymphoma. Sensitizing these cancers was achieved by shutting down the drug-resistant pumps. This impressive age-old anticancer spice was also shown to protect normal tissues and organs, such as the liver, kidney, mouth, and heart, from the damaging effects of chemotherapy and radiotherapy.

An impressive study led by Madhwa Raj, PhD, research professor in obstetrics and gynecology at LSU Health Sciences Center, New Orleans, found that a cocktail of six natural compounds, including curcumin, killed 100 percent of sample breast cancer cells with no toxic side effects. The results published in the *Journal of Cancer* revealed the combination of curcumin, EGCG, indole-3-carbinol (from crucifer-ous vegetables), and others dramatically reduced multidrug-resistant cancer cells; prevented invasion and metastasis; and activated specific genes in the cancer cells, leading to their death.

Guidelines to Using Nutraceuticals During Your Cancer Care

Both the diagnosis of cancer and the rigors of going through chemo-therapy are emotionally draining and nerve-racking. Knowing chemo-therapy is very toxic—with its host of side effects and the notion that it may or may not work—leaves you feeling out of control. As you try to navigate all this, you also need to decide whether to use nutraceuticals while going through chemo- and radiotherapy. To help you make a de-cision, here are three options on the table:

ONE: REFRAIN FROM TAKING ANY NUTRACEUTICALS DURING CANCER CARE. As you consider this option keep in mind that since there is little to no research to show that nutraceuticals interfere with chemo, this action may leave you open for the toxic effects of the anticancer agents and radiotherapy.

TWO: TAKE CONCENTRATED NUTRIENTS SIMULTANEOUSLY WITH CHEMO AND RADIOTHERAPY UNTIL YOUR CANCER CARE IS FINISHED. It is quite clear that the aforementioned plant-based nutrients do not interfere with the cytotoxic effects of chemo; they enhance the therapeutic effects of the chemo by "sensitizing" cancer cells to the drugs. The nutrients will pro-tect the body from damage as a consequence of chemo toxicity.

THREE: TAKE NUTRIENTS AND ANTIOXIDANTS AT TARGETED TIMES. In this option, you take the nutrients that enhance the function of the chemo at the same time chemo is administered. These include vitamin D, EGCG, and curcumin. Then take the rest of the nutraceuticals the day after the infusion of anticancer agents. These include enzymes, aloe, glutamine, vitamin C, OPCs, EGCG, and vitamin D. Taking nutrients at specific times should enhance the chemo and reduce toxicity and side effects without interfering with the functions of the chemo and radiotherapy.

As each person responds differently to anticancer agents and supplements, be sure to consult a qualified health provider to create exact dosing for supplements. The anticancer efficacy of plant-based compounds results from their individual use, as well as their use in combination with chemotherapy. Individual nutrients widely used in preclinical cancer prevention and treatment studies have been shown to have a robust effect on the various mechanisms of cancer, including chemo-resistance.

The reality is that there are countless phytochemicals found in plant-based foods that have the same effects as the nutraceuticals mentioned here. If you are going through cancer care, it's an absolute must that you create a nutrient-dense food plan to provide cancer-killing nutrients that will also enhance the function of chemo and radiation. To get started, check out the "Food Substitutions" list on page 173 or download the list of "Foods to Avoid" from my website. To emphasize this point again: make sure to eat plenty of plant-based foods throughout the day, including garlic and onion (alliums) and cruciferous vegetables (broccoli, cauliflower, Brussels sprouts, kale, and bok choy). Make sure also to eat wild-caught fish that provides fish oils and anti-inflammatories, as well as mushrooms to support immunity.

Z NOTE: According to the journal *Cytokine*, chemotherapy-induced peripheral neuropathy (CIPN) is the most common reason for patients halting their cancer treatments. CIPN is a painful condition of the hands and feet brought on by the toxicity of certain chemotherapy drugs. Emerging data reveal that nerve toxicity created by anticancer agents occurs due to inflammation. Chemo causes the release of those annoying and destructive inflammatory cytokines (IL-6, TNF) that are partially responsible for the tingling and burning pain of CIPN. To combat the peripheral neuropathy, focus on reducing inflammation by eliminating refined sugars, grains, dairy products, synthetic salts, and partially hydrogenated fats. You should also design your personal rebuild food plan to include plenty of plant-based foods and fatty fish containing anti-inflammatory omega-3 fatty acids. Research has also found the amino acid L-glutamine to be helpful with CIPN.

NUTRACEUTICALS TO REBUILD FROM AUTOIMMUNE DISEASE

As you learned in chapter 1, the immune system is a network of cells, tissues, and organs that defends the body against infections and other diseases. One arm of the immune system—Th2—produces specific proteins known as antibodies that identify, attack, and destroy unwanted substances, including bacteria, viruses, fungi, and other damaging proteins like gluten. The second arm—Th1—is involved in directly killing foreign invaders, cancer cells, and cells that are infected with viruses and bacteria.

The body's immune system is considered balanced when there is constant movement and communication between the Th1 and Th2 immune states. Sometimes the immune system becomes misdirected and attacks specific proteins, tissues, and organs of the body. This is called autoimmunity. In the case of autoimmune disease, one of the two arms of the immune system, either Th1 or Th2, becomes dominant, resulting in the body's immune system attacking *itself*.

Typically, pharmaceuticals, including chemotherapy, biotherapies, anti-inflammatories, and steroids, are prescribed to combat an imbalanced immune response; these treatments are focused on managing symptoms and achieving "remission." While most, if not all, drugs can have adverse side effects, they are not meant to balance and rebuild the immune system. Rather, they are meant to target one compound or protein in the mixture of inflammation.

Many studies show that balancing the chemical messengers (cytokines) that come from the Th1 and Th2 arms of the immune system can have a profound effect on creating a more balanced immune response. Research also reveals improvements in either arm of the immune system through the use of plant-based compounds, which are inexpensive and readily available.

If you decide to take plant-based nutrients to affect your immune system, including echinacea, mushroom extracts, or ginseng, the goal remains to address the underlying cause of the imbalanced immune system. Typically, these natural immunodrugs will balance the immune system but won't fix a leaky gut, high cortisol, stressed adrenal glands, low vitamin D, or an inflammatory diet loaded with allergens, and so on—all potential causes of autoimmune disease.

The immune system is complex and flexible, able to handle invaders with accuracy and remarkable efficiency. While our defense system has vulnerabilities, there are ways to support, enhance, and regulate immune function. In addition to uncovering the cause of autoimmunity, proper immunonutrition is vital to immune cell function. As you read through different sections in the book, you will gain a greater understanding and get the tools you need to create a plan to rebuild your immune system for improved health.

Plant-based compounds that stimulate Th2 when Th1 is dominant:
EGCG
Pycnogenol
Curcumin
Quercetin
Lycopene

Epigallocatechin-3-gallate (EGCG)

Research from the journal *Molecular Aspects of Medicine* states that the compound EGCG found in green tea reduced the pro-inflammatory actions of Th1. According to the *Annals of Clinical and Laboratory Science,* and the *Journal of Pharmacognosy and Phytochemistry,* green tea suppressed the production of IgE antibodies from the Th2 arm of the immune system while at the same time creating harmony in the immune system by balancing both Th1 and Th2.

Pycnogenol

Pycnogenol (pine bark extract) acts as a powerful antioxidant and modulator of the immune system. According to a study in *Nutrition Research and Practice,* Pycnogenol was found to shift immune patterns by decreasing Th1 cytokine production and increase Th2 cytokines, thus causing a more balanced immune response.

Curcumin

The yellow chemical compound curcumin, extracted from the popular yellow spice turmeric, was also found to be a powerful anti-inflammatory in those with the autoimmune dysfunction colitis. Curcumin was found to be more powerful than the strong steroid dexamethasone at decreasing the expression of Th1 cytokines and increasing the expression of Th2 cytokines, causing a shift from Th1 to Th2. Data found in the *British Journal of Pharmacology* indicate that curcumin was effective at reducing Th1 cytokines and could be used as a therapeutic approach to Th1-mediated autoimmune diseases.

Quercetin and Lycopene

Both quercetin from apples and lycopene from tomatoes were found to turn off the orchestrator of inflammation NF-kB and create a more balanced Th1/Th2 immune response.

Plant-based compounds that stimulate Th1 when Th2 is dominant:
Ashwagandha
Maitake, reishi, and shiitake mushroom extracts
Astragalus
Echinacea
Ginseng

Ashwagandha

Ashwagandha is an adaptogenic herb (one that restores balance) known for its effects on thyroid and adrenal function. It has also been shown to activate and enhance Th1 immunity. A study from the journal *Vaccine* showed that ashwagandha caused an increase in T cell numbers and the cytokines that come from them, demonstrating its usefulness as an immune stimulant.

Mushroom Extracts

Of all the natural immune-enhancing foods we can eat, nothing compares to the almighty mushroom. The fruiting body of the maitake mushroom contains a carbohydrate called beta-glucan that, for years, has been known to enhance immune function. As an immunostimulating agent, the beta-glucan in maitake mushrooms acts through several mechanisms to enhance our defense system. For one, beta-glucan activates the function of white blood cells through the receptors found on immune cells after being digested. This carbohydrate is also released by those white blood cells and taken up by other immune cells, leading to various immune responses. The end result is improved immunity. In *Biological and Pharmaceutical Bulletin*, researchers showed that beta-glucan triggered the Th1 arm while shutting down antibody production from B cells (Th2), thus establishing Th1 dominance when the immune response was Th2 dominant.

The beta-glucans from reishi and shiitake mushrooms also had profound effects on the immune system and created a more balanced Th1 and Th2 response. Studies in the *Journal of Agricultural and Food Chemistry* and *Mediators of Inflammation* state that both reishi and shiitake, including other edible fungi, provide major substances with immunomodulatory and antitumor activity. The carbohydrates and proteins found in these mushrooms have been shown to suppress autoimmune disease and the allergic response, while defending against cancer through proper immune modulation. This said, certain mushrooms and their extracts can induce a Th1 response, whereas others favor a Th2 response. Because autoimmune conditions are complex immune disorders, it's imperative to consult with a qualified health professional to evaluate the differences in activities among various mushroom extracts and their isolated ingredients (metabolites) to determine if mushroom products will benefit your specific immune challenges.

Astragalus and Echinacea

The traditional Chinese herbs astragalus and echinacea were also found to reduce inflammation, stimulate Th1 cells, and suppress an overactive Th2 response. Studies found in both *Biochemistry and Cell Biology* and the *Chinese Journal of Integrative Medicine* reveal a significant reduction in chronic inflammation seen in asthmatics—a Th2-dominant condition. Astragalus was shown to improve Th1 cytokines and reduce Th2 cytokines, thus creating a more balanced immune response. The herb echinacea has always been noted for its ability to enhance immune function. Researchers have showed that echinacea enhanced immune function primarily through the activation of Th1, creating a synergistic effect between Th1 and Th2 responses.

Ginseng

Korean researchers found that a carbohydrate in the herb *Panax ginseng* caused the production of Th1 cytokines and the production of natural killer cells. Ginseng's ability to enhance Th1 immunity was also stated to be effective as an anticancer agent. Data from the *Journal of Ginseng Research* also indicate that ginseng was found to have immune-stimulating effects in the Th1 arm of the immune system.

> **NOTE:** Stressing the importance again, vitamin D deficiency is a major cause of autoimmune disease. Whether you are challenged by either Th1 dominance or Th2 dominance, get your vitamin D measured. If your vitamin D level is below 50ng/ml, increase your sun exposure, eat foods high in vita-

min D (salmon, sardines, cod liver oil, shrimp, eggs), and supplement with vitamin D.

Z NOTE: Practitioners are increasingly using low-dose naltrexone (LDN) to treat autoimmune diseases. Originally used to treat those with drug addiction, LDN blocks opioid receptors in the brain, preventing people from feeling high after using opioid drugs. LDN has also been found to regulate T-regulatory cytokines creating a more balanced Th1 and Th2 response. LDN was also shown to boost levels of endorphins that modulate the immune system by orchestrating the activity of T lymphocytes—those involved with autoimmune disease.

NUTRACEUTICALS TO REBUILD FROM DIABETES

If you recall, there are two forms of diabetes, type 1 and type 2. Both types create dysglycemia—abnormal blood sugar. Type 1 diabetes, also known as insulin-dependent diabetes, is a smoldering autoimmune condition, in which the immune system attacks the beta cells of the pancreas, resulting in a deficiency of the hormone insulin. Type 2 diabetes, also known as non-insulin-dependent diabetes, is a chronic condition in which your body doesn't produce enough insulin, or your body ignores the effects of insulin, causing less sugar to move into your cells. Consequently, your blood sugar remains chronically high. Where type 1 diabetes is a condition of a lack of insulin, type 2 is not the result of insufficient insulin production. Instead, it's actually the result of too much insulin produced on a long-term basis due to eating a high-carb, high-sugar, and high-fat diet.

While eating a healthful diet and exercising regularly is necessary to manage your blood sugar naturally, the assistance of targeted nutritional support is also a key component to achieving healthy blood sugar levels. Regarding type 2 diabetes, there is no magic-bullet pharmaceutical to treat it, and there is no single nutrient that will reverse it. However, there are nutrients that, when added to your personal rebuild, can assist in fixing blood sugar problems. Specific nutrients work to support your body's ability to use insulin, thus helping you maintain healthy blood sugar levels.

Magnesium

Magnesium is a mineral needed for more than three hundred biochemical reactions in the body, including helping the body digest and metabolize fat, carbs, and protein, and aiding in the production of energy and regulation of blood sugar levels. However, for many reasons, from plants being grown in nutrient-depleted soils to the overconsumption of alcohol, magnesium deficiency is becoming epidemic. Public health concerns regarding type 2 diabetes and the role of magnesium in blood sugar have led researchers to investigate the relationship between type 2 diabetes and magnesium.

The result of a meta-analysis of thirteen observational studies published in *Diabetes Care*, including 536,318 people and 24,516 new cases of diabetes, found that higher magnesium intake was associated with a lower risk of type 2 diabetes. From the *European Journal of Clinical Investigation*, a randomized, double-blind, placebo-controlled trial was conducted on ninety-seven individuals with severely low levels of magnesium (hypomagnesemia) and without diabetes. The experimental group received 50 ml magnesium chloride for three months, all with improved function of pancreatic beta cells resulting in lower fasting blood glucose and insulin levels. Another study, published in *Diabetes, Obesity and Metabolism*, found that supplementing with 365 mg/day of magnesium for six months reduced insulin resistance in 47 overweight individuals, all of whom had normal magnesium levels.

It's clear that low magnesium levels are associated with insulin resistance, impaired glucose tolerance, and decreased insulin levels. Basically, the pancreas needs magnesium to secrete enough insulin, and magnesium is needed to sensitize cells to insulin in order to allow sugar into the cells. This process is even controlled by a magnesium-dependent enzyme called tyrosine kinase. If you are dealing with type 2 diabetes and uncontrolled blood sugar, it's important to eat plenty of dark green leafy vegetables and other foods high in magnesium. If you are battling blood sugar issues, it's important to supplement with magnesium.

Vitamin D

Vitamin D (the "sunshine vitamin") plays an important role in countless biological processes and has also been found to regulate blood sugar. Similar to magnesium deficiency, vitamin D deficiency is a serious problem. Also like magnesium deficiency, vitamin D deficiency is an epidemic. Statistics from the *Archives of Internal Medicine* reveal that three-quarters of the U.S. population is deficient in vitamin D. Extensive research has shown that a deficiency in vitamin D is linked to the development of a variety of cancers, such as colon, prostate, and breast; heart disease; autoimmune disease; arthritis; and diabetes.

There is growing evidence that a vitamin D deficiency could be contributing to your diabetes—whether type 1 or type 2. Evidence indicates that vitamin D deficiency leads to poor insulin output and abnormal blood sugar levels. After conducting a meta-analysis and review of the impact of vitamin D on blood sugar control, researchers concluded that low vitamin D levels hindered blood sugar control by interfering with the actions of insulin. An observational study from the Nurses Health Study, which included 83,770 women, found that those with low vitamin D had an increased risk of type 2 diabetes; a daily intake of 800 IU of vitamin D combined with 1,000 mg of calcium reduced their diabetic risk by 33 percent. A study out of *Diabetes Care* involving seventy type 2 diabetics over the age of seventy found that those with vitamin D levels lower than 20 ng/ml had double the risk of developing type 2 diabetes.

Vitamin D is needed to regulate the immune response in those with type 1 diabetes. In an amazing cohort study conducted over a one-year period in northern Finland, researchers collected data on 10,821 children regarding vitamin D supplementation and its association with the bone disease rickets. What they found was remarkable: children who took 2,000 IU of vitamin D daily were 80 percent less likely to develop type 1 diabetes. In addition to avoiding foods with gluten and dairy (containing the destructive protein casein—linked to type 1 diabetes), it may be crucial for all children to take vitamin D early on to prevent the development of type 1 diabetes. Although the role of vitamin D in helping to regulate blood sugar is still in study, it seems quite clear that it plays a role in the prevention of both type 1 and type 2 diabetes.

Certain vitamins are synergistic with one another, meaning each enhances the effect of the other. Vitamin D and magnesium are synergistic. Adequate levels of magnesium are needed for the absorption and metabolism of vitamin D. Because magnesium is needed to turn vitamin D into its active form calcitriol, it's best to take magnesium and vitamin D at the same time.

Green Tea (EGCG)

A number of studies have demonstrated the role of green tea and the EGCG it contains in patients with type 2 diabetes, insulin resistance, and poor glucose management. In general, the results of these studies show a favorable response in markers of glucose metabolism and insulin resistance. In one study, researchers reviewed seventeen trials comprising 1,133 subjects to assess the impact of green tea on blood sugar control. Analysis of the data revealed that green tea "significantly" reduced fasting blood sugar levels, hemoglobin A1c, and fasting insulin.

A study published in *PLOS ONE* involved ninety-two subjects with diabetes and high LDL-cholesterol and triglycerides who were divided into two groups. One group received 500 mg of EGCG three times a day for sixteen weeks. The control group received a capsule of cellulose (a placebo) three times a day for the same sixteen weeks. The results of this study revealed a reduction in insulin resistance in those taking the EGCG and, as a bonus, a significant increase in high-density lipoprotein (HDL).

It appears that green tea polyphenols, including EGCG, are effective at lowering blood sugar. EGCG was found to influence the way glucose passes from the intestine into the bloodstream. When you eat starchy foods, the enzyme amylase is needed to break down the starch into simple sugars so these sugars can be absorbed. Green tea polyphenols such as EGCG inhibit amylase activity and reduce elevation of glucose and insulin.

Additional Nutrients

In addition to magnesium, vitamin D, and green tea, other nutrients have shown promising effects on blood sugar control. Chromium is a trace element that has been shown to reduce insulin resistance and glucose metabolism. Foods high in chromium include broccoli (a number one healthful food choice), green beans, tomatoes, romaine lettuce, Brazil nuts, and shellfish. Alpha-lipoic acid is a powerful antioxidant that has been shown to improve insulin sensitivity and symptoms of diabetic neuropathy. Biotin, a B vitamin, is needed to process glucose. Foods high in biotin include almonds, sweet potatoes, eggs, onions, tomatoes, carrots, walnuts, and salmon.

AS WITH ALL biochemical reactions in the body, vitamins, minerals, and other cofactors are needed for proper glucose metabolism and insulin signaling. Deficiencies in any of these micronutrients can impair blood sugar levels and cause insulin resistance. The evidence is clear: deficiencies of specific nutrients such as magnesium and vitamin D increase the risk of diabetes. On the flip side, taking these specific nutrients can help reverse and correct abnormal blood sugar and insulin resistance.

While taking nutraceuticals will assist the body in regulating sugar and "re-sensitize" cells to insulin, nothing replaces a high-fiber, nutrient-rich food plan when you are rebuilding from diabetes. The *Rebuild* food plan is designed to help you quickly regulate your blood sugar by providing the countless nutrients and phytochemicals that regulate blood sugar, including the powerhouses vitamin D, magnesium, and EGCG.

> **Z NOTE (SUMMARY):** Optimal doses of nutrients for any specific conditions have not been established by the FDA or any other governing health authority at this time. It's up to you and your doctor to decide what amount works best for you.

What goes hand-in-hand with eating nutrient-dense foods and supplements to rebuild from disease, prevent recurrence, and get lean? Exercise. You are probably thinking, *Ugh, now I have to exercise,* or *Exercising takes too long.* Would you be interested in a method of exercise that has been scientifically proven to change your body composition and reverse disease in less than 30 minutes a day? How about a type of exercise that causes fat burning to continue for hours or days later? Exercising to rebuild your health, get lean, and burn fat is about working smarter, not harder.

In the next chapter you will read about the most powerful method of exercise for rebuilding from disease and getting rid of dangerous fat. No gimmicks, just proven steps to cut your workout time in half and create a lean, disease-free body.

4

Re-action #2
Exercise with Periods
of Intensity

You have learned that unhealthful foods and a lack of nutrient-dense foods are the major reasons behind ill health. What we eat can cause disease and make us overfat by turning on hormonal switches that push the body to make fat and store it. An unhealthy body composition—high body fat, low lean muscle—is another major driver for serious diseases, including cancer, heart disease, diabetes, autoimmunity, and more. Now that you know how to turn the right switches in your body on and off, you'll have a better understanding of this next section.

Your Body Composition

In my office I use a device called a bioelectrical body composition analyzer to measure body fat and lean muscle. The good news is that you don't need a machine to measure yourself. With a few simple calculations, you can determine your body mass index—the relation of your weight to your height. That, along with your basal metabolic rate and body fat percentage, which you calculated in chapter 3, will give you a starting point from which to track your fat loss and muscle-building progress along the way.

BODY MASS INDEX CALCULATION

Body mass index (BMI) is a tool that shows if you are at a healthy weight for your height. It is also a way to calculate the health risk associated with your body composition—the ratio of lean tissues to fat. Determining your BMI is a simple calculation.

To calculate your BMI, divide your weight in kilograms by your height in meters squared. The basic formula is:

$$\text{BMI} = \text{Weight (kg)} \div \text{Height in meters (m)}^2$$

Let's use a person who weighs 160 pounds and is 5 feet 8 inches in height as an example.

First convert the pounds to kilograms by dividing the weight by 2.2.

160 pounds ÷ 2.2 = 73 kg (72.72 rounded off)

Now let's convert the inches to meters: Multiply the height in inches (5 feet 8 inches = 68 inches) by 2.54, then divide the total by 100.

68 inches x 2.54 = 173 (172.72 rounded off) ÷ 100 = 1.73 meters

Multiply the resulting number by itself.

1.73 x 1.73 = 2.99

Now let's combine those two numbers to get the BMI.

73 kg ÷ 2.99 m = 24 (24.414 rounded off)

This person has a body mass index of 24. A BMI of 18.5 to 24.9 is considered a normal weight. A BMI of 25 to 29.9 is considered overweight, and anything 30 or above is obese. Calculate your own BMI, record it on the worksheet on page 354, then check your score in the table below. Calculate and record your BMI again every four weeks to track your progress.

BODY MASS INDEX CLASSIFICATIONS

Classification	Risk	BMI Score
Underweight	Moderate	Less than 18.5
Normal	Very low	18.5–24.9
Overweight	Low	25.0–29.9
Obese Class 1	Moderate	30.0–34.9
Obese Class 2	High	35.0 39.9
Extreme Obesity	Very high	More than 40.0

NOTE: Someone who is classified as overweight by their BMI may not necessarily be "overfat." A 5-foot-5, 250-pound couch potato and a 5-foot-5, 250-pound body builder have the same BMI. Why? BMI is merely a ratio of weight to height and doesn't take into account whether that weight is fat or muscle. That is why you need to know your body fat percentage (see page 177) in addition to BMI.

TAKE YOUR MEASUREMENTS

Along with your BMI and body fat percentage, physical measurements of your body will provide additional points of change and progress to keep you motivated. The best way to measure is without clothes. If you need someone to help you, you can wear a tank top and thin shorts, or something like that, to cover up. If you measure with clothes, remember to wear the *same* clothes each time you measure so your values will be consistent.

CHEST: Measure around your chest, across the nipple.
WAIST: Measure around your waist, across your belly button.
HIPS: Measure around your hips and buttocks at the widest part.
BICEP: Measure the upper arm around the widest part of your *unflexed* bicep.

Record these measurements on the worksheet on page 354, and take them again after four, eight, and twelve weeks to see how your body composition is improving. Continue recording your progress until you are satisfied with your results.

In addition to tracking your measurements, there's nothing better than before-and-after pictures to show your progress. Think of how proud you are when you renovate a room—or the whole house—and compare the wonderful changes to what was there before. Taking photos of yourself before you change will definitely be your best motivation not to go back. I suggest you take the photos three ways: from the front, from the side, and from the back. The pictures will be the proof of all your hard work.

You should also record your weight on the worksheet on page 354, because it is an important additional marker of progress. Remember, though, that the goal is to focus on losing fat while maintaining the lean muscle—not just on shedding pounds.

Transforming Your Body

To transform means to change in appearance, form, or structure. By implementing the steps in this book, you will transform your mind, your body, and your life. Remember my acronym DIET—for Decide, Indulge, Enjoy, and Transform (see page 10)? Tracking your medical test results and taking pictures of yourself before and after will be evidence of your **decision** to get rebuilt. Having the before-and-after pictures shows that **indulging** in a variety of nutrient-dense, low-calorie foods has ignited the change in your body composition from being overfat to having the body you want and the health you deserve. Improvements in your health and body composition will give you a sense of **enjoyment** and happiness, and enable you to see the fruits of your efforts. Finally, improvements in your test scores and your before-and-after pictures will show that you were able to **transform** yourself—inside and out.

Transforming is a process that requires several different states of mind. David Bliss, the retired CEO of a management and consulting company, describes the "states of change" a person goes through in order to transform from "now" to a place in the future. The transformation happens in three stages: your current state; the future state, which is where you want to be; and the transition state, which is the time between where you are now and where you want to be.

THE CURRENT STATE

Having to deal with a chronic and serious health condition, along with being unhappy with your body and the way you feel, is most likely the reason you chose this book. You must believe that staying the way you are—whether you are overfat, fatigued, or dealing with chronic health issues—is no longer an option for you. In your current state, you may be thinking, *Now what?* Ask yourself why you want to transform. Perhaps you fear a recurrence and the future health issues you might face if you don't change. Are you modifying your lifestyle—your habits and daily rituals—so you'll be around longer for your children? Whatever your reason, you have to *feel* the reason—not just know it intellectually, but feel it in your heart. Once you have done this, you will set in motion the steps to rebuild your health and improve your body composition.

THE TRANSITION STATE

In this state, you are no longer content with prior unhealthful habits, but you are not yet where you want to be. As you travel along your journey—changing the way you eat, putting in place an exercise schedule, and improving your lifestyle—sometimes you hit bumps in the road. To keep yourself going strong, you will need support, motivation, reinforcement, measurements of progress, and celebration of the small victories along the way. Let's talk about these important factors.

SUPPORT: It's okay to share your fears and struggles with your spouse, friends, and family members as you go through your personal rebuild. Sometimes it's hard to open up and share because that makes you vulnerable. Look for people who are nonjudgmental, who make you laugh and boost you up when you need a lift, and who are also looking to rebuild their health.

MOTIVATION: Nothing matches the feeling you have when someone pumps you up, gives you strength, and helps provide the motivation to succeed. Look to those with whom you can exercise, cook, and share meals and recipes for constant motivation.

REINFORCEMENT AND MEASUREMENT OF PROGRESS: These go hand in hand. Change can be difficult and frustrating, but it can also be rewarding. When your internal terrain and your body composition change, that is a measurement of progress. Measuring your progress can also be done by recalculating your BMI, basal metabolic rate (BMR), and body fat percentage. What about your health progress? An improvement in your health can be seen with new blood work, hormone profiling, or any other method of testing that was used initially to diagnose your condition (see chapter 8, Testing the Disease Terrain). Testing can also provide a prognosis for your condition. Perhaps your inflammation markers—C-reactive protein and erythrocyte sedimentation rate—have improved, or your fasting blood sugar and hemoglobin A1c (markers of diabetes) are back to normal. Whatever the markers were to diagnose your condition(s), retest them to monitor your progress. These measurable changes will show you that your efforts are paying off. That deserves a "Great job!" Positive reinforcement is also a key supportocol to keeping you from falling off the wagon.

CELEBRATION: As you meet your short-term goals, reward yourself by doing something that makes you feel good. Perhaps you buy a new pair of shoes, a new exercise outfit, or a new mobile device you can load with heart-pumpin' music. Maybe enjoy a night on the town or a quiet, relaxing weekend away. Reward yourself with whatever makes you feel good, whatever keeps you motivated to get you through the transition state.

THE FUTURE STATE

You must have a clear, motivating picture of the future you want to create. You have to create an exciting vision for what you want to achieve. This vision and ideal must be emotionally felt and owned by you; someone can't just tell you it would be good for you. What does the future look like in your mind's eye? A newly built body? Getting off medications and the reversal of your health issues? Maybe you dream of walking into your favorite store to buy that outfit you've always wanted. Or maybe you want to live a healthful life so you can be a more active parent. Whatever this future state looks like for you, you must feel it. Going through change because your spouse or family has been nagging you is not sustainable. What's *your* motivation for change? What's *your* mental finish line?

Lose the Fat, Save the Muscle—at Any Age

Let's get into your body composition and the type of movement you need to adopt to rebuild your body. Weight loss has always been synonymous with size. The weight-loss industry spends zillions of dollars advertising the "get thin, lean, and sexy" mind-set. Of course, in order to do this, you must buy some product or program. While being lean is important for a multitude of reasons, the goal of healthy weight management is better body composition. It's about losing fat. From today on, divorce yourself from the notion of "weight loss" and focus on *fat loss.*

You may have noticed that throughout this book I have made the distinction between weight and fat. We all think we know the difference between fat and muscle. Yet many people trying to lose fat surely don't act that way. In order to take full advantage of the exercises outlined later in this chapter, it's worth making sure you do understand what you're working for. That's the best way to change your shape.

WHAT IS FAT?

Fat (adipose tissue) is the body's built-in battery; its main role is to store energy. Along with providing energy, it insulates and cushions the body. Fat can be classified as subcutaneous (under the skin) or visceral (surrounding the organs—for a reminder of the dangers of visceral fat, turn back to page 40). Believe it or not, fat is a hormone-producing tissue. It can produce hormones like leptin (which helps control appetite) and adiponectin (which helps burn fat). Fat also makes estrogen—do you recall aromatase? (If not, see page 47.) It is also a source of inflammation, which causes your immune system to wage war on your body and could ultimately lead to chronic disease.

WHAT IS LEAN MUSCLE?

Muscles are the body's motors; they produce force and cause motion by contraction (shortening). Muscle tissue is biologically active and requires a lot more calories to fuel itself than fat tissue does. The more lean muscle you have, the faster your metabolism is, which allows you to burn more calories in a day. There are two types of muscles in the body—smooth and skeletal. Smooth muscle makes up the heart and is found in the walls of organs and in blood vessels. We will focus on skeletal muscle, which drives your metabolism and is a major component of body composition

Real "dieting" is about body composition—decrease the body fat and increase the lean muscle. When people lose weight rapidly, they not only lose fat; they lose muscle, too. That's not healthy. I will show you how to get rid of the fat and preserve your muscle. Wouldn't it be nice if that could be accomplished without much effort? Is it possible? Yep! This is done by combining highly nutritious, fat-burning foods with the right kind of exercise.

Body Types

Being overfat is a major risk factor for the most serious diseases. A simple measurement to determine your risk for illness is your waist circumference; when your waist increases in size, so does your risk of disease. A waist circumference of 40 inches or more for men and 35 inches or more for women is a red flag for cardiovascular disease and diabetes. But research shows that the waist-to-hip ratio is a far better measurement for determining risk for serious disease than just the waist measurement alone.

To get your waist-to-hip ratio, turn to page 354, where you recorded your body measurements (if you haven't done it yet, now's the time to get out the measuring tape!) and note what you wrote down for your waist and hips. Divide your waist measurement by your hip measurement to get your waist-to-hip ratio. For men, any number at 1 or above indicates disease risk; for women, any number 0.8 or above is a significant risk.

ACCUMULATION OF FAT IN THE ABDOMEN: The "apple-shaped" body or "potbelly" is characterized by accumulated fat—subcutaneous fat and visceral fat—in the midsection, and is linked to higher instances of heart disease, diabetes, gallbladder disease, high blood pressure, and stroke. This body type is more common in men, but frequently develops in postmenopausal women. Research suggests that a buildup of fat around the midsection poses a higher risk for disease than fat buildup around the hips. This body shape is also associated with increased likelihood of insulin resistance, type 2 diabetes, and high blood lipids like cholesterol and triglycerides.

ACCUMULATION OF FAT ON THE HIPS AND BUTTOCKS: This body type is sometimes referred to as a "pear body," characterized by hips that are wider than the shoulders. This extra fat around the hips poses less risk for serious illnesses. A pear-shaped body is associated with higher likelihood of high levels of estrogen, a state called estrogen dominance.

REGARDLESS OF THE location of adipose tissue, excessive body fat is unhealthy. It can trigger diabetes, heart disease, and internal inflammation, which can set off certain cancers. That's another reason using the supportocols in this book is so important for your health.

> ### WARNING:
> ### YOU CAN'T OUT-TRAIN A CRAPPY DIET
>
> Before we get to different exercises you might want to try, I should make one point clear. You're fooling yourself if you think you can out-train a diet of high-calorie, low-nutrient, processed foods. If you continue to eat the same unhealthful foods and your exercise doesn't burn the calories you've eaten, you're going to increase your body fat. And if you eat those foods late in the day, your body is going to convert into fat the sugar and calories you don't burn off before bed. When you combine exercising with eating healthful foods, you'll get a healthy, lean body composition.

Before we talk about exercise, I'd like to outline the dangers of being sedentary. Our physical, social, and economic environments have caused an increase in sedentary behaviors and reduced our physical activity. We spend too much time watching TV, working or playing on the computer, sitting at our desks, and driving, and this has become a serious health hazard. Physical inactivity and sedentary behavior increase your risk of developing chronic diseases, including heart disease, stroke, cancer, obesity, type 2 diabetes, and high blood pressure, and can worsen those conditions if you already have them.

According to *Exercise and Sports Sciences Reviews*, TV viewing time was associated with metabolic syndrome, a condition characterized by increased body fat, abnormal blood sugar and insulin levels, high blood pressure, and high blood fats. The authors of the study also found that for every hour someone spent watching TV (sitting time), there was an associated 18 percent increased risk of all-cause mortality, including cardiovascular mortality independent of other risk factors like diet, smoking, and high blood pressure. A study published in *Medicine & Science in Sports & Exercise* concluded that riding in a car for more than ten hours a week increased the likelihood of death from heart disease by 48 percent. Finally, data from the *American Journal of Preventive Medicine* revealed that sedentary behavior was associated with higher levels of inflammation produced by fat. Remember adipocytokines from chapter 1? When your fat gets angry, it spits out the inflammatory agents leptin, TNF-alpha, and IL-6, which are linked to serious disease. Sedentary behavior was found to be associated with unfavorable levels of these inflammatory compounds.

Rebuild from Disease with High-Intensity Interval Training (HIIT)

Extensive research has proven that regular exercise has a wide range of health benefits, including improved cardiovascular function, improved muscle mass, and bone health. Exercise has also been shown to help the immune system fight disease, reduce free radical damage, reduce inflammation, regulate blood sugar, and prevent excessive body fat.

As noted in the *Scandinavian Journal of Medicine and Science in Sports*, exercise can be used as therapy for a wide range of disorders, such as insulin resistance, type 2 diabetes, hypertension, obesity, heart disease, osteoporosis, depression, and cancer. *Circulation*, the journal of the American Heart Association, states that long-term physical exercise improves relaxation of the blood vessels through the release of nitric oxide, the chemical that relaxes blood vessels and allows for less restricted blood flow, thus improving conditions of the heart and reducing high blood pressure. Additional research from the journal *Acta Biomed* indicates that regular exercise has been shown to reduce visceral fat, help insulin sensitivity, and improve glucose levels, blood pressure control, and blood lipid profiles. It further goes on to say, "For these reasons, regular aerobic physical activity must be considered an essential component of the cure of type 2 diabetes."

Can exercising improve brain function and other conditions associated with the brain? *Clinical Practice & Epidemiology in Mental Health* has found that exercising can significantly fight depression and can be used as an alternative to medications for depression.

Z NOTE: Depression is a severe medical condition with multiple manifestations and factors that play a role, including genetics; brain biology and chemistry; emotional events such as trauma, loss of a loved one, difficult relationships, and early childhood experiences; and inflammation. The immune system, particularly a type of white blood cell called a macrophage, plays an important role in the pathology of depression. Data from the journals *Biological Psychiatry, Neuroscience and Biobehavioral Reviews*, and *Pharmacological Reports* indicate that under normal conditions, the immune system reacts to any disturbances in the nervous system. Physical and mental stressors can activate the immune system to release pro-inflammatory compounds IL-6 and TNF, which are responsible for disturbances in the production of neurotransmitters, including serotonin, glutamate, GABA, and dopamine, all of which are implicated in the cause of depression. As Dr. Kelly Brogan states in her book *A Mind of Your Own*, depression is not a disease; it's a symptom. It's no wonder why so many people who are put on mind meds to treat their symptoms don't respond to them. They don't resolve the physical cause of the depression.

So now it's time for the third and final Dr. Z Rule. Only three rules you have to keep in mind. That's tough, right? Do you think you can follow them to achieve that new you?

Z RULE #3. DO HIGH-INTENSITY INTERVAL TRAINING

Extended periods of endurance exercise have long been associated with burning fat. Gyms are filled with people running, oscillating, and climbing stairs for hours on end in the hope of melting off body fat. Yet, for most people, lengthy exercise with moderate intensity comes up short in producing fat loss. Research is finding that high-intensity exercise done in short periods improves fat oxidation (burning) better than high-volume endurance training.

Endurance training involves exercising at a steady pace for 20 minutes or longer. This type of exercise is usually performed at a gym or at home on machines like a treadmill, elliptical machine, stair-climber, or any other machine found in the cardio section of the gym. Long-distance running and bike riding are also considered endurance exercises. Hard-core endurance junkies engage in major long-distance cycling and triathlons. Endurance training has always been associated with heart health. However, research is showing that hard long-term endurance exercise is linked to damage to the right ventricle of the heart and a weakened immune system. Periodic aerobic exercise can strengthen the heart, improve circulation—allowing more oxygen to get into the body—and improve skeletal muscle strength.

High-intensity interval training (HIIT) typically involves exercising with all-out intensity for a short period, followed by a period of low-intensity exercise or rest. A great example of this is sprinting—explosive movement for a short time, followed by a walk or rest. The most used program in the research is the Wingate protocol, which involves high-intensity sprinting for 30 seconds with hard resistance. This is done four to six times separated by 4-minute rest periods, and performed three times a week for two to six weeks. Although this routine may seem simple, it is very effective. Other researchers have created modified high-intensity protocols, all of which are very effective at getting rid of fat and greatly improving metabolism. I have included a very effective HIIT routine that takes little time and has a major impact. You won't believe the results.

THE RESEARCH BEHIND HIIT

In the *Journal of Applied Physiology*, researchers found that seven sessions of HIIT over a two-week period improved whole-body fat oxidation (burning) as well as the capacity for skeletal muscles to burn fat. Studies from different sources all show that HIIT is a very effective way to reduce not only subcutaneous fat but also visceral fat. According to the journal *Metabolic Syndrome and Related Disorders*, short-term, high-intensity aerobic exercise reduced visceral fat in overweight adults.

An article in *Cancer Research* states that women who exercised with moderate intensity five times a week for forty-five minutes not only reduced their body fat by 2 percent but also had a significant reduction in serum estrogen. Why is this important for women and men? Because body fat creates estrogen, which is a major spark for cancers of the breast, endometrium, and ovaries in women, as well as the prostate in men.

Research found in the *British Medical Journal* and *Acta Oncologica* revealed that high-intensity exercising improved cardiopulmonary (heart and lung) function, muscle strength, aerobic capacity, and emotional well-being, as well as reduced fatigue in those being treated with chemotherapy for advanced cancers. A study published in *Physiological Reviews* found that intense exercising for short periods increased the activity of natural killer cells—a type of white blood cell that kills cancer—for hours after exercising. Perfect. HIIT: a self-induced cancer treatment.

For heart disease, HIIT is also superior to aerobic exercise with moderate intensity. Data found in *Australian Family Physician* and *Circulation* indicate that HIIT reduced LDL cholesterol, while increasing

HDL cholesterol. HIIT was also found to improve endothelial function, blood pressure, left ventricular function, and glucose regulation. High-intensity training was shown to be safe for those with preexisting heart disease and those who had already suffered a heart attack. Furthermore, research published in *Australian Family Physician* found that periods of exercising with intensity were beneficial for those with stable angina and post-cardiac stenting, and after coronary artery grafting. In the journal *Metabolism*, researchers found that HIIT was far better for getting rid of subcutaneous fat than exercising at a constant pace with moderate intensity. HIIT, according to a study in the *International Journal of Obesity*, is a very efficient way not only to burn fat but also to reduce its formation in the body and improve metabolism.

HIIT is also the exercise mode of choice to regulate insulin, growth hormone, and glucagon. In studies published in the *European Journal of Applied Physiology*, the *Journal of Applied Physiology*, and the *Journal of Nutrition and Metabolism*, exercising with intensity was shown to increase the release of growth hormone and help balance insulin and glucagon. If you remember, insulin stores fat and glucagon burns fat. Growth hormone, released after exercising, helps build muscle and, like glucagon, causes the body to burn fat for fuel.

EXERCISE SMARTER, NOT HARDER!

As we get into specific workout plans, please stop to consider what you are able to do physically, and ensure that you have no health issues to prevent you from exercising or that may be exacerbated by this workout. Before beginning, you may want to consult an experienced health care practitioner—one who understands how exercising benefits the body. If you are not used to exercising, you may want to adopt a low-intensity exercise program first and then increase the frequency and duration of the exercise as you become able to train with more intensity.

You may have seen different high-intensity workouts like the Wingate protocol (see page 245), but I'd like to share the effective one I use, which requires only 20 minutes per session. As an example, I will describe my high-intensity aerobic training on an at-home treadmill that I use during inclement and cold weather. If you have a treadmill, it's time to remove the boxes and jackets thrown on it and give it a dusting.

After turning on the machine, I start with a low-intensity (level 2) walk for 2 minutes. While walking, I'm getting a feel for the machine, and I'm warming up my legs. After those 2 minutes, I increase the speed on the treadmill to a moderate intensity (level 4 or 5). This takes me from a nice-paced walk to a super-fast walk or slow jog. I continue this pace for 1 minute. Then it's time for the high-energy, high-intensity run. I increase the speed on the machine to level 8 or 9. I run at top speed for 1 minute. My heart rate elevates, and my muscles feel as though they are starting to get pumped. Once the minute is up, I quickly slow down back to the low intensity I started with for 2 minutes. Following the 2 minutes, I speed back up to a level 4 or 5 of moderate intensity for 1 minute, then again at level 8 or 9 at all-out exertion for 1 minute, followed by throttling down to the 2-minute low intensity.

NOTE: For many, going all-out for 1 minute is tough. If you need to, just start off at 30 seconds. As you get more conditioned, go to 45 seconds and then to 60 seconds, if you can. Your high-intensity set may be only 30 seconds; that's okay. Everybody is different. You need to find the level that challenges you enough to burn the fat and increase your metabolism.

I repeat this sequence five times, and then cool down with a 3- to 5-minute walk at low intensity, or just walk around for a bit off the treadmill until I'm somewhat rested. Following this sweat session, I know that I'm burning fat for hours to come. This sequence takes roughly 20 minutes; the cool-down is another 5. It will make you feel as if you've worked out for much longer than 20 minutes. I'll sometimes do this routine on a stationary bike indoors; I use a road bike when I'm training outside.

When you're just beginning to exercise with intensity, start by walking, riding, or moving on a treadmill, elliptical machine, or stair climber for 4 to 5 minutes just to get your head into it. Once you are used to a workout that fits you, you may not need to spend time doing this. Once you condition yourself, start the 2-minute low-level intensity as soon as you begin. Your ability to exercise with intensity is probably different from mine.

Your "level 9" is based on your fitness level. Don't stress by comparing yourself to others or get frustrated because you think you should train like an Ironman. Once you start your own HIIT program, you can test your initial abilities and change them as you progress.

If you are a runner, sprint on hills for the high-intensity set, or just sprint on a level surface if you're not near a hill. If you're a cyclist, cycle up a steep hill with intensity; if you are on a stationary bike, you can increase its resistance, or stand up to increase the intensity. Whatever the sport, figure out how to exercise with periods of low intensity, moderate intensity, and then high intensity.

Don't worry if you are not a sprinter. HIIT can be performed on a bike, treadmill, oscillating machine, any other exercise machine, or just on your own two feet. What's the right type of HIIT exercise for you? That's hard to say, because I don't know your abilities, disabilities, access to exercise equipment, environmental restrictions, and/or health issues that may hinder your ability to exercise with intensity. Pick any aerobic exercise, as long as you can increase your intensity in intervals. You can create a HIIT program using TRX suspension training, kettlebells, or boot-camp style exercises. The great news is that HIIT involves less learning and less time. You don't have to spend all day at the gym, or exercise for hours on end until you're exhausted. Twenty minutes of high intensity allows for maximum fat burning and disease recovery!

WHEN IS THE BEST TIME TO EXERCISE?

I realize everyone has a busy schedule, so finding time to exercise can sometimes be challenging. The good news is that you require short periods of HIIT to rebuild from a health crisis, burn fat, and maintain your muscle. The answer to the question "When is the best time to exercise?" is more variable. First, here are some things to consider.

Whether it's HIIT, weight training, or some other form of resistance exercise, you should not work out on an empty stomach. A safe time to exercise is about one to four hours after eating a small meal. Why? The delay allows the stomach to empty. By that time, your blood sugar has risen and insulin has stored it in the muscle as glycogen.

Pre-exercise eating is very important. Let's say you get up, swill down a cup of coffee, and head off to the gym. Because you haven't eaten since the night before, your blood sugar is low. If you exercise with no fuel, your body reaches for your muscle sugar first. Then it depletes your liver sugar. After that, your body depends on hormones to break down muscle in order to provide you with the blood sugar for continued exercise. This is not what you want to do. Remember body composition. Lose the fat, build the muscle. Exercising without fuel can cause you to lose valuable muscle.

It's worth going back over what cortisol does inside your body. As you remember, cortisol is a hormone released from the adrenal glands during times of stress. Cortisol is an anti-inflammatory hormone, which means it helps control any allergic responses as well as helping to regulate blood sugar. However, when your blood sugar is low, cortisol can have an adverse effect. The brain's only fuel source is glucose, so when blood sugars are low, cortisol breaks down muscle, turning it into glucose for the brain's survival. Muscles require sugar in order for them to perform during exercising. If you don't eat before exercising, you may not have the right amount of fuel to work out. Cortisol will break down the muscle, and at the same time it will maintain the fat, because the brain can't use fat as a fuel source.

Cortisol follows a circadian rhythm; it is highest in the morning and lowest at night. Some research studies have found that exercising in the afternoon is best; others advise exercising in the morning. My opinion is that you should work out in the morning or at some point during the day one or two hours after you've eaten something. Try to avoid working out in the evening; it will raise your cortisol and disrupt your sleep. Choose the time of day that works for you, and plan to eat a snack or a small meal with protein and some form of complex carbohydrate at least an hour before that. If you eat too much or too soon before exercising, you may get nauseated. That's because your body is trying to digest the food and at the same time manage your muscles and heart during the activity. So wait at least one hour after eating before you exercise.

Definitely eat a serving of protein with a serving of carbs *after* the workout to prevent the effects of cortisol, and to load your muscles with glycogen (muscle sugar) again.

Let me point out again that you can't out-train a crappy diet. If you are exercising until exhaustion thinking that you can burn off a pizza you ate the night before, you're sadly mistaken. Eating a healthful diet coupled with HIIT is the best strategy to burn fat and get lean. Since lean muscle eats excessive calories and burns fat, creating it or having more of it has a big impact on a healthy body composition. Building a lean and muscular body is best done with high-intensity and resistance training (strength training) that you can do right at home or at your local gym.

NOT SEEING THE RESULTS?

There are many reasons why people can't get rid of fat—from not knowing what to eat, how much to eat, and when, to uncontrollable, emotional eating. There can be undiscovered physical reasons behind failed attempts in the fat-loss arena. Those physical or biological issues not only prevent fat loss but can also lead to discouragement. Eventually, you may give up on "diets," thinking they don't work. Let's not forget the frustrations about exercise; too much or too little can prevent you from achieving better body composition. If you are running into obstacles along your fat-loss journey, it will help to know the obvious, and not so obvious, reasons why your body composition is not changing.

DON'T JUST WING IT. What you eat, combined with your activity level, determines how well your metabolism functions. Your unique metabolism is based on your body's systems (e.g., heart and circulation, digestion) and muscular structure. Your caloric calculation is meant to stop the production of fat, burn existing fat, and maintain lean muscle. If you are overeating or undereating, you will be either making fat or holding on to it. Major calorie restriction also causes the release of the hormone ghrelin, which increases appetite and eventually causes overeating.

THE GOOD, THE BAD, AND THE UGLY. What you eat is just as important as how much. Eating 1,300 calories of pizza, fast food, soda, and ice cream is completely different from eating 1,300 calories of healthful proteins, greens, starchy vegetables, nuts, seeds, and fruit. Food is information. It not only gives us energy; it provides the nutrients that keep us free of disease. High-calorie processed foods will not only create disease but also increase insulin, the hormone that makes you fat.

EXERCISE AVERSION. "It takes too long." "It's too much effort." These are thoughts that may prevent you from getting started. Good news! Exercising to burn fat, rebuild from disease, and prevent disease takes only 20 to 30 minutes a day, or even every other day. Spending a day at the gym is a waste of time and actually may hinder your fat-loss goals. Exercising with intensity rather than duration is the best way to get rid of flab on the abs. On the other hand, deciding to blow off exercise will definitely slow down your fat-loss goals. Remember not to overtrain or push too hard right out of the gate. You want to build up gradually so you stay the course, rather than hitting it hard, which might leave you sore and discouraged.

BAD MOON RISING. When the sun goes down and the moon comes out, that is a sign to reduce your food consumption. You should eat during the day when you're active, not when you're getting ready for bed. If you eat most of your calories at night, you are definitely storing fat and increasing internal inflammation. Calories from food are meant to be burned during the day, not stored as fat while you sleep. If you have to eat in the evening, choose green or other colorful vegetables and a small piece of protein. This will have little effect on the hormones that store fat while you're snoozing.

TAKING THE WRONG APPROACH. How you approach the challenge of changing your body composition and your health starts with a decision. For some, the "all or nothing" approach works; others prefer setting small, realistic goals. Perhaps start with a walk every day until you are ready to engage in more strenuous exercise. Likewise, substitute coconut milk ice cream for regular ice cream. Making small changes will ease the transition into a regular pattern of more healthful eating and exercising, which will serve not only your body composition but also your long-term health.

SLEEP ISSUES. Sleep is important, not just for overall health but also to get rid of the bulge. Poor sleep patterns create simple-sugar cravings during the day, which is counterproductive for fat-loss goals. Poor sleep can be caused by many things, including life stressors, progesterone deficiency, eating late at night, and alcohol consumption. Make it a priority to discover and resolve the culprit behind your sleep problems. Read about the benefits of good sleep in chapter 7.

STRESS. Stress increases cortisol, which causes fat to be stored in the belly. Stress can also trigger overeating. When we are burned out from a stressful day, we tend to overeat refined, high-calorie foods, the ones that create that unwanted muffin top. These simple-sugar foods relax us temporarily, causing a boost of serotonin, which makes us feel good in the short term. Identify your stressors and find a way to deal with them that won't make you sick or fat. See chapter 5 for more on stress.

SELF-DEFENSE. A strong connection exists between obesity and sexual abuse or other serious emotional trauma. It is natural to protect yourself when you have been traumatized or violated in any way. Subconsciously, being overfat can make you less attractive to others. It also may shut down sexuality and keep your libido in check. If you have been traumatized in any way, seek help from a counselor, one who specializes in recovering from sexual abuse and posttraumatic stress.

DON'T GIVE UP ON YOURSELF. If you miss exercise one day, or eat something you shouldn't, don't stress. Just dust yourself off and get back on track the next day. Having a bad day does not mean you "can't do this" or "all is lost." Reconnect with the real reason you have chosen to rebuild yourself—the emotionally felt reason. That will guide you back to a pattern of consistent behavior and help you avoid feeling guilty when you have an off day. Remember, if you give up on your body, it will give up on you.

Strength Training

I know the words *strength training* and *weight lifting* can be intimidating to some. I get it. Images of climbing onto big machines, or trying to push massive plates of steel, can be nerve-racking. So don't do that. Leave the giant plates of steel to the people who body build and strength train for competition and sports. Strength training with weights can be done at any age, by any gender. Weights can range from one pound to hundreds of pounds, just as resistance training with machines can be simple or complex, depending on your body composition goals. You may think you will get big and bulky if you start on a strength training program. This is actually far from reality. Forget those images of overmuscled body builders. Training with weights is not just for football players and body builders; it is one of best ways to get rid of fat, tone and build your muscles, and regain your health.

Why? Because strength training plays a key role in changing your body composition and reversing disease. It causes your muscles to push against some force, or resistance. Probably the best example of this form of exercise is weight lifting. Using weights to lift or machines to push against increases the strength and size of the muscles involved. Other examples of strength training are resistance bands, sand bags, kettlebells, TRX, and Bowflex machines.

Coupling HIIT with strength training is the ultimate way to rebuild your body after disease. In the *Journal of Applied Physiology*, researchers found that resistance exercise with weights burned fat throughout the body, specifically belly fat. Other documented benefits include regulating blood sugar and insulin, slowing down the aging process of our cells, and improving strength and endurance. Lean muscle is the fountain of youth.

First, make sure you are physically able to train with weights or use resistance devices. Next, develop a resistance-training protocol for yourself; this depends on your abilities. When you exercise with resistance or weight, you do it based on your fitness level. At the start, pick weights that allow you to do 10 to 12 repetitions. As you get stronger, you can increase the amount of weight you are using per exercise.

Here's an example of combining HIIT with strength training using weights: a shoulder exercise like a seated dumbbell press. I will usually start with 50 pounds as my first set. I press the dumbbells for 10 reps, a comfortable range and weight for me. Once I'm done with that set, I look at my watch and rest for the next minute or minute and a half. I then grab the 60-pound weights and press them for 8 reps. Again, I rest for a minute or minute and a half, then press the 70-pound dumbbells for a set of 6 reps. After another minute to minute and a half of rest, I press 80-pound dumbbells for 4 reps. For my last set, I drop the weight back down to 50 pounds and go back to doing 10 to 12 reps. This is the HIIT set. Once completed, I cool down for a couple of minutes.

I use 50-plus-pound weights because I can, but there is no contest here. You may use 10 or 15 pounds, and that's perfectly fine. Make sure you are comfortable with the weights you use so you don't hurt yourself. Try working out with someone who can spot you. An experienced trainer can also instruct you in technique to maximize results and prevent injury.

Exercise Schedule

On pages 270–271, I've included an exercise log for you to keep track of your workout schedule, including the upper-body and lower-body exercises you do. When designing your own personal workout schedule, look at the weekly schedule on page 257 to get a game plan started. Maybe you prefer to do HIIT a few days a week and then do a few days of strength training. There is no right or wrong here. You just need to choose what works for you. There are many ways you can build on this program, such as using a trainer or searching online for specific types of exercise.

These charts show my exercise schedule; I alternate resistance with HIIT aerobic exercises. Allowing yourself sufficient recovery time is just as important as the training, so sometimes I take one or two days off during the week to let my body recover. After the recovery, start where you left off. If your last training was 20 minutes of aerobic exercise, start with either upper- or lower-body strength training. If you did weight training before the recovery time, start with 20 minutes of aerobics.

Monday	Tuesday	Wednesday	Thursday	Friday	Saturday	Sunday
Upper-Body Weights	20 Minutes HIIT Aerobics	Lower-Body Weights	20 Minutes HIIT Aerobics	Upper-Body Weights	20 Minutes HIIT Aerobics or Off Day	Off Day

Monday	Tuesday	Wednesday	Thursday	Friday	Saturday	Sunday
Lower-Body Weights	20 Minutes HIIT Aerobics	Upper-Body Weights	20 Minutes HIIT Aerobics	Lower-Body Weights	20 Minutes HIIT Aerobics or Off Day	Off Day

If you train using some other form of anaerobic exercise, like kettle-bells, cable machines, body-weight training, or sand bags, create a program that encompasses multiple sets with increasing difficulty, then a high-intensity set at the end. Remember: Figure out what weights and exercises you can do based on your ability. Then exercise. If you are already training for endurance, ramp up the fat-burning and muscle-building by adding two or three days of HIIT with weights. This will increase not only your strength but also your VO2 max, a measurement of how well the body uses oxygen during exercise; it is used to determine how fit you are, and good VO2 max is needed for long endurance training.

You may be thinking, *Wait, I don't belong to a gym* or *I'm not comfortable going to the gym*. That's okay. The first ten exercises I'm going to show you can be done at home. Because I don't recommend lifting bags of cement, or throwing yourself over the back of the foot board on your bed, you will need a few items for doing these exercises at home. You may want to purchase some hand weights that you can manage. Buying a single bench that can be used for many exercises is a good idea. Last, you may want to get a yoga mat so the exercises that require you to lie or kneel on the ground aren't uncomfortable.

You can find lots of exercises to tone and build your muscles, but I think these top ten "build and burn" exercises are excellent for starting at home.

Dr. Z's Top 10 Build-and-Burn Exercises

1. Push-Up

Push-ups build both muscle and strength in the upper body, including the chest, arms, and shoulders, and they don't require machines or weights to perform. Push-ups look easy, but for some, they pose a challenge. As with any exercise, there is a technique to performing them correctly. Poor push-up technique can cause injury to your low back and shoulders.

THE TECHNIQUE

Get into the push-up position with your elbows in a locked position.

Place your hands slightly wider than shoulder width. Keep your abs and butt (glutes) tight to avoid too much extension in your low back. Keep your head and neck in a straight line with your body. Don't look forward; keep facing down.

Lower yourself by bending your elbows until your chest almost touches the floor. Now push yourself back up to the starting position.

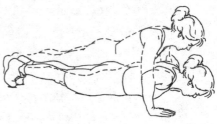

This exercise can also be done with a stabilization ball or yoga ball. This may be slightly more difficult because your feet are up, and you have more weight coming through your chest and arms.

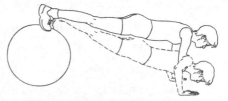

Use the same technique here regarding hand placement and head and neck position, and tighten up those abs and glutes.

Repeat for the desired number of reps.

DR. Z SAYS . . . "For a more challenging push-up, contract your abs and tighten your core by pulling your belly button toward your spine. While you tighten your abs, inhale as you lower yourself, and exhale as you push up off the floor."

2. One-Arm Dumbbell Row

The one-arm dumbbell row is an excellent exercise to strengthen, tone, and build your lats—the muscles that give the V-shape to your back. It also works the mid-back and rear shoulders. The picture shows the position of the dumbbell perpendicular to the bench. You can also position the weight and your hand to be parallel with the bench.

THE TECHNIQUE

Position yourself on the right side of the bench with your left knee and hand resting on the bench.

Pick up the dumbbell with your right hand while securing the right foot on the ground. Now pull your shoulder blade back while keeping your arm straight. This becomes the starting position.

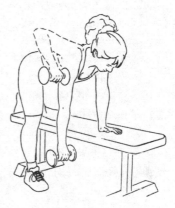

Pull the dumbbell up to your side until it just about makes contact with your ribs. Lower the weight until the arm is fully extended and the shoulder is stretched downward.

Repeat for desired number of reps, then repeat on the other side.

DR. Z SAYS . . . "Another way to hold the weight is with the palm of your hand facing your torso. This may be more comfortable and will prevent you from brushing the weight against your side."

3. Seated Dumbbell Press

One basic shoulder exercise stands above the rest—the seated dumbbell press. Strong and shaped shoulders not only look good in a dress, suit, or on the beach; strong delts (shoulders) will give you a strong competitive edge in sports and assist in other forms of training.

THE TECHNIQUE

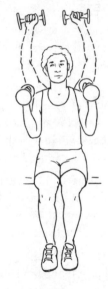

Sit on a stable bench or chair with your feet firmly planted on the ground and your back against the back of the chair. Lift the weights up to the starting position seen in the picture. If the weights are heavier than you can lift straight up to your shoulders, place them on your knees, and use your legs to assist in lifting them.

From the starting position, push the weights while rotating them to the finished position. Once completed, slowly lower the dumbbells to the starting position.

Repeat for desired number of reps.

> **DR. Z SAYS . . .** "The shoulder contains three joints surrounded by small muscles that can be injured with improper form, so don't get sloppy."

4. Standing Dumbbell Curl

The upper arm, or biceps, is the most famous muscle in the body. When I ask you to "make a muscle," what's the first muscle you think of? The biceps. The best exercise to build and shape the biceps is the standing dumbbell curl.

THE TECHNIQUE

Grab two dumbbells and hold them down at your sides with the palms of your hands facing your body.

Start the movement with one palm facing the body, and when the dumbbell clears your side, begin to rotate it so at the end of the movement, your palm is facing up.

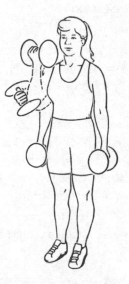

As you lift the weight, feel the biceps contract all the way to the top. Now slowly lower the weight, again with your palm facing up. When you reach your side, the dumbbell and your palm should be facing your body.

Then curl with the other arm. Repeat for desired number of reps.

DR. Z SAYS . . . "Try not to cheat by swinging your body or swinging your arm through the movement. Stand still while you curl."

5. Triceps Kickback

The triceps are made up of three heads: the long, lateral, and medial head. The lateral head is the part of the triceps that is really visible, when you extend the arm. The kickback is excellent for isolating the triceps, and it will help prevent the back of your arm from jiggling when waving good-bye.

THE TECHNIQUE

Kneel over your bench while supporting your body with one arm. With your left knee down, and your left hand and arm supporting you, grab a dumbbell with the right hand.

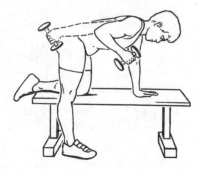

Now position your upper arm parallel to the floor. Extend the arm by contracting the triceps, until the arm is straight. Return your arm and repeat the movement.

Repeat for the desired number of reps, and then change arms.

DR. Z SAYS . . . "Make sure your elbow is positioned at your side, high enough to get the full movement. To prevent poor range of motion here, have your elbow slightly higher than your shoulder. Now kick back . . . you should feel it."

6. Dumbbell Squat

The squat is a superb exercise that not only targets the upper thighs (quads) and the buttocks (glutes) but also works the whole body. The major bonus with this exercise is that it burns a lot of calories and burns fat. Second, squats can improve your overall strength, your endurance and balance, and your flexibility.

THE TECHNIQUE

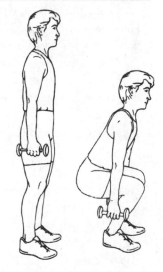

Stand with dumbbells to your sides.

Slightly point your feet out so when you bend, your knees are facing the same direction as your feet.

Bend your knees forward while allowing your hips to bend back behind. As you lower yourself, keep your back as straight as you can and, again, your knees pointed in the same direction as your feet.

Lower yourself until your thighs are just parallel to the floor. Now push up and extend your knees until your legs are straight.

Through the full movement, keep your head straight, back straight, and chest high. Also keep your feet firmly planted on the floor.

Repeat for the desired number of reps.

DR. Z SAYS . . . "There really is no other single exercise that can improve strength, flexibility, coordination, and bone-density health than the squat. Regarding technique, it's important to stay upright. There is a tendency to lean forward here, so shift your shin bones forward and keep your heels down."

7. Lunge

The lunge is really just a large step. Try taking a large step, then push yourself back up to the standing position. You will get a sense of which muscles are working and which ones will get toned with this exercise. Lunges are the quintessential quad, hamstring, and glute exercise; they are also excellent for your core.

THE TECHNIQUE

Stand with the dumbbells to your sides. Now lunge forward with the first leg. As you lunge, land on your heel, then your forefoot. Once you are stable on your foot, lower your body by bending at the knee and the hip until the rear knee almost touches the ground.

Return to the original standing position by forcibly pushing back with the forward leg. Repeat the lunge with the opposite leg.

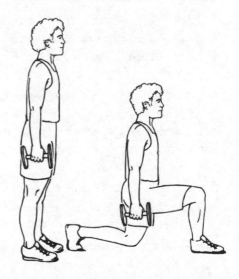

DR. Z SAYS . . . "Keep your torso straight and your abs in as you push through your foot back to the starting position."

8. High-Knee Step Up

We all want toned and well-shaped glutes (the muscles that form the buttocks) and hamstrings (the muscles on the back of the leg). You can improve the shape of your back end by the right diet, high-intensity training, and resistance training. For keeping fat off your seat, and having shapely hams, the high-knee step up is a great exercise.

THE TECHNIQUE

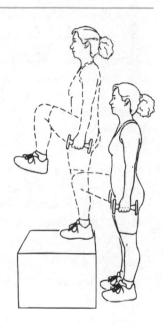

Stand with your feet parallel about hip-width apart while holding dumbbells in your hands. Start with a light weight to get a feel for the movement and the level of difficulty.

Now step to place your right foot on a platform, placing your foot firmly on the platform while keeping good posture. Now push off with your left foot to raise your body onto the platform. As you come up onto the platform, continue to raise that left knee higher than the left hip, and then place that foot back down next to the right one.

On the downward phase, step backward with the left foot and place it on the ground in its starting position. Let your body lean slightly forward during the step back to create balance. Now follow with the right foot, putting it down next to the left.

Repeat these steps for the opposite side, and repeat for desired number of reps.

DR. Z SAYS . . . "Try to avoid moving your foot and ankle (swaying in or out), because this will make you lose your balance. Don't make it too easy. Using a box or platform that's only a few inches tall won't challenge your hamstrings and glutes."

9. Dumbbell Calf Raise

Nothing stands out on your legs like muscular calves. The calves are tough to build because they are in constant use all day, keeping us standing and moving. The muscles that make up the calves are the soleus and the gastrocnemius muscles. They need more than just walking to get shapely and muscular. The calf raise is *the* exercise to build buff calves. The calf raise can be done multiple ways. Here is one exercise using dumbbells.

THE TECHNIQUE

You're going to need a small board like a 2x4 to do this exercise. Grab your dumbbells and put the balls of your feet on a stable wooden board. Your heels should be touching the floor. This is your starting position.

Point your toes straight ahead, and raise your heels off the floor by contracting the calves. As with all exercises, exhale through the movement. At the top of the contraction, hold for a second or two.

Lower yourself to the starting position. Repeat for desired number of reps.

Option 2: To provide more stability, use one dumbbell at a time. Hold a dumbbell in your right hand as you exercise the right calf. You can lean against a wall or post with the left hand for stability. Then switch hands and do the left side.

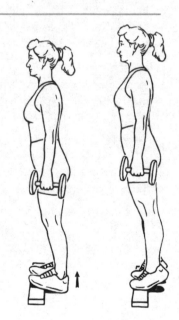

DR. Z SAYS . . . "If you find the 2x4 too wobbly, or it's flipping on you, get a step platform at a gym equipment store or online. This will definitely give you stability on your toes."

10. Crunch

You can have a toned and flat stomach or a six-pack if you choose. There are two things to remember here: you have to exercise and train your abs and, most important, get rid of the fat overlying the muscle. A great exercise to start building your abs is the crunch.

THE TECHNIQUE

To do a perfect crunch, lie down on the floor on your back and bend your knees. Place your hands across your chest, not behind your neck or head. By putting your hands behind your head, you tend to pull your head and neck forward, which will do your abs no good, and you may hurt your neck.

While pulling your belly button back and keeping your back flat against the floor, contract your abs, bringing your shoulders about 3 to 5 inches off the floor. Exhale while you come up, and keep your feet on the floor.

At the top of the movement, hold for a few seconds and then slowly lower yourself back down. Start again.

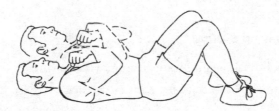

DR. Z SAYS . . . "Exhale while you come up, and squeeze those abs. See if you can do 15 to 20 reps for four to five sets."

For Serious Exercise

You are probably hungry for more build-and-burn exercises after reading through the Top 10. On page 272 I provide a chart you can use to pick exercises to incorporate into your strength training. You can copy these pages and use them to record the exercises you choose and the weights you use. Here's an example of a schedule that may work for you. Depending on your personal schedule, figure out how to get in a few days of intensity training and strength training. It's always a good idea to take a day off to recover and give your body a break.

Monday	Tuesday	Wednesday	Thursday	Friday	Saturday	Sunday
Upper-Body Weights	20 Minutes HIIT	Lower-Body Weights	20 Minutes HIIT	Upper-Body Weights	20 Minutes HIIT	Off

Remember these tips:

- When exercising aerobically, use the HIIT principles. Start the exercise at a low intensity for 2 minutes, then increase to a moderate intensity for 1 minute, and finally, go to high level of intensity for 30 to 60 seconds.
- Alternate aerobic training with strength training.
- Train your upper body one day, then your lower body the next time you train with weights.
- When strength training, perform five sets of an exercise, increasing the weight each set. Start with 12 repetitions, then 10, then 8, then 6 reps, then a high-intensity set.
- Allow 1-minute rest periods between sets.

Here are sample routines for the upper body and lower body to get you started. On Monday, start with the upper body; on Wednesday, train your lower body. As described on page 268, each exercise consists of five sets: 12, 10, 8, 6 reps, plus a final set of 10 to 12 reps as your high-intensity set.

Chest	Barbell Bench Press
Back	Lat Pull-Down
Shoulders	Seated Dumbbell Press
Triceps	Triceps Push-Down
Biceps	Dumbbell Curl
Quads	Barbell Squat
Hamstrings	Lying Leg Curl
Glutes	High Knee Step-Up
Calves	Smith Machine Calf Raise

See page 272 for an additional list of exercises to choose from.

REBUILD EXERCISE LOG

UPPER-BODY EXERCISES

EXERCISE—choose one from each group			Reps	Weight Lifted
CHEST	Barbell Bench Press Barbell Incline Press Dumbbell Bench Press	Incline Dumbbell Bench Press Dumbbell Fly Flat Bench Fly	x12 x10 x8	
	Chosen Exercise		x6	
	Intensity Set		x12	
BACK	Pull-Up Lat Pull-Down One-Arm Dumbbell Row	Seated Cable Row Back Extension Superman Stability-Ball Extension	x12 x10 x8	
	Chosen Exercise		x6	
	Intensity Set		x12	
SHOULDERS	Seated Dumbbell Press Barbell Military Press	Rear Dumbbell Raise Barbell Upright Row Dumbbell Front Raise	x12 x10 x8	
	Chosen Exercise		x6	
	Intensity Set		x12	
BICEPS	Standing Dumbbell Curl Standing Barbell Curl	Preacher Curl Concentration Curl Cable Curl	x12 x10 x8	
	Chosen Exercise		x6	
	Intensity Set		x12	
TRICEPS	Seated Triceps Ext. Barbell Lying Triceps Extension Triceps Kickback	Triceps Push-Down Dip Dumbbell Triceps Extension	x12 x10 x8	
	Chosen Exercise		x6	
	Intensity Set		x12	

REBUILD EXERCISE LOG

LOWER-BODY EXERCISES

EXERCISE—choose one from each group		Reps	Weight Lifted
QUADRICEPS	Dumbbell Squat Leg Press	Leg Extension Barbell Squat	x12	
			x10	
			x8	
	Chosen Exercise		x6	
	Intensity Set		x12	
HAM-STRINGS	Lying Leg Curl Lunge High-Knee Step Up		x12	
			x10	
			x8	
	Chosen Exercise		x6	
	Intensity Set		x12	
GLUTES	Lunge High-Knee Step Up Squat		x12	
			x10	
			x8	
	Chosen Exercise		x6	
	Intensity Set		x12	
CALVES	Standing Calf Raise Dumbbell Calf Raise Seated Dumbbell Calf Raise		x12	
			x10	
			x8	
	Chosen Exercise		x6	
	Intensity Set		x12	
ABS	Crunch Medicine Ball Crunch	Stability Ball Crunch Abdominal Oblique	x12	
			x10	
			x8	
	Chosen Exercise		x6	
	Intensity Set		x12	

UPPER-BODY EXERCISES

CHEST

Barbell Bench Press	Incline Dumbbell Bench Press
Barbell Incline Press	Push-Up
Dumbbell Fly	

BACK

Back Extension	Pull-Up
Lat Pull-Down	Seated Cable Row
One-Arm Dumbbell Row	Superman

SHOULDERS

Front Raise	Seated Dumbbell Press
Military Press	Upright Barbell Row
Rear Dumbbell Raise	

BICEPS

Cable Curl	Standing Barbell Curl
Concentration Curl	Standing Dumbbell Curl
Preacher Curl	

TRICEPS

Dip	Triceps Push-Down
Lying Triceps Extension	Seated Triceps Extension

LOWER-BODY EXERCISES

QUADRICEPS

Dumbbell Squat	Leg Press
Leg Extension	

HAMSTRINGS

High-Knee Step-Up	Lunge
Leg Curl	

GLUTES

High-Knee Step-Up	Squat
Lunge	

CALVES

Dumbbell Calf Raise	Standing Calf Raise
Seated Dumbbell Raise	

ABS

Abdominal Oblique	Medicine-Ball Crunch
Crunch	Stability Ball Crunch

Barbell Bench Press

The barbell bench press is probably the most popular iron-pumping exercise in the gym. It is a tried-and-true exercise for building and toning your chest (pecs), the front of your shoulders, and the back of your upper arms (triceps).

THE TECHNIQUE

Lie with your back flat on the bench and your feet firmly placed on the ground.

Grab the barbell above you with the grip slightly wider than your shoulders. Lift the barbell off the rack and in a slow, controlled movement, lower it to your chest about nipple height.

Just before the barbell touches your chest, press the bar upward to a locked elbow position.

Repeat the desired number of reps.

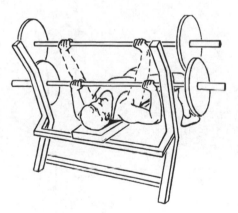

DR. Z SAYS . . . "Keep your feet flat on the ground and don't arch your back. Doing so may result in sprain/strain issues in the lower back."

Dumbbell Bench Press

The dumbbell bench press is a great chest toner and builder. Besides building the muscles that fan across the chest—the pectoralis (pecs)—the press is a great exercise to strengthen other stabilizing muscles involved in daily activities.

THE TECHNIQUE

Sit at the end of the bench with the dumbbells resting on your lower thigh. In one motion kick the weights up as you lie down on the bench. Position the dumbbells to the sides of your chest with your arms bent under each dumbbell.

Now press the dumbbells up with the elbows until the arms are extended—where the weights now almost touch.

Lower the weights to the sides of the upper chest until you feel the pecs (chest) stretch. Repeat for the desired number of reps.

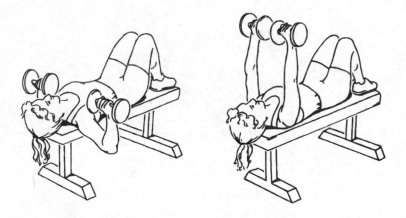

DR. Z SAYS . . . "Use a full range of motion here. When you are done, don't drop the weights. Instead, twist the dumbbells so your palms are facing each other. Now, while lying, lift your knees up and place weights on your knees. Push your upper body up while pressing weights into your thighs. This creates momentum to get up without dropping the weights."

Incline Dumbbell Bench Press

Just like the flat-bench dumbbell press, the incline press is fantastic for chest development, more specifically the upper chest (pecs).

THE TECHNIQUE

Sit at the end of the bench with the dumbbells resting on your lower thigh. In one motion kick the weights up as you lean back on the bench. Position the dumbbells to the sides of your chest with your arms bent under each dumbbell.

Now press the dumbbells up with your elbows until your arms are extended—where the weights now almost touch.

Lower the weights to the sides of the upper chest until you feel the chest (pecs) stretch.

Repeat for the desired number of reps.

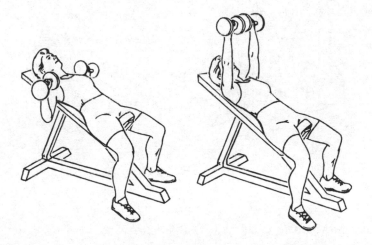

DR. Z SAYS . . . "When you're finished, don't drop the dumbbells; this foolish move may damage the rotator cuffs in your shoulders. Instead, turn the weights so your palms are facing each other, put the weights on your thighs, and then stand up."

Flat Bench Fly

Flat flies are definitely one of my favorites for toning and building the outer, middle, and lower parts of the chest. This exercise really forces the chest muscles to work.

THE TECHNIQUE

Sit at the end of the bench with the dumbbells resting on your lower thighs. In one motion kick the weights up as you lie down on the bench. While lying on the bench, support the weights above you with your hands facing each other.

Lower the dumbbells out to your sides until the pecs are stretched, with the elbows in a slightly bent position. Once at the bottom, repeat for the desired number of reps.

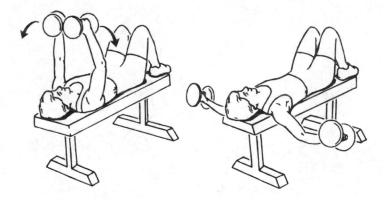

DR. Z SAYS . . . "After your last rep, with the dumbbells now above you, bring up your knees. In one motion, drop your legs and sit up at the same time, placing the dumbbells on top of your thighs. This is a safe way to get up when you are lifting heavier weights."

Lat Pull-Down

If you want to build a nice-looking, muscular, strong back, the lat pull-down is a key exercise. This exercise works the latissimus dorsi or "lats," which are responsible for giving the back a "V" shape. This movement also works, to a lesser extent, the shoulders and arms.

THE TECHNIQUE

Sit on the seat and work your knees under the thigh pads so you fit comfortably underneath them. The thigh pads prevent the weights from pulling you off the seat.

Grab the cable bar with a medium to wide grip. You should just about reach the bar when seated. If you can't, try adjusting the thigh pads before sitting. Grip the bar at your desired width and then let your body weight pull you down into the seat with your knees sliding under the thigh pads.

Keeping your back straight, pull the bar down to the upper part of your back. Slowly return the bar to the original position, while feeling your arms stretch up.

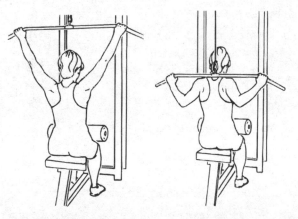

DR. Z SAYS . . . "When pulling the weight down, try not to push your head forward. This puts stress on the neck and joints of the shoulders. Try the same pull-down with the bar in front of your upper chest."

Pull-Up

Okay, pull-ups are hard to do. But, just like the lat pull-down, the pull-up is an excellent exercise for building and strengthening your back. You can use the other back exercises to condition yourself in order to get going on the pull-up bar. Having too much weight to your body and not enough strength creates frustration when trying to do pull-ups. Get rid of the fat, and build and strengthen your body so you can add this to your routine.

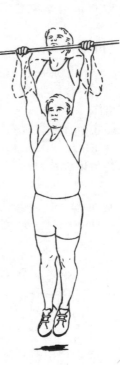

THE TECHNIQUE

This is pretty straightforward.

Grab the pull-up bar with your hands placed about shoulder-width apart and your palms facing away from you.

Pull yourself upward until your chin is over the bar. Complete the exercise by slowly moving to the hanging position, so your arms and shoulders are fully extended.

Repeat for the desired number of reps.

DR. Z SAYS . . . "Accomplishing a pull-up is empowering. Strive to do not just one but sets of them that are part of your routine. Gyms have pull-up assisted machines to help you get strong enough to do them on your own. As Nike says . . . just do it!"

Seated Cable Row

The seated cable row is another one of those "must do" exercises for training the muscles of the back. Like the squat for your legs, the cable row is a great compound exercise. Compound exercises are multijoint movements that involve action and stability from many muscle groups. The cable row hits the lats, postural muscles, rear shoulder muscles overlying the shoulder blades, and muscles in the arms.

THE TECHNIQUE

Sit on the bench with your hips back and your knees slightly bent, with your feet vertical on the platform. Now reach for the handles of the bar or cable attachment. You will feel a slight stretch in your hamstrings and low back.

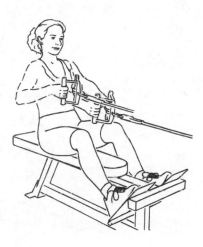

Pull the cable attachment to your lower chest and at the same time straighten yourself up—all in one movement. While pulling, pull your shoulders back and push your chest forward while slightly arching your back.

Return the cable attachment back to the starting position so your arms are extended, your shoulders are stretched, and your low back is flexed forward.

Repeat for desired number of reps.

DR. Z SAYS . . . "Try not to hyperextend when pulling back or round your back when extending your arms. This can put unnecessary force into the joints of your spine and aggravate any back problems you may have."

Superman

The Man of Steel is not the only one who can have great posture. This is a great exercise to strengthen the muscles of the lower back, as well as to tone your glutes and hamstrings. Don't be fooled; this exercise is harder than it looks, but it is a must-do.

THE TECHNIQUE

Lie facedown on the floor with your arms extended and your legs together—also extended. Keep your head and neck in a neutral position.

Keeping your limbs straight and your upper body stationary; simultaneously lift your arms and legs up toward the ceiling, forming a curve with your body. Exhale as you lift your legs and arms. Hold for a count of 10 and don't forget to breathe. Inhale and lower your limbs to the ground to complete a rep.

Repeat for the desired number of reps.

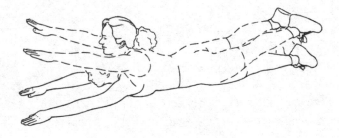

DR. Z SAYS . . . "This is a great exercise for anyone suffering from back problems. It helps to restore normal joint movement and strengthens the muscles that support the spine, making it a great therapeutic exercise."

Stability Ball Extension

An alternative to the Superman exercises is extension on a stability (or yoga) ball. This exercise strengthens the back of your shoulder (or rear delts) and the muscles of the middle back. This is another great posture builder.

THE TECHNIQUE

Kneel on the ground and lean over an exercise ball while grabbing dumbbells placed next to the ball. Raise your torso away from the ball; at the same time, lift your arms up and away from the ball.

Return your torso (upper body) to the ball and repeat for the desired number of reps.

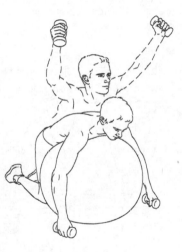

DR. Z SAYS . . . "When lifting your arms, rotate your hands so your palms are facing down holding the weights in a horizontal position. The obvious hazard here is letting the ball roll away from you during the exercise. Pay attention. To prevent the ball from rolling away from you, wedge a pair of shoes under the front edge."

Back Extension

Just like the Superman exercise, back extension on a bench is a great way to strengthen your lower back and postural muscles.

THE TECHNIQUE

Before getting on the bench, set the height of the pads no higher than the top of your pelvis (bones of your waist).

Get yourself into position on the back-extension bench by standing in front of the pads, then resting your thighs on the pads while securing your feet behind you. Ask for assistance if you are unsure.

Start with your back and spine straight. Slowly lower your upper body down until your upper body is pointing to the ground. Now raise yourself back up to the starting position using the low-back muscles in a slow, controlled movement.

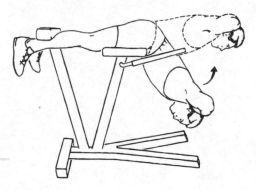

DR. Z SAYS . . . "Don't force yourself up too far, forcing an exaggerated curve in your low back. To do so may stress the joints in your low back, causing a sprain/strain issue and pain."

Barbell Military Press

One of the best exercises for shoulder development and strength is the military press. For many years, the press was a measure of your upper-body power, and it still is today. When effectively executed, the military press works mainly the shoulders, and secondly the triceps (back of the arm) and your abs.

THE TECHNIQUE

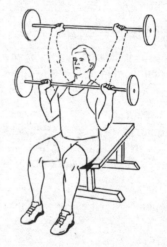

Grab a barbell with an overhand grip slightly wider than your shoulders and sit on a bench. Position the barbell in front of your upper chest.

With your feet firmly planted on the ground, press the bar upward until your arms are extended overhead. Exhale as you lift. Lower the bar back to the chest. To give yourself a little more strength through the lift, tighten up your abs.

Repeat for the desired number of reps.

DR. Z SAYS . . . "You can perform this standing, or seated in front of a Smith machine (see page 298). If you have lower back problems, you are better off doing this one seated."

Dumbbell Front Raise

Along with looking good, the front of the shoulders (or "front delts") are involved with activities of daily living like lifting a grocery bag or briefcase. The key to this exercise is form, so use light weights and slow, controlled movement.

THE TECHNIQUE

Grasp dumbbells in both hands and position them in front of the upper legs with your elbows straight or slightly bent.

Raise the dumbbells forward and upward until your arms are above horizontal. Exhale as you lift. Then, slowly lower the weight back down to the starting position.

Repeat for the desired number of reps.

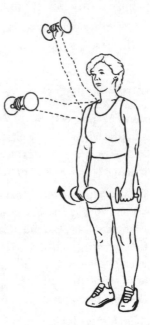

DR. Z SAYS . . . "Focus on moving only your shoulders, and avoid swinging the weights. That can injure your shoulders and low back."

Rear Dumbbell Raise

Not all shoulder exercises are created equal. Most people train the front and the side deltoids, neglecting the rear deltoid. There are three heads to the deltoid muscle—front, medial, and posterior. All three need to be trained equally if you want nice, well-rounded shoulders.

THE TECHNIQUE

Grab dumbbells and sit at the end of a bench with your feet placed beyond your knees. While bent over with your torso on your thighs, position the dumbbells behind your feet. Grip the dumbbells with a slight bend in your elbows and your palms facing down.

Begin by raising your arms to the sides until your elbows are at shoulder height. Maintain the fixed position of your elbows, and keep the upper arm perpendicular throughout the movement.

Lower and repeat for the desired number of reps.

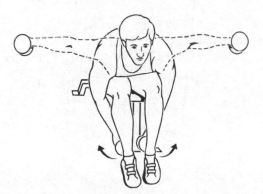

DR. Z SAYS . . . "Keep your torso against your thighs. If you position your torso at, say, 45 degrees, you are not targeting the rear deltoid. Keep your body down and your feet forward, forcing your torso down on your thighs."

Barbell Upright Row

The upright row is one of the best compound exercises emphasizing the upper traps (the "massage my shoulders" muscles) and the deltoids. The upright row can help you fully develop the shoulders and trapezius muscles evenly.

THE TECHNIQUE

With an overhand grip, pick up a barbell with your hands shoulder-width apart.

Keep your back straight and eyes facing forward. Now lift the barbell straight up with your elbows leading. Allow your wrists to flex as the bar rises.

Lower and repeat for the desired number of reps.

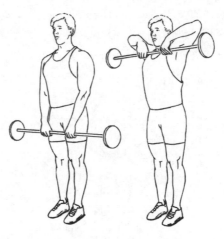

DR. Z SAYS . . . "Focus on keeping your elbows higher than your forearms. Also, don't lean forward or back, because the movement of your body makes the exercise easier. At the top, pause and squeeze the traps and shoulders for a little more intensity."

Barbell Curl

The barbell curl is the meat-and-potatoes exercise for your biceps, and it is a favorite exercise because of the high visibility your upper arms get. As it sounds, the biceps are composed of two heads—the short head and the long head.

THE TECHNIQUE

While standing upright, grip a barbell with palms up, just beyond shoulder width, and elbows to your sides.

While holding your upper arm stationary, curl the bar up until it is at shoulder level. Exhale as you lift.

When the bar is being lifted, you should feel the front of your upper arm or biceps contract.

Once completed, slowly lower the bar to the starting position for the next repetition.

Repeat for the desired number of reps.

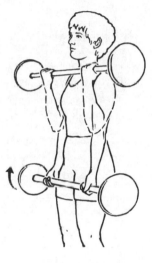

DR. Z SAYS . . . "Form is key here! To help lift the weight, many people sway during the lift, which can injure your lower back. To prevent this, tighten up your abs during both lifting up and lowering down of the bar."

Concentration Curl

The concentration curl is a fantastic exercise for isolating just the biceps. It is the exercise of choice for maximum biceps stimulation, as well as to build the peak of the biceps. Because you can isolate the biceps, you can use it to resolve any asymmetries in your arms, for example, if one arm is bigger than the other.

THE TECHNIQUE

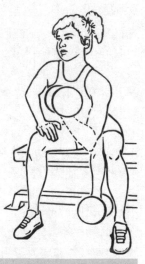

Sit on a bench with feet apart. Grasp a dumbbell between your feet while placing the back of your left upper arm to your left inside thigh.

Raise (curl) the dumbbell to the front shoulder. Then lower the dumbbell until the arm is fully extended.

Repeat for the desired number of reps, then switch arms.

DR. Z SAYS . . . "Breathe out when curling the weight. At the top of the contraction, hold the position for a second as you squeeze the biceps. Avoid swinging motions at any time."

Preacher Curl

The preacher curl is a variation of the barbell curl that you do sitting on a curl bench. This is also a great exercise to isolate the biceps for strength and building the upper arm. As a variation, this can also be done with single dumbbells.

THE TECHNIQUE

Set up your barbell on the preacher bench. Sit on the bench and grab the bar, palms up and hands shoulder-width apart.

Raise (curl) the bar until the forearms are vertical; at the same time, squeeze the biceps. Now slowly lower the barbell until your arms are fully extended.

Repeat for the desired number of reps.

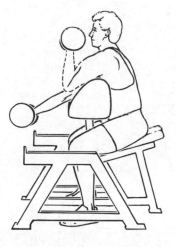

DR. Z SAYS . . . "When lowering the barbell, be careful not to overextend your elbows. This can cause stress on the lower biceps tendon where it attaches near the elbow. Right at the bottom of the movement, leave a slight bend in your arms to take away the physical stress put on the tendons."

Triceps Push-Down

The triceps push-down is one of the best exercises to build the back of the arm (triceps). Like it sounds, the triceps is composed of three different heads that give the classic "horseshoe" appearance when the arm is extended. This is a great exercise to help "turkey arm" syndrome.

THE TECHNIQUE

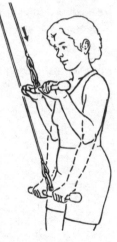

While facing the triceps machine, grasp the cable bar with an overhand grip. The starting point is about chest level.

Keep your feet at or slightly wider than shoulder width, and keep your elbows to your sides.

Start with light weights to see how this exercise works.

Brace your body by tightening up your stomach (abs). Now push down on the handle until your elbows are fully extended.

Allow the bar to come back to a starting point with a controlled movement.

Repeat for desired number of reps.

DR. Z SAYS . . . "Bend your knees slightly while you push down on the bar, and stay upright as much as possible. Try not to bend forward too much while pushing down, as this might be rough on your shoulders and lower back."

Barbell Lying Triceps Extension

The lying triceps extension is one of the best triceps builders there is. Period. During this exercise, most people have a tendency to let their elbows flare out. Before you start, remember to keep your elbows in, and don't lock your elbows at the top of the movement. By doing so, you take tension away from the triceps, the muscles you are trying to build.

THE TECHNIQUE

Lie on your back on a bench so your head is at the end of the bench. With a barbell on the ground at the head of the bench, reach back and grasp the barbell with palms facing up. Lift the barbell up so it's positioned over your forehead with your arms extended.

With the arms fully extended, lower the bar by bending the elbows. As the bar comes close to your head, bring it back slightly so it just clears the curvature of your head. Now as the bar clears your head, extend the arms fully. Repeat for the desired number of reps.

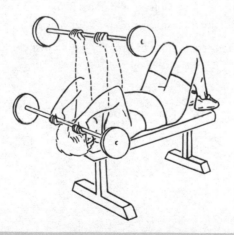

DR. Z SAYS . . . "Inhale as you lower the bar by bending at the elbows, and exhale as you push the bar up to an extended-arm position. Only your forearms should move; your upper arms should remain stationary."

Dumbbell Triceps Extension

Here's another triceps isolation exercise. Among all the triceps exercises to choose from, this particular movement is sure to tone and build the back of your arms. The key to getting the benefits out of this exercise is form.

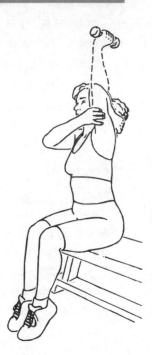

THE TECHNIQUE

Sit on a seat or bench. While holding a dumbbell in your left hand, position the dumbbell overhead with your arm straight up or slightly back. At the same time, take your opposite hand and support the back of the arm to be extended. This helps prevent movement of the whole arm when extending.

Lower the dumbbell behind the neck or shoulder while maintaining your upper arm's vertical position throughout the exercise. Extend the arm until your arm is straight.

Repeat for the desired number of reps, and then switch arms.

DR. Z SAYS . . . "When you lower the dumbbell, let it pull your arm down and back to get a nice stretch in the triceps. If done correctly, you should feel this only in the triceps."

Dip

The dip is a great compound movement that works multiple muscles in the upper body, like the chest, shoulder, and triceps. You can use the dip to build your chest muscles, or you can use it as a triceps exercise.

THE TECHNIQUE

Get up on the parallel bars with your torso perpendicular to the floor. This will isolate the triceps. If you lean forward, you will emphasize your chest and shoulders.

While supporting yourself, bend your knees and cross your feet behind you. Slowly lower your body until your shoulder joints are just even with your elbows. Now push back up until your elbows are nearly straight but not locked.

Repeat for the desired number of reps.

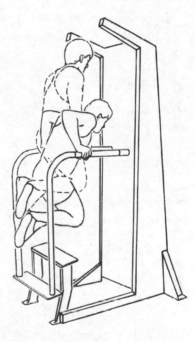

DR. Z SAYS . . . "For some, this may be tough on the shoulders and pecs. If you are feeling pain with this movement, consider another exercise. If you have no pain or pre-existing shoulder problem, the dip is superb for the triceps, chest, and shoulders."

Barbell Squat

If you're not squatting, you're not training. The squat is a superb exercise that targets not only the upper thighs (quads) and the buttocks or glutes; it works the whole body. The major bonus with this exercise is that it not only burns a lot of calories; it burns fat. Squats can be done with a barbell as seen, on a Smith machine, or holding dumbbells or kettlebells.

THE TECHNIQUE

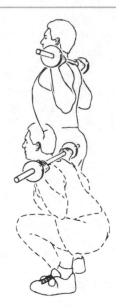

Place the barbell just above your shoulders, resting it on the upper-back or trapezius muscles. If that is uncomfortable, wrap a towel around the bar to protect your upper back.

Stand with your feet roughly shoulder-width apart and slightly turned out.

Bend your knees and lower into a squat position. Stop when your knees are at 90 degrees. Try to keep the natural curve in the low back.

Stabilize the bar with your upper body, and push with your legs and glutes to a standing position while keeping your knees in line with your toes.

Repeat for the desired number of reps.

DR. Z SAYS . . . "Always start light; you can add weight as you learn good form and get stronger. Make sure your knees line up with your feet, which are slightly pointed out. When coming down, try to maintain the curve in your low back. If the weight is too heavy, it will force your back into an unnatural position."

Leg Press

The leg press is a compound movement to strengthen your quads (thighs) and glutes (butt). This is a great exercise to prepare you for all sports, including skiing, biking, sprinting, and all other activities that require lower-body strength.

THE TECHNIQUE

After putting weighted plates on the machine, sit with your back on padded support. Place your feet on the platform. The higher you place your feet, the more hamstring and glute involvement; the lower your foot placement, the more quad involvement. Push with your feet, extending your hips and knees. Release the dock (support) lever and grab the handle to the sides.

Lower the sled by flexing your hips and knees until your knees are close to your chest. At the bottom of this movement, push to extend your knees and hips.

Repeat for the desired number or reps.

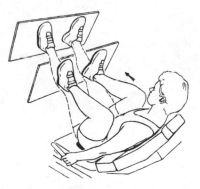

DR. Z SAYS . . . "To prevent excessive stress on your knees and low back, avoid lowering your legs too close to your torso. Allow your thighs to touch the outside of your lower ribs."

Leg Extension

If you are looking to build and shape the front of your thighs, leg extensions will get the job done.

THE TECHNIQUE

Sit on the machine with your back against the padded support. Place the front of your lower legs under the padded lever. The back of your knees should be positioned at the front end of the seat. Grasp the side handles for support and to keep yourself on the seat.

Extend your legs until your knees are straight. Hold that for a count of three, then slowly return the padded lever to its original position by bending your knees.

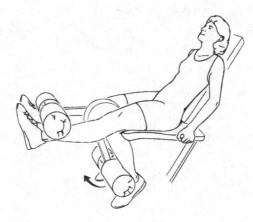

DR. Z SAYS . . . "To avoid issues with your knees or low back, make sure your back is firmly pressed against the seat back. While lifting, don't wobble or sway side to side. Adjust the lower limb pads so they are not too far up your shins. Don't do this exercise if your knees hurt."

Lying Leg Curl

Having great thighs doesn't mean a thing if you don't have nice hamstrings. The lying leg curl is an isolated exercise used to tone and build the backs of your thighs. The hamstrings are the legs' biceps.

THE TECHNIQUE

Position your body on the leg-curl machine facing down. Adjust the leg pads, so they are at the lowest part of your calves.

Grab the handles on the bench, and pull the weight up toward your body. Feel the hamstring contract, and squeeze at the top position.

From the top position, slowly lower the weight back down to the starting position.

Repeat for the desired number of reps.

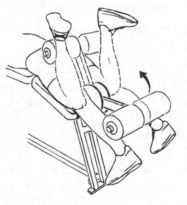

DR. Z SAYS . . . "Use the full range of motion here, by curling the weight as high as possible—almost until the pads are touching your buttocks. Allow yourself the full stretch at the bottom."

Standing Calf Raise

Calves—either you got 'em or you don't. Those who didn't inherit the calf gene are going to need to do a little work. The calf muscles—gastrocnemius and soleus—are tough to develop and, therefore, require very specific training. The standing calf raise is the gold standard in calf development.

THE TECHNIQUE

Standing calf raises can be done on a Smith machine (as shown), on a standing calf machine, off a step, or by holding dumbbells. When executing Smith machine calf raises, set the bar on the Smith machine to shoulder height. Put a step or calf block below the bar.

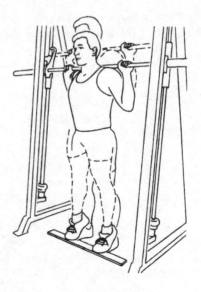

Step on the block and position the balls of your feet on the edge, pointing your toes slightly inward. Get yourself under the Smith bar, so the bar is across your shoulders. Now push the weight off the rack, and drop your heels down as far as possible. Slowly raise your heels as high as you can go, squeezing your calf muscles at the top. Slowly lower your heels back to the starting position.

Repeat for the desired number of reps.

DR. Z SAYS . . . "When lowering your heels, don't bounce or come down too hard, as this may put too much stress on the Achilles tendon. Squeeze your calves at the top for maximum effect."

Seated Dumbbell Calf Raise

The calves contain a deep muscle (soleus) and a superficial muscle (gastrocnemius), which you see when the calves contract. The soleus gives the calf width, while the gastrocs give the calf the diamond shape. The seated dumbbell calf raise is the best way to add some girth to your calves.

THE TECHNIQUE

Sit on the edge of a bench and place the balls of your feet on a 2x4 or a step platform. Place a pair of dumbbells on top of both knees. Lower your heels as low as you can to feel the stretch. Push off with your toes, lifting your heels while contracting the calves.

Lower your heels to the starting position again.

Repeat for the desired number of reps. If you need heavier weights, find the seated calf bench.

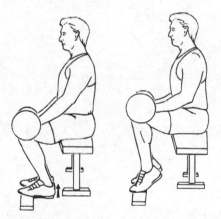

DR. Z SAYS . . . "The calves are dense and super strong, so make sure you stress them. When dropping your heels, go slow and don't bounce. To do so may injure your Achilles tendon."

Medicine Ball Crunch

Here's another variation of the crunch for your abdominals. This is a little more challenging because you are holding a weighted medicine ball. Try this with a 4-, 6-, or 8-pound ball.

THE TECHNIQUE

Hold a small medicine ball against your chest. Position yourself with feet flat on the ground and knees about shoulder-width apart.

Contract your abs while holding the ball against your chest; at the same time, exhale. As you exhale, really squeeze your abs; hold for a second or two, then slowly lower yourself back down.

Repeat for the desired number of reps.

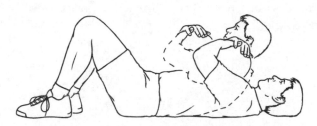

DR. Z SAYS . . . "Again, form is key here. When raising your chest, contract those abs while exhaling. You are sure to get a good 'burn.'"

Stability Ball Crunch

For those with lower back issues, this is a great alternative to floor crunches.

THE TECHNIQUE

Secure an exercise ball with foam wedges or sneakers to prevent it from rolling back. Sit back on the ball, keeping your feet and knees shoulder-width apart, and interlock your fingers behind your head.

While holding yourself in place on the ball, contract your abs, raising yourself about 30 degrees. Exhale on the way up, and inhale on the way back.

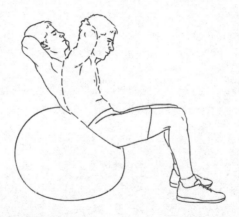

DR. Z SAYS . . . "When performing the crunch, keep from moving on the ball. Just use it to support yourself. Exhale when you crunch, and inhale on the way back."

Abdominal Oblique

To tone and develop sexy abs, you need to work the muscles on the sides of the abdominals (the obliques). If you have "love handles," that fat has covered this important muscle group. If you are a woman looking for the hourglass figure, or a gent who wants that "V" shape, get to work on your obliques.

THE TECHNIQUE

Sit on an exercise ball. Walk forward with your feet to position the ball in the middle of your back. At the same time, interlock your fingers and place your hands behind your head. Your head should be positioned horizontally to your body.

In this position, contract your abdominals and flex at the waist. At the same time, twist slightly, bringing your left elbow toward the opposite side of your body.

Repeat for the desired number of reps, changing sides. The crunches can also be done alternating: left to right, right to left.

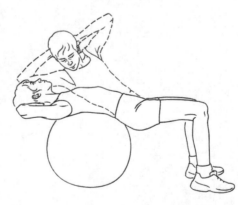

DR. Z SAYS . . . "Don't pull on your head or neck; use your abs. To really work your abs and obliques, try holding a weight or medicine ball (5 to 10 pounds) against your chest. Holding the weight, contract your abs while exhaling."

Summary

Before you start your exercise program, here is a summary of the steps you should follow to rebuild yourself using high-intensity interval training. Make sure you remember to eat a serving of protein and complex carbs at least 60 to 90 minutes before your workout. If you don't get your blood sugar up and glycogen stored in your muscles, your body will release cortisol, which breaks down muscles to produce fuel for the brain. Second, eat protein, complex carbs, and some fruit after the workout to help quickly refuel the muscles with glycogen.

HIIT involves starting at a slow pace for 2 minutes, speeding up the exercise to a moderate level for 1 minute, and going all-out for 1 minute. After this high-intensity set, throttle down and start the process again at a slow pace for 2 minutes, speed up to a moderate pace for 1 minute, and, again, exercise with maximum effort for 1 minute. Following the high-intensity set, throttle back down to the slow level. Do this routine five times for a total of 20 minutes.

Every other day, do the same high-intensity program with weights. On one day, train the upper body, the next day the lower body. Take off a day or two to recover. Without recovery time, you may be prone to aches, pain, sprains, and strains, so let the body heal. During this healing time, make sure you eat very clean foods, including protein, complex carbs, fats, vegetables, and low-sugar fruits loaded with anti-oxidants (blueberries, blackberries, and strawberries).

By incorporating high-intensity training into your daily habits and rituals, you will experience an incredible change in your body composition. Exercise and HIIT will also help you quickly rebuild your health and improve your internal terrain to prevent a future recurrence and any other chronic health issues, which is the true prize. I hope your transformation creates changes in all aspects of your life—mind, body, and spirit.

5

Re-action #3
Hit the Brakes on the Stress Response

Okay, stress: How bad can it be? At one point I thought I was on top of the world. I had just received board certification in neurology, and my practice was the busiest it had ever been. My patients were getting well, and referrals were at an all-time high. The fruits of my work allowed me to purchase a new home and still sock away money for a rainy day. I was also involved in a relationship that was moving in the right direction, or so I thought.

Then my world began to implode. At the busiest time of my career, I discovered that a trusted employee was stealing from me and her insurance company to support a very well-hidden drug habit—heroin addiction. In the midst of major renovations on my new house, my relationship turned sour. Dealing with stress both at the office and at home—day after day, week after week, month after month—became the norm.

I plugged along in the office and at home, but I kept my thoughts and emotions bottled up, my usual MO. It never occurred to me that stress could contribute to a life-threatening situation. Months later, long after those crises were over, I began to feel "off." My strength in the gym wasn't quite right, and I was often reaching for a little extra caffeine and B vitamins to help boost my energy.

Around that time, a friend asked if I was intentionally losing weight.

As time passed, I began to feel more tired than usual, as though I had the flu or was fighting an infection. I began to get major headaches when bending over, which I'd never had before.

One night I was awakened by a sheet-drenching sweat. I was startled to feel the bed soaked, as if someone had hosed me down in the middle of the night. Now I knew something was seriously wrong. That week I had my blood tested, and found that my lactate dehydrogenase, a biomarker indicating tissue destruction, was off the charts. I called a radiologist and had an X-ray of my chest done. As we viewed the result, he pointed to the film and said, "You have a giant tumor in your chest."

We often hear stress is dangerous, but to my mind, here was the disturbing proof.

The Deadly Effects of Stress

Stress and the stress response have multiple effects, and have been implicated in a wide variety of health issues, from cancer and heart disease to a leaky gut and slow wound healing. Stress adds to your internal environment a psychological factor that can cause disease.

Think about it: our busy lives are full of deadlines, frustrations, and demands. We live in stressful times; for many people, constant high stress is a way of life. You are sitting in an audience, and the speakers blast a high-pitched squeal—you cringe. You take your eye off the traffic light for a second, and the impatient driver behind you blasts the horn. An hour before that important exam, your stomach churns, and you head for the bathroom. Sound familiar? We've all had a physical response to some experience. The experience is the stressor; the physical response is the stress reaction.

Stress is a perception of a momentary threat, which creates an adaptive response in the body to ensure survival—for example, shivering when you get cold, or sweating when you get too hot. The stressor can be physical (an infection, toxin, or trauma) or emotional (abuse, anger, guilt, fear, loss of a loved one). The stress reaction is the body's way of preparing itself for "fight or flight." Stress becomes a health hazard only when stressors are constant and the physical stress response doesn't stop. When we don't return to a normal pre-stress set point, the result is disease.

Stress has always been considered in a negative light; in reality, it helps to maintain the natural workings of the body. There are positive stimuli that are considered stressors; exercise is the best example. This form of stimulus causes changes in the body to adapt to the demands of the physical activity. This form of stress has beneficial effects. The heart rate goes up; hormones are released to maintain blood sugar; and blood vessels dilate to send blood to the skeletal muscles, supplying them with oxygen and glucose. This type of stress is natural. Once the physical activity stops, the body returns to a normal state of functioning.

Negative stimuli, like emotional stressors, also create physiological changes in response to a specific event. Under emotional stress, the brain and body release targeted hormones, along with other brain chemicals, in response to the perceived threat. These acute stress reactions and ensuing hormones are temporary. Once the threat has passed, the body should come back to the normal state.

Let's take a look at your stress hormones. The three that contribute to the creation and progression of all chronic disease are adrenaline (epinephrine), noradrenaline (norepinephrine), and cortisol. All three come from the adrenal glands, located above your kidneys.

ADRENALINE: Under stress, adrenaline causes an increased heart rate and constriction of blood vessels; it dilates your air passages and increases your energy.

NOREPINEPHRINE: Norepinephrine helps to provide energy, and increases your heart rate, as well as oxygen to the brain and blood flow to the muscles.

CORTISOL: Cortisol helps to increase blood sugar while the body is under stress; aids in the breakdown of protein, fat, and carbohydrates, which provide us with energy; and acts as an anti-inflammatory.

The stress reaction in the body is vastly complex, involving different organs, metabolic systems, and hormones. Momentary stressors cause a quick squirt of stress hormones into the bloodstream to prepare for the threat. Typically, the physical symptoms of stress include aches and pains, dizziness, diarrhea or constipation, chest pain, and rapid heartbeat. Emotional symptoms of stress include anxiety, moodiness, irritability, and agitation.

The danger occurs when your stressors cause the constant release of hormones, similar to a dripping faucet. The long-term stress reaction becomes maladaptive. This is when stress causes disease. So how bad can stress be? Let's start with the gut.

STRESS AND LEAKY GUT

As an acute threat, stress can have both a short- and long-term influence on the function of the gastrointestinal tract. Under stressful situations, the hormones cortisol, adrenaline, and norepinephrine communicate with the immune system, causing the release of histamine and prostaglandins. These compounds create the miserable symptoms of seasonal allergies. They also increase intestinal permeability, causing leaky gut. As you remember, leaky gut allows harmful substances to pass from the gut into the body, setting the stage for a major immune dysfunction. Studies found in the *Journal of Gastroenterology and Hepatology* paint a clear picture of the influence of the stress reaction, gut function, and disease. Long- and short-term stressors cause leaky gut, reduced water, sodium and calcium absorption, and reduced blood flow into the gut. Stress has also been shown to contribute to reflux, dyspepsia, and stomach ulcers.

Everyone perceives and reacts to stress in different ways. They also have different ways to deal with stress. Some people eat foods high in sugar, salt, and fat, while others drink alcohol or smoke cigarettes to take the edge off. Some patients I see choose meditation, yoga, and exercise. Not all forms of exercise are beneficial, however. Quite often we think more is better when it comes to healthful activities. This is not the case with long durations of exercise. A study published in the *Journal of Applied Physiology* looked at athletes competing in a triathlon consisting of a 2.4-mile open-water swim, followed by a 112-mile bicycle ride, and finishing with a 26.2-mile run. At the end of the event, the athletes were given a sugar solution containing lactulose and rhamnose to drink. Researchers found these sugars leaked through the athletes' gut into the blood.

STRESS AND INFLAMMATION

When we think of inflammation, it brings to mind swelling, redness, pain, sunburn, or a sprained ankle—all local inflammatory responses. Systemic inflammation, on the other hand, is a state where the immune system is releasing chemical messengers into the blood, which can change normal functions and contribute to disease processes.

Cytokines are small chemical messengers that transmit information from cell to cell. Cortisol, adrenaline, and norepinephrine are released when we are under stress. Those hormones then stimulate the immune cells to secrete inflammation-promoting cytokines, such as interleukin 1 (IL-1), interleukin 6 (IL-6), and tumor necrosis factor (TNF). Yes, here they are again. These active compounds play a role in the process of inflammation—the driving force behind chronic disease.

STRESS AND THE IMMUNE SYSTEM

Cortisol, the "stress hormone," has multiple effects in the body. It acts as an anti-inflammatory, helps regulate blood sugar, and aids in the metabolism of fat, protein, and carbs. However, when your cortisol level gets too high for long periods of time, it can suppress your immune system and decrease your ability to fight bacteria and viruses. The immune system is your internal armed services. When an invader, like a virus, enters the body, the body responds by sending out a type of white blood cell called a natural killer (NK) cell. Its role is to seek and destroy cells infected by viruses and cancer cells. Under prolonged stress, cortisol suppresses the function of the NK cell, thus allowing viruses to take hold and cancer cells to survive in the body. Individuals under constant stress often have outbreaks of shingles and/or cold sores; for some, stress causes the onset or return of cancer. Data published in *Nature Reviews* indicate that elevated cortisol can increase susceptibility to infectious agents; influence the severity of infectious disease; diminish the strength of immune responses to vaccines; reactivate latent herpes viruses; and slow the healing of wounds.

A study in *Health Psychology* followed 276 volunteers to measure how quickly they would get sick from the common cold virus after acute and chronic stressful life events. The study found that individuals who experienced severe acute stressful events lasting less than a month long were less likely to develop colds. Those who experienced chronic stressors lasting a month or longer were more prone to getting colds.

STRESS AND WOUND HEALING

Multiple studies show how wound healing is affected by stress. A study in the *Lancet* found that in women who took care of a relative with Alzheimer's disease, a 3-millimeter wound took 24 percent longer to heal than in those in the control group. Additional research found in *Psychosomatic Medicine* showed that a common stressor—academic exams—caused small wounds on the hard palate (roof of the mouth) to heal 40 percent slower than the same wounds healed during summer vacation. This collective research shows that psychological stress increases cortisol and reduces certain chemical messengers needed for tissue repair and healing.

STRESS AND THE CANCER MICROENVIRONMENT

Stress plays a major role in all steps of the development and progression of cancer. A study published in *Nature Reviews* found that the release of stress hormones can compromise DNA repair mechanisms, leading to the development of cancer. As cancer develops into a tumor, the hormones cortisol, adrenaline, and norepinephrine have a major impact on the biology of the tumor and its surrounding environment.

NK cells and cytotoxic T (CT) cells, another group of cancer-killing white blood cells, recognize cancer cells by a certain ligand (flag) on the cells' surface and target them for destruction. Like NK cells, CT cells attach to the cancer cell and inject powerful enzymes into it, eventually leading the cancer cell to cause its own cell death. Cortisol, adrenaline, and norepinephrine reduce the ability of NK cells and CT cells to "see" cancer cells and tumors. Research in the *Lancet* found that the stress-induced suppression of NK cell activity caused tumor development.

Adrenaline and norepinephrine have been shown to increase angiogenesis, the development of blood vessels to feed tumors. These hormones were also found to protect cancer cells from their programmed cell suicide (apoptosis).

Last, when cancer cells metastasize from their original site, they can survive only if the environment favors their survival. A research study published in *Cancer Research* demonstrated epinephrine not only suppressed the immune system when cancer cells were on the move but also removed any roadblocks regarding movement and migration of cancer cells, allowing the process of metastasis to happen.

I'm just scratching the surface of the role of the stress reaction on the cancer microenvironment. The stress reaction is also fueled by a secondary source: cytokines and inflammation. The pro-inflammatory cytokines IL-1, IL-6, and TNF all contribute to the development of tumors. The role of IL-6 in cancer cell proliferation and survival is well documented. The *Journal of Clinical Investigation* states that IL-6 plays a pivotal role in the development of Kaposi's sarcoma and multiple myeloma. IL-6 has also been found to contribute to other cancers, such as colon cancer, lymphoma, and breast cancer. IL-1 was found to increase tumor invasiveness and metastasis. At the site of tumor development, IL-1 caused the tumor to adhere to healthy tissue, and it assisted malignant cells in invading distant tissues.

In the same research study, tumor necrosis factor (TNF), another cytokine involved in inflammation, was shown to enhance tumor progression, stimulate angiogenesis and metastasis, and impair the immune system by suppressing the white blood cells responsible for killing cancer cells.

STRESS AND HEART DISEASE

Emotional stress has been linked to increased deaths in those with coronary artery disease and the progression of atherosclerosis. Under stress, the brain fires signals to the adrenal glands, which then spit out cortisol, adrenaline, and norepinephrine. This reaction happens so fast, most people are not aware it's happening. According to a study in *Circulation* and the *Journal of Clinical Endocrinology & Metabolism*, the blast of stress hormones in the body has multiple effects on the coronary arteries and the heart.

Endothelial function was studied in healthy male subjects who were exposed to a mental stress test. Dilation of the arteries (controlled by the endothelium) was measured with high-resolution ultrasound immediately before the mental stress test, as well as 30, 90, and 240 minutes after its completion. Their findings revealed that momentary mental stress and the surge of stress hormones caused a rapid impairment of the endothelium for four hours after the stress diminished. These findings show that short-term emotional stressors—the ones we have every day—have an adverse reaction on the heart.

Mental stress was also shown to cause myocardial ischemia (reduced blood flow to the heart). A study published in *Circulation* followed 196 patients with existing coronary artery disease to determine the effects of mental stress on the oxygen supply to the heart. Participants underwent bicycle exercise and psychological stress testing with radionuclide imaging to compare exercise-induced ischemia to the reduced blood flow to the heart due to the stress reaction. They found mental stress proved to be a more potent stimulus for reducing oxygen to the heart. Their data also revealed patients who had ischemia during mental stress also had an increased mortality rate.

Additional studies regarding the stress reaction and coronary artery disease show cortisol, adrenaline, and norepinephrine all had deleterious effects on the heart. Anger can result in left-ventricle dysfunction and reduced output of blood from the left side of the heart, damage to the arteries, and increased blood pressure. Mental stress elevates cortisol. Cortisol was shown to accelerate atherosclerosis by increasing toxic body fat, thereby causing inflammation and insulin resistance.

STRESS AND DIABETES

It's widely recognized that stressed people with diabetes have a hard time regulating their blood sugar. When you have type 2 diabetes, stress may make your blood sugar go up and become more difficult to control. As a result, you may need to take more diabetes drugs or insulin. Here is where the problem lies: higher levels of cortisol cause cells to become resistant to insulin. The pancreas then struggles to keep up with the high demand for insulin. Your cells don't get the sugar they need, and the cycle continues. High cortisol = ineffective insulin = high blood sugar.

Constant emotional stress and frustration caused by dealing with abnormal blood sugar can wear you down and cause you not only to neglect your diabetes but also to continue eating junk and processed foods, drinking more, or smoking. Sometimes stress and blood sugar changes can be the things that cause you to realize you have a diabetic condition.

STRESS AND BODY COMPOSITION

The prolonged release of cortisol can cause sleep issues, anxiety, muscle wasting, immune suppression, and an increase in belly fat. According to a study in *Obesity Reviews*, chronic stress "inhibits the secretion of growth hormone, testosterone, and 17 beta-estradiol (estrogen), all of which counteract cortisol's effects. The net result is an accumulation of visceral fat." In another research article, from the journal *Psychosomatic Medicine*, researchers found that high cortisol levels cause circulating fat to be deposited deep in the abdomen as visceral fat, the dangerous fat.

Visceral fat has high concentrations of cortisol receptors. When cortisol is high, any circulating fat cells or fatty acids get stored in visceral fat. Visceral fat can wreck your liver. Researchers from the Wake Forest University School of Medicine found that the stress reaction, with its destructive hormones, caused fat cells to be released from the visceral fat and end up in the liver, contributing to glucose intolerance and high insulin.

Finally, cortisol is involved in blood sugar/insulin dysfunction. High blood sugar levels and insulin suppression lead to cells with no energy. No energy causes increased appetite and sometimes eating too many high-calorie foods. Unused energy is stored as fat.

SUSAN'S STORY

Susan K. is an extremely active mother of two who works long hours and enjoys running and cycling. Prior to a scheduled orthopedic surgery, she came to see me with pain in her right shoulder and lower-right back. She also expressed frustration with fatigue, poor sleep, and difficulty dropping some unwanted body fat. Following her consultation, I ordered hormone testing and performed a physical and neurological exam on her to determine the cause of her pain. The hormone testing revealed high cortisol levels throughout the day and into the night. This explained her fatigue, poor sleep, and difficulty losing the fat. Although her diet was pretty good, we redesigned it to fit her lifestyle better. To control the cortisol and get her body to release glucagon, we increased her protein intake to three or four servings a day. She replaced less desirable carbs with high-fiber carbs that didn't spike her blood sugar. Next, she ate before exercising and right after to replenish her energy—keeping her cortisol under control. Finally, she decreased the time she spent exercising and increased the intensity for shorter periods.

As a result, Susan was able to control her cortisol and increase her glucagon levels. In eight weeks she dropped 17 pounds of body fat, had more energy, and started to get a good night's sleep. Her shoulder pain and lower back pain were caused by unresolved muscle imbalances that required joint manipulation and therapeutic exercises. In less than four weeks, she was 90 percent symptom-free, and she canceled the unneeded surgery.

Stress and Autoimmune Disease

Psychological stressors are also implicated in the development of autoimmune disease. In fact, a study in *Autoimmunity Reviews* states that up to 80 percent of those who developed an autoimmune disease reported having uncommon emotional stress beforehand. It is presumed the surge of cortisol, adrenaline, and norepinephrine lead to immune dysregulation and increased cytokine production, resulting in autoimmune disease.

The stress response has also been known to cause an imbalance of inflammatory and anti-inflammatory cytokines. Cortisol, adrenaline, and norepinephrine have been shown to alter the balance between Th1 and Th2 white blood cells and their specific cytokines, tipping the immune response from defense to attacking one's own body—autoimmune disease.

Dr. Z's Tips to Control Stress

How do you deal with stressors? Do you overreact to situations because that's the way you grew up? Do you obsess over situations? Can you compartmentalize the stressors? If you are rebuilding from a major disease, you have to change your perception of stress. The best way of dealing with stress is to manage it as it occurs. Try these methods to prevent the health issues associated with long-term stress.

CHANGE YOUR PERCEPTION. Life is filled with frustration, pain, disappointments, and unpredictable actions of others. You can't change this endless loop, but you can change your perception of the stressor. By doing so, you can minimize the release of cortisol, adrenaline, and norepinephrine, as well as the destructive effects they have on the body.

RELAX. Relaxation is the opposite of stress, and it can create a sense of feeling calm. This can be accomplished by simply sitting quietly doing slow, relaxed breathing or participating in a few sessions of relaxing yoga.

GET A GOOD NIGHT'S SLEEP. Eight hours of sleep each night increases healthy hormones, such as growth hormone. It helps to repair the body and regulates other hormones that control appetite. This is important because, without proper sleep, we tend to eat empty-calorie foods (simple carbohydrates) with no nutritional value.

EAT HEALTHFUL FOOD. Food has a limitless supply of macro- and micro-nutrients to power us throughout the day, but most of us barely tap into this resource. We can all become more efficient eaters in order to function at our best. When we're stressed, it's easy to eat on the run or eat junk food or fast food. However, under stressful conditions, the body needs vitamins and minerals more than ever! For the sake of variety and health, a moderate diet consisting of green vegetables, low-sugar fruits, lean protein, complex carbohydrates, and good fats appears to be better in the long run. Frequent small meals allow a constant source of fuel for the body, as well as energy to power you through your day.

GET REGULAR EXERCISE. Research shows that regular exercise reduces stress hormones. Regular exercise boosts the immune system, increases healthy hormones, lowers blood pressure, and decreases the risk for developing cardiac disease, diabetes, and obesity. Different types of high-intensity exercise can be done for varying lengths of time, depending on how strenuous the activity is. These exercises include dancing, skating, skiing, running, walking, bicycling, stair climbing, weight lifting, boot-camp training or circuit training, and swimming. Basically, any physical activity you can do with resistance, at intervals of low, moderate, and high intensity, will help to reduce stress.

ELIMINATE NEGATIVITY. Create thoughts that build you up and give you abundance. Focus on situations you can control, and get rid of the negative people and talk in your life. Epigenetic research shows we are the product of our thoughts; what we focus on affects the physical body and environment. So think positive, and create your destiny.

MEDITATE. Meditation is a powerful tool for self-transformation. Scientists have found evidence that meditation has a biological effect on the body, changing the state of the brain and the autonomic (involuntary) nervous system. Researchers believe that these changes account for meditation's positive effects. The National Institutes of Health reports that regular meditation can reduce chronic pain, anxiety, blood pressure, substance abuse, posttraumatic stress response, and the blood levels of stress hormones.

TRY GUIDED ACTIVE BREATHING. A new method of therapy has emerged that combines traditional talk therapy with guided breathing, while surrounded by relaxing and emotion-provoking music to help in the "emotional retraining" session. The method involves a skilled professional who gives breathing instructions (which involve you actively) while helping you process your stressors and hidden emotions or memories through talk and soft touch. As a composer conducts an orchestra, the coach guides and moves you through the session, instructing you on the depth and speed of breath while helping you process your thoughts and emotions, until you uncover, process, and pull out that stuck mental splinter. For more information on guided active breathing, check out the work of my wife, Holly Bliss (www.beinbliss.com).

Summary

"Stress kills" is not just a statement found on bumper stickers or thrown around at the local coffee shop. Stress is a real, very combustible fuel that creates and contributes to chronic diseases. Learning to manage stress is a lot more important than finding a way to mask it. Covering up stress with a crutch (i.e., alcohol, medication, and destructive behavior) to alleviate the outward symptoms will do little to improve the situation. It's never too late to learn tools to put stressors in their place.

6

Re-action #4
Reboot Your Internal Clock

I used to think sleeping was meant just to recharge your batteries after a long day. I often thought it was a waste of time. After all, if you sleep away part of the day, there's not enough time left to get everything done. As a society we associate sleeping late with laziness and a poor worth ethic, whereas waking early is equated with success and worth.

However, a poor night's sleep not only makes you feel tired and fatigued; it also increases your risk for developing disease. When you are rebuilding from a chronic health issue, a loss of sleep will hinder your ability to do so, and it may increase your chances of recurrence or an exacerbation of that condition. New research is uncovering the link between sleep deprivation and heart disease, cancer, diabetes, immune dysfunction, obesity, and increased mortality. Sleep is anything but a waste of time.

Sleep Loss and Disease

How much sleep is the right amount? Seven to eight hours per night. Anything less is generally considered to be sleep loss. Too much sleep, or not enough, may be an indication of a more serious health issue. The main symptoms of sleep loss are excessive sleepiness during the day, fatigue, poor memory and concentration, irritability, and often a depressed mood. Not enough sleep can also delay reaction time, and make you distracted, causing mistakes (like spilling scalding coffee on your foot!).

There are many causes of sleep loss; some are self-inflicted, while others have an organic or physical reason.

- External factors that cause sleep loss include your job (e.g., long work hours, jet lag, shift work) and lifestyle behaviors, such as watching TV or spending time online to all hours of the night.
- Emotional stressors that activate the stress response, thus increasing levels of cortisol, norepinephrine, and adrenaline, are known to disrupt the circadian rhythm and sleep clock.
- Food can disrupt sleep. Carbs and high-glycemic refined foods influence blood sugar and insulin, which interfere with the release of melatonin and growth hormone.
- Excessive use of alcohol and other stimulants can interfere with sleep.
- Hormone imbalances, such as low progesterone and high cortisol, can interrupt the sleep cycle.
- Exercising late will increase cortisol and adrenaline—a momentary stress response.
- Sleep apnea from insulin resistance and blood sugar dysregulation will awaken the sleeper throughout the night.
- Conditions, including insomnia and restless leg syndrome (also known as a magnesium deficiency), interfere with getting restful sleep.

Basically, sleep is a reversible period of physical and mental inactivity, whereby we are less responsive to external stimuli. When your mind and body are "offline" during sleep, the body goes through physical changes, including reduction in blood pressure, body temperature, respiration, and heart rate. However, while certain functions of the body slow down during slumber, other activities increase. For example, as soon as you fall asleep, your brain releases growth hormone (GH), which stimulates cell growth and activates cellular regeneration. GH helps regulate metabolism, deflates fat cells, helps regulate blood sugar, and promotes protein synthesis in cells.

Your body has its own internal clock to control its natural sleep-and-wake pattern. This clock also controls how much of the sleep hormone melatonin is produced. Melatonin is secreted into the blood in a rhythmic manner, peaking in the dark hours of the night and dropping during the day. Exposure to light abruptly suppresses the release of melatonin in the body.

During sleep and the release of growth hormone and melatonin, cells are busy repairing themselves, wounds are healing, and the brain is trucking out metabolic waste products at a rapid pace. Unfortunately, because of our fast-paced world, sleep loss has increased in recent years, causing numerous behavioral and physiological changes. Recent studies have reported associations between sleep loss and inflammatory responses as well as the progression of heart disease, cancer, diabetes, obesity, and other chronic health crises.

SLEEP DEPRIVATION AND INFLAMMATION

Inflammation is the key physiological catalyst in all chronic diseases. A high-calorie, nutrient-deficient diet, too much body fat, stress, and a toxic environment all increase levels of inflammation. Research is revealing that partial or total sleep loss increases the inflammatory agents IL-1, IL-6, TNF, and CRP.

Studies in *Brain, Behavior, and Immunity* and the *Archives of Internal Medicine* state that sleep disturbance turns on genes that cause inflammation. During the inflammatory response, white blood cells produce inflammatory messengers called cytokines. Some cytokines communicate with other white blood cells to join in the inflammation; others, including IL-6, TNF, and CRP, are associated with a greater risk of developing heart disease, diabetes, certain cancers, obesity, and other inflammatory diseases, such as rheumatoid arthritis and Crohn's disease. In the journal *Practice & Research Clinical Endocrinology*, researchers showed a reduction of sleep by just two to four hours a night increased levels of IL-6, TNF, and CRP.

According to a study in the *Journal of Allergy and Clinical Immunology*, sleep loss produced significant increases in blood levels of TNF-alpha and IL-6—messengers that affect the nervous, hormonal, and immune systems. In a study found in *Best Practice & Research Clinical Endocrinology*, investigators also found each hour of reduced sleep (which is not much) increased circulating levels of disease-promoting cytokines. Last, a study in *Biological Psychiatry* showed that a single night of sleep reduced by 50 percent resulted in the activation of NF-kB, the orchestrator of inflammation. When turned on, NF-kB causes the increase of pro-inflammatory agents, thus setting the stage for disease.

SLEEP DEPRIVATION AND HEART DISEASE

Coronary artery disease is an inflammatory condition involving an interaction between free radicals and the immune system in the walls of the arteries that supply blood to the heart. Data from the *Journal of Pineal Research* showed melatonin to be cardio-protective by reducing cellular damage and preventing oxidation of LDL. Several studies, including a study out of the *Lancet*, also showed that people with coronary artery disease and hypertension have significantly lower melatonin levels. In fact, they found that the lowest levels of melatonin correlated with increased severity of disease.

Another study in *Best Practice & Research Clinical Endocrinology* found sleep deprivation to increase blood pressure and cause alteration in the endothelium. Since the endothelium is the barrier between the circulating blood and the artery itself, dysfunction of the endothelium allows white blood cells and unwanted material to pass into the wall of the artery. In addition, endothelial dysfunction will cause unwanted platelets to stick to the wall of the artery and cause constriction, leading to high blood pressure.

Last, research published in the *European Heart Journal* found that short and long durations of sleep are predictors of cardiovascular outcomes. The data the authors gathered showed that short sleepers (fewer than seven to eight hours per night) have a greater risk of developing coronary artery disease and stroke, whereas those sleeping five hours or fewer should be considered at high risk for cardiovascular disease and mortality.

SLEEP DEPRIVATION AND CANCER

Researchers continue to study the biological effects of sleep deprivation on diseases like cancer. Sleep loss has been shown to disrupt immune function and increase inflammation, both of which promote the development of cancer. Melatonin secretion, which is stimulated by darkness and decreased by light, has multiple effects on the cancer microenvironment. Studies discussed in the *Journal of Medicine and Life* showed that melatonin had profound effects on tumor biology. It was found to reduce cell proliferation and tumor growth, and to inhibit blood vessel development to tumors. Melatonin also participates in activating the immune system needed to prevent tumor development. Fascinating evidence reveals this powerful sleep hormone prevents cancer cell metastasis and invasion into other tissues.

Melatonin was also found to protect against estrogen-driven breast cancer. Estrogen is involved in many aspects of the malignant process, including cellular proliferation, angiogenesis (blood vessel development), and metastasis. A study in the *Journal of Biological Chemistry* showed that melatonin blocked the stimulating effects of estrogen on breast cancer cells. Additional studies demonstrate that melatonin levels are diminished in breast cancer, and peak nighttime blood concentrations of melatonin are dramatically lower in breast cancer patients.

Quality sleep is important to healing and proper immune function, making it essential to get no less than seven to eight hours of sleep. For those dealing with cancer, sleep loss is a serious hazard. Studies in recent years have shown the link between sleep loss and the top forms of cancer. Research from *Cancer Epidemiology, Biomarkers and Prevention, Cancer,* and *Breast Cancer Research and Treatment* all found that those who experienced loss of sleep were more likely to develop colorectal, prostate, and breast cancers. The studies also showed that women who chronically lost sleep not only were at a greater risk for developing breast cancer, but developed a more aggressive type of breast cancer.

Many types of cancer are created by DNA damage from ionizing radiation, toxins, or a lack of nutrients. When DNA is damaged, specific tumor-suppressor and DNA-repair genes become active, producing protein to repair the broken DNA material. For a multitude of reasons, these repair mechanisms fail to do their jobs, and cancer develops. Sleep and the circadian rhythm are another backup system that helps in the repair. The circadian rhythm gene NPAS2 has been shown to help in DNA repair, and it acts as a tumor suppressor.

Emerging evidence suggests that disruption in sleeping and the circadian rhythm increases the risk of developing cancer. The hormone melatonin appears to be a key factor in preventing carcinogenesis and all stages of cancer progression. Sleep loss disrupts the circadian rhythm and the release of melatonin, setting us up for the development and progression of cancer.

SLEEP DEPRIVATION, DIABETES, AND OBESITY

Sleep loss is linked clearly to the development and progression of both heart disease and cancer. It can also lead to impaired glucose tolerance and diabetes. While you sleep, your body must maintain normal circulating blood sugar levels so your brain can continue to function in the absence of food. When you sleep less than seven to eight hours, you increase your chances of developing diabetes. A study in the *Archives of Internal Medicine* found that those who did not get a full seven to eight hours of sleep, as well as those with interrupted sleep, developed impaired glucose tolerance and an increased incidence of diabetes. It has been proposed that a lack of sleep acts as a stressor, causing the release of the stress hormone norepinephrine. Norepinephrine causes the release of fatty acids from fat cells, which can lead to insulin resistance and unmanaged blood sugar. Sleep deprivation was also found to alter growth hormone and cortisol secretion, both of which interrupt normal blood sugar levels.

When you fall asleep (assuming you haven't just eaten a big load of carbs), there is less circulating insulin and less sensitivity to insulin, making cells less tolerant to glucose. As the night progresses, glucose tolerance begins to improve, and blood sugar levels begin to decrease before waking. Sleep loss and interrupted sleep both disrupt insulin function and blood sugar regulation. Another association between blood sugar issues and sleep loss is inflammation. Sleep loss increases the inflammatory cytokine IL-6, which has been shown to contribute also to insulin resistance and abnormal blood sugar.

Sleep deprivation can contribute directly to the development of insulin resistance and diabetes by causing problems of glucose regulation, and indirectly through changes in appetite that can lead to being overfat or obese. Obesity is a major risk factor for insulin resistance and diabetes. There are two major hormones that regulate appetite: ghrelin and leptin. Ghrelin, from the stomach, will make you feel hungry, while leptin from your fat cells makes you feel full. When you don't get enough sleep, your level of ghrelin goes up, and your level of leptin goes down. This can lead to changes in your appetite where you feel hungrier when sleep-deprived than you do when well-rested, causing you to overeat and increasing your risk of becoming overfat or obese.

A study from the *American Journal of Nutrition* found sleep loss caused people to eat excessive high-energy snacks rather than meals.

While higher ghrelin and lower leptin levels were found, those who did not get enough sleep were also physically less active. Both increased appetite and lack of physical activity also play a major role in the development of an unhealthy body composition. Basically, not enough sleep increases your appetite, thus causing you to overeat high-calorie foods with higher carbohydrate content. Consequently, you become physically less active, which ultimately throws off your energy balance and leads to higher body fat and obesity.

Beyond an unhealthy body composition, high body fat increases inflammatory cytokines (IL-6, TNF) that are implicated in all chronic disease. High body fat increases insulin resistance, a major contributor to the development and progression of cancer. Overeating high-calorie, high-sugar foods can also mean eating fewer nutrient-dense foods, which is proven to cause disease.

Rebuild with a Good Night's Sleep

Getting to sleep can sometimes be a challenge. Here are some strategies to improve your quality of sleep and ensure you are getting enough sleep. To start, make sure your bedroom and your bed are comfortable, then use these tips:

- Get to bed at the same time every day.
- Avoid stimulants, including caffeine, nicotine, and excessive alcohol.
- Don't exercise five to six hours before your normal bedtime. Exercise will increase cortisol and adrenaline, which will disrupt your normal sleep cycle and circadian rhythm.
- Try to sleep only when you are sleepy.
- Make sure your room is dark and all electronics are off.
- Listen to relaxing music, and read 15 to 30 minutes before bed.

Reading at night is a powerful sleep aid for me. Try reading in bed in low light for quicker shuteye. By the way, you may not want to read the best-selling murder mystery or page-turner that keeps you up all night.

- Do not eat high-energy foods after dinner. Good options include low- to no-carb vegetables (cucumber, tomato, bell peppers). The idea here is not to disrupt your natural balance of growth hormone, insulin, and cortisol. Eating high-energy, high-carb foods may increase your energy and make it difficult to fall asleep.

- Eat healthful protein for dinner, such as turkey, chicken, eggs, and wild game. These food sources are high in tryptophan, which will increase levels of serotonin and melatonin needed for a good night's sleep.

- Avoid dairy products, including cheese. Dairy is high in L-tyrosine, an amino acid that helps to produce energy.

- Manage your stressors. Environmental stressors that activate the stress reaction and the release of the stress hormones cortisol, adrenalin, and norepinephrine will certainly keep you awake or cause a poor night's sleep. See the stress section, and try to change your perception of stressors so you stop the flood of stress hormones that are keeping you awake.

- Get eight hours of sleep. You feel terrible when you haven't gotten a good night's sleep, right? Well, there are a lot of benefits to be gained from a good night's sleep. When you fall asleep, your body releases growth hormone to help rebuild; it also helps to burn fat. Sleeping improves the immune system's ability to fight infection. It also reduces stress by lowering blood pressure and levels of stress hormones, elevated by our fast-paced lives. Sleep has also been shown to regulate blood sugar, which can reduce your chance of developing diabetes.

Summary

A good night's sleep is not only one of the most satisfying experiences; it is also crucial to good health. A solid seven to eight hours of uninterrupted sleep help you maintain normal mental function and energy levels, promotes rebuilding and repair of cells and tissues, improves immunity, and staves off disease.

However, less than seven to eight hours of sleep per night makes it rough to get through the day, and will cause the development and progression of the most serious diseases, including heart disease, cancer, blood sugar issues, and diabetes. Sleep loss will also increase inflammation and cause you to overeat high-calorie foods, thus contributing to being overfat and prone to disease.

Last, with our fast-paced lives and drive to get things done, on top of exposure to too much indoor and outdoor lighting, many of us suffer from low levels of melatonin. Since melatonin protects us from disease (and not producing enough can cause disease), we need to follow the strategies listed previously in order to get adequate sleep so our bodies can rebuild from disease.

7

Re-action #5
Reduce Contamination

Everyday toxins can be a serious hazard. From the foods we eat and the water we drink to a wide range of environmental chemicals, we are contaminated every day with unregulated substances with known and unknown toxicity. At high enough levels, toxins are poisonous to our cells, tissues, and organs. These compounds can be water-soluble and quickly eliminated through the urine, or fat-soluble and hide in the fat tissues of the body for long periods of time. Regardless, toxins alter the internal terrain and ultimately can threaten our health, increasing our chances of developing cancer, diabetes, obesity, and other chronic diseases.

Heavy metals, such as mercury found in fish, cause neurological dysfunction as well as heart and kidney damage. Bisphenol A (BPA), a chemical from plastics, mimics hormones like estrogen that can stimulate cell growth and tumor development. Casein, a protein found in dairy products, can elicit an immune response that can lead to the development of diabetes.

Rebuilding from a disease requires you to find alternatives to foods and beverages that may be loaded with toxins that will slow down or even prevent your personal rebuild. This doesn't mean you should obsess over your food choices. Just be aware of and informed about the potential hazards of everyday food toxins so you can make the best choices when selecting what to eat and drink.

Since there is an overwhelming amount of information regarding food toxins and environmental contaminants, I will break down the toxicity/disease connection into two parts: toxins in our food and environmental toxins linked to serious chronic conditions.

Toxins in Our Food

In the section "Three Foods That Kill," we learned that bread, dairy, and sugar pose serious health issues when consumed every day. Grains containing gluten can cause leaky gut, a condition in which the barrier in the gut is breached, allowing unwanted proteins to enter the circulation. Gluten can cause an immune response that creates health-threatening disease. Dairy contains growth factors and inflammatory proteins, including casein, that can also increase gut permeability, thus setting the stage for autoimmune diseases, heart disease, the neuro-developmental condition autism, and the brain disorder schizophrenia. Refined sugars, including table sugar (sucrose) and high-fructose corn syrup, are proven to cause diabetes, insulin resistance, and obesity. High insulin and inflammatory conditions trigger the development of certain cancers and coronary artery disease.

Toxins called lectins and phytates, found in grains and legumes, can also have ill effects on our health. Lectins and phytates are chemicals that protect plants from the harsh environment and the attack of insects. Lectins have been shown to contribute to unwanted intestinal permeability and to trigger immune reactions that create autoimmune disease and allergies. Phytates are considered antinutrients and mineral magnets, which bind to and remove minerals, such as iron, from the body. Experiments show that phytates in wheat-based foods block absorption of about 90 percent of the iron. Phytates also remove the minerals calcium, zinc, magnesium, and copper, which are crucial in countless metabolic reactions in the body. However, taking vitamin C or eating vitamin C–rich foods with high-phytate foods can improve mineral absorption.

Peanuts carry a dangerous mold, which produces the toxin aflatoxin. Aflatoxin is a potent carcinogen produced by the *Aspergillus flavus* and *Aspergillus parasiticus* molds, which grow on peanuts, corn, and cottonseed, and are even found in milk. Aflatoxin can cause liver damage and cancer, gastrointestinal dysfunction, decreased appetite, and decreased reproductive function.

Heavy metals are other food-based hazards with serious health implications. Mercury, lead, nickel, and cadmium cannot be degraded or destroyed; they enter our bodies through food, drinking water, and air. Heavy metals are a big deal, as they can accumulate in the body over time due to their slow elimination. They get into our water supply from industrial waste (power plants, pulp mills, waste incinerators) and acidic rain that can wash these metals into streams, lakes, and rivers. Organic mercury (methylmercury) is the form found in seafood. Basically, methylmercury is found in the aquatic microorganisms and sediment on the ocean floor. That sediment is consumed by small fish, which are then eaten by larger fish. The mercury works its way up the food chain until we are eating unhealthful amounts in our favorite Friday-night fish dinner. According to the Natural Resources Defense Council, dangerous levels of mercury are found in king mackerel, marlin, shark, swordfish, tilefish, and bigeye tuna. High mercury is also found in bluefish, grouper, Chilean sea bass, albacore, and yellowfin tuna.

Mercury toxicity has been shown to damage the central nervous system, peripheral nervous system, gastrointestinal system, kidneys, and heart. Data published in the *Journal of Cardiovascular Disease & Diagnosis* showed that mercury had multiple detrimental effects on the cardiovascular system, including endothelial dysfunction, vascular smooth-muscle dysfunction, and high levels of oxidation—all steps involved in the creation of atherosclerosis. The clinical consequences of mercury include coronary artery disease, high blood pressure, cardiac arrhythmias, increased carotid artery thickness, left ventricular hypertrophy, and heart attacks. Mercury toxicity has also been shown to cause autoimmune disease. A study in *Environmental Health Perspectives* found that at low levels, methylmercury caused autoantibody production and immune dysregulation, leading to subclinical (without signs and symptoms) autoimmune dysfunction. Additional studies in *Environmental International* showed the link between elevated mercury levels and high levels of thyroid antibodies in women.

If that's not bad enough, heavy metals have been found to interfere with normal gene expression and DNA repair, setting the stage for the development of cancer. Heavy metals have also been implicated in neurodegenerative diseases, such as Alzheimer's disease, Parkinson's disease, and Lou Gehrig's disease (ALS).

The good news is that your body can rebuild from heavy-metal toxicity through powerful detoxification systems and the detoxifying protein metallothionein, which binds to those metals and transports them to the liver, where they are processed, detoxified, released into the gut, and eliminated through stool.

Fish is not the only protein source that can be toxic; meat also has potential hazards. Cooking at high heat levels, as you do when grilling, for example, kills bacteria and other food-borne pathogens, and it also causes protein in meat to produce compounds called heterocyclic amines. These compounds can be carcinogenic when the meat is burned, blackened, and charred. (See page 99 for more information on this topic.) You should also completely avoid processed and cured meats, including the conventional cold cuts, sausage, and bacon that typically are served at popular delis and well-known sandwich franchises. Under certain conditions, the nitrites added to these foods as preservatives can morph into molecules called nitrosamines, which can cause cancer. Processed meats also contain a whole bunch of other nasty compounds that can affect your health. Meat doesn't naturally come in a block wrapped in plastic, so avoid all processed meats. Stick to free-range grass-fed meats as a healthful protein source.

As I work with patients guiding them on proper nutrition, I am frequently asked about artificial sweeteners like NutraSweet (aspartame) and Splenda (sucralose). A dieter's dream is to continue eating sweet things without all the calories or all the guilt. For many, replacing table sugar with artificial sweeteners is a common strategy for getting rid of body fat. Rewarding yourself with something sweet without the sugar may reduce your calories, but putting an unnatural substance in your body makes you a test subject for the "swallow it and see what happens" experiment. Artificial sweeteners pose a threat to our health.

Aspartame is made up of aspartic acid and phenylalanine (both amino acids) and methanol (wood alcohol). Aspartic acid can pass the blood/brain barrier and act as an excitotoxin, causing the overstimulation and death of neurons. For individuals who ingest too much phenylalanine, or have an inability to break it down, the side effects can include headaches, dizziness, seizures, and brain damage. Once aspartame enters the small intestine, the methanol is released and absorbed into the body. Methanol is then broken down into formaldehyde (embalming fluid, the kind found in the jars where frogs are kept before dissection) and formic acid, which is the toxin from the sting of red ants. Methanol toxicity can cause dizziness, vision problems and blindness, headaches, nausea and gastrointestinal disorders, weakness, fatigue, memory loss, and behavioral problems.

Another popular artificial sweetener is sucralose, a chemical made by adding chlorine atoms to sucrose. The chlorocarbons that make up sucralose have a similar structure to that of pesticides. Is sucralose safe? Well, as of 2006, only six human trials on Splenda had been published; most of the studies on Splenda were done on animals. Although the health problems in animals were significant, the Splenda researchers downplayed the adverse health effects in the animals to make sucralose appear safe rather than making sure people weren't harmed.

Toxins in the Environment

Persistent organic pollutants (POPs) are chemicals that persist in the environment, get into the food chain, and end up accumulating in human fat tissue. POPs contribute to the development of disease and hinder your ability to rebuild from your health crisis. They include:

- Bisphenol A (BPA)—found in metal containers and cans, and plastic bottles
- Polychlorinated biphenyls (PCBs)—found in fish, including bluefin tuna, rockfish, sole, rainbow trout, farmed salmon, white croaker, and shellfish. When eating fish, make sure you trim the fat and remove the skin, as PCBs are stored in the fatty parts of the fish. PCBs are also found in dairy.
- Phthalates—found in plastics such as plastic bags, household paints, nail polish, and glues
- Organotin compounds—found in pharmaceuticals, herbicides, fungicides, pesticides, plastics, and disinfectants
- Perfluorinated compounds (PFCs)—found in microwave popcorn bags, pizza boxes, Teflon cookware, shampoos, denture cleaners, paints, adhesives, and insecticides
- Polyvinyl chloride (PVC)—found in vinyl shower curtains, pill coatings, and fragrances
- Dichlorodiphenyltrichloroethane (DDT)—found in fish and shellfish, insecticides, and aerosols

It's a well-known fact that pesticides and herbicides are sprayed on our produce. PCBs are found in the soil and water supply, along with dioxins, BPAs, and phthalates from plastic household products. POPs have been shown to damage cellular DNA, destroy the immune system, promote tumor growth, and make cancers more aggressive. These chemicals are also commonly referred to as endocrine disruptors; they interfere with the hormonal system and thus produce adverse reproductive, developmental, neurological, and metabolic effects.

Growing evidence published in *Environmental Health Perspectives* has recently linked type 2 diabetes with DDT and PCB. Researchers found that these POPs impaired glucose metabolism and insulin sensitivity and increased abdominal obesity, which led to high blood sugar and a higher risk of developing type 2 diabetes. These toxins are also known carcinogens. Research published in the *American Journal of Epidemiology* and *Advances in Breast Cancer Research* found that these chemicals acted as weak estrogen, which made cancers of the breast and prostate more aggressive.

Another important way toxins cause cancer is the attachment of the chemical to a cell's DNA; this is called a DNA adduct. DNA adducts can cause mutations, interfere with DNA repair, and damage genes responsible for regulating cell growth and proliferation—all necessary steps in the development of cancer. Research found in the journal *Carcinogenesis* reveals that pesticides, herbicides, heavy metals, chemicals from cigarette smoke, and the chemicals from processed foods all act on DNA. The chemotherapeutic agents cyclophosphamide and cisplatin are also known DNA adducts that have been shown to cause secondary cancers. The toxic compounds found in cigarette smoke damage the DNA-repair gene p53, which, in addition to repairing genetic damage, is the gene responsible for activating a cell's self-destruct mechanism (apoptosis) when the genetic damage is too extensive.

Obesity is now a global problem, not only for individuals but also for the health care system and the economy. High-calorie, nutrient-poor foods, combined with a lack of physical activity, are the major causes of this pandemic. However, recent findings published in the journals

Endocrinology and *Environmental Health Perspectives* have found a third culprit behind the obesity issue. They report that endocrine disruptors like DDT, BPA, PCB, and organotins (metallic compounds containing lead, tin, and mercury) can increase the number and size of fat cells and alter the hormones involved in appetite, satiety, and food preferences. In combination with processed foods and physical inactivity, these obesogens (chemicals that make more fat) are becoming a major factor in the development of obesity.

Toxicity has also been linked to infertility, neurological disorders, attention deficit disorder, and other learning challenges.

Detoxification

Toxicity, your body's response to a toxin, depends on the built-in detoxification system found in the liver. Efficient detoxification depends on a series of reactions that bind toxins to specific molecules to escort them out of the liver and into the gut for elimination. The liver's detox system depends on specific amino acids and nutrients such as cysteine, selenium, and zinc derived from foods.

If your internal terrain has become toxic from years of processed foods, too much alcohol, and the overuse of prescription drugs, the liver's detoxification system fails to do an efficient job at removing harmful substances. You have no way to protect yourself and rebuild quickly and effectively if you are exposed to toxins and unable to detoxify and discard them quickly. An overtaxed liver; nutrient deprivation (from nutrient-deficient foods); and the constant exposure to toxic chemicals in our foods, air, and water can create serious disease.

Enter glutathione. Glutathione is one of the most important antioxidants in the body. It is needed for the detoxification of toxins, including heavy metals. Found in every cell of the body, glutathione protects our cells from free radical damage by recycling the other antioxidants, including vitamin C and vitamin E. Formed from the amino acids glutamic acid and cysteine, glutathione is the major ingredient the liver needs to break down and eliminate toxins from food and the environment. Glutathione owes much of its strength to the amino acid cysteine. Cysteine is rich in sulfur, which is abundant in eggs, garlic, and onion. These foods and cruciferous vegetables (broccoli, cauliflower, kale, Brussels sprouts, and cabbage) help restock glutathione levels.

Glutathione doesn't come in a pill; it is created by nutrients found in different food sources. This is another reason to eat a variety of whole foods that provide the basic ingredients for proper function, including detoxification. Nutraceuticals, including N-acetylcysteine, niacin, alpha-lipoic acid, and CoQ10, can also help replenish glutathione stores, thus improving your detoxification so you can rebuild from a health crisis and prevent its return.

Summary

In order to rebuild from disease and prevent recurrence, you have to eliminate processed foods that contain additives, preservatives, refined grains, dairy, and sugar, as well as reduce your exposure to the POPs found in everyday products, including plastic bottles, metal food cans, detergents, flame-retardants, food, toys, cosmetics, and pesticides.

To help reduce the burden of toxins that you ingest, as well as their potential health risks, you have to become a modern-day hunter-gatherer and forage for natural foods, grass-fed meats, and fish that don't contain high levels of mercury. Consider buying organic produce from your local farmers' market and farm stands. Aslo, clean your produce with a vegetable and fruit wash. You may also want to look for household products that are free of BPA, phthalate, and dioxins. These chemicals are hazardous not just to bugs—they pose a real threat to us.

8

Testing the Disease Terrain

In order for you to rebuild yourself and prevent another health catastrophe, you need to understand what in your internal terrain may have contributed to the development of your disease or chronic health issues. In this chapter, I've given lists of biomarkers and medical tests that can uncover the reasons for your poor health.

What are biomarkers? They are biological clues that can be measured through blood, saliva, or urine, and are used to evaluate normal physiological function; a pathological (disease) process; and your response to drug or supplement therapy. Biomarkers identify your potential for developing disease, as well as the current state and severity of disease, and they help predict future disease and probabilities for recurrence. Testing for certain biomarkers will provide information that will allow you to take appropriate action so you can rebuild. In addition to tests that will provide clues to the origins of your poor health, you will find specific tests that will give you information about your active disease—the current state of your condition. Identifying the specific clues outlined here will enable you to identify the dysfunction in your physiology and then create the best plan of action to resolve those issues, allowing you to rebuild your health.

Most chronic diseases have common threads and common causes. For example, inflammation is a core reaction in the body and a major player in the development of chronic disease. Abnormal blood sugar levels (dysglycemia) and high insulin (hyperinsulinemia) are markers of another important disease process linked to cancer, heart disease, dementia, Alzheimer's, and other chronic diseases. High blood sugar and high insulin levels are also implicated in the onset of endocrine (hormone) disorders, including polycystic ovary syndrome (PCOS). If you are dealing with or rebuilding from coronary artery disease or cancer— or if you are concerned about Alzheimer's disease—you should read the diabetes section. For any of the major diseases, definitely read the section on obesity and metabolic syndrome. The specific clues in the biomarkers will enable you to identify the dysfunction in your physiology, allowing you create the best plan of action to rebuild your health.

ALEX'S STORY

Alex is a college student who came in with her parents looking for causes for her weight gain, amenorrhea (absence of menstruation), increased body hair, and acne. She was also dealing with anxiety and obsessive-compulsive behaviors. Alex had been told by another doctor that her behavioral issues were caused by multiple tick-borne infections, including Lyme, babesiosis, and ehrlichiosis. She took four different drugs for six months to combat these infections. I asked what that doctor had told them would indicate that Alex was getting better. Her parents responded, "When the babesiosis marks turn white." Babesiosis marks? I'm not an infectious-disease expert, but that sounded very odd. I asked to see the marks on her skin, and I was shocked to see everyday stretch marks. That doctor had convinced Alex and her parents that the stretch marks on her waistline were due to a tick-based infection, and the lightening of her stretch marks (often pink to reddish in color) was due to a response to the drugs. When I showed them similar stretch marks on countless images from a Google search, they were surprised and angered. Alex immediately stopped all the drugs she had been prescribed for Lyme, babesiosis, and ehrlichiosis.

To me, rapid weight gain, amenorrhea, and more abundant body hair all sounded like polycystic ovary syndrome (PCOS). Using saliva testing and whole blood or capillary blood to assess hormones, I found that Alex was low in progesterone and estrogen and that her testosterone was slightly elevated. In addition to hormone testing, general blood work revealed elevated blood sugar. This pattern is often seen in young women with PCOS. To help regulate her blood sugar, I worked with her to eliminate all bread, dairy, and processed sugars from her diet while providing substitutions, including healthful plant-based carbs and dairy alternatives. I also gave her nutrient supplements to help her with her hormone deficiencies and the PCOS. Within three months, she had lost weight (body fat) and started a more regular menstrual cycle.

Z NOTE: Polycystic ovary syndrome (PCOS) is a common hormonal disorder among women of reproductive age; it is characterized by chronic lack of ovulation (anovulation) and the elevated androgen testosterone. Small cysts develop in the ovaries because of chronic elevated blood sugar and insulin levels. Hyperinsulinemia (elevated insulin) has been shown to maintain elevated androgens (male hormones), including testosterone, which can cause increased body hair and acne, as well as abnormal or absent menstrual cycles. The key to improving or resolving PCOS is controlling blood sugar and insulin.

While you rebuild yourself, you and your health professional can use these tests to assess your current health status and how your health is improving over time. You should test these biomarkers—depending on your health issue—at the beginning of and during your personal rebuild. Some of these biomarkers may be familiar, but many may not. No worries. Talk to your doctor or find a specialist in functional medicine who will get these tests done for you and help you interpret the results. Where applicable, I have listed labs that test specific biomarkers.

The Cardiovascular Terrain

If you are rebuilding from heart disease or want to prevent another heart event, testing the cardiovascular terrain and your potential for developing coronary artery disease must include biomarkers for inflammation, heart muscle damage, and potential root causes of atherosclerosis.

TESTING FOR ARTERIAL INFLAMMATION

This first set of biomarkers provides information regarding inflammation in the arteries. Since atherosclerosis is an inflammatory condition in the wall of the artery—not the accumulation of cholesterol—these biomarkers can provide information about the potential for plaque rupture and a pending heart attack or stroke. Testing arterial inflammation must include:

- Oxidized LDL
- Myeloperoxidase (MPO)
- hs-CRP
- Lp-PLA2
- F2-isoprostanes
- Microalbumin/creatinine ratio
- Asymmetric dimethylarginine (ADMA)
- High-sensitive cardiac troponin T (hs-cTnT)

These tests should be your first priority. After all, for many, the first sign of coronary artery disease is sudden death.

TESTING FOR HEART MUSCLE DAMAGE

This set of biomarkers will tell you if the muscle of the heart has been damaged after a heart attack:

- Troponin
- Creatine phosphokinase (CK)
- Creatine kinase MB isoenzyme (Ck-MB)
- B-type natriuretic peptide (BNP)
- High-sensitive cardiac troponin T (hs-cTnT)

TESTING THE CARDIOVASCULAR TERRAIN

Damage to the endothelium, the layer of cells that lines the arteries, is the first step in developing heart disease. The following biomarkers provide the clues to how the endothelium got damaged, why you developed atherosclerosis, and what to test for to prevent recurrence or regression of the disease:

- Fasting glucose and hemoglobin A1c
- Vitamin D (25[OH]D)
- Thyroid hormones (free T3 and free T4)
- hs-CRP
- Lipid panel (cholesterol, LDL, HDL, triglycerides)
- Complete blood count with differential
- Comprehensive metabolic profile
- Advanced lipid panel (ApoA1, ApoB, ApoB/ApoA ratio, lipoprotein[a])
- Uric acid
- Homocysteine

CLINICAL NOTE: High homocysteine indicates a risk for atherosclerosis and coronary artery disease, as it can oxidize LDL. A vitamin B_{12} or folate deficiency can cause elevated homocysteine. To determine if you have a B_{12} or folate deficiency, check the health of the red blood cells in a complete blood count. A true deficiency of either B_{12} or folate will cause an elevation in mean corpuscular volume (MCV) and mean corpuscular hemoglobin (MCH). MCV is a measurement of the average size of a red blood cell, and MCH is a calculation of the average amount of hemoglobin inside a red blood cell. Most blood panels test these levels, but check with your doctor to confirm. Elevated homocysteine levels are also seen in people with a common genetic variant called methylenetetrahydrofolate reductase (MTHFR). This defective gene leads to high homocysteine levels in some people who inherit the MTHFR variant from both parents. Blood testing can be done to determine if you have mutations in the MTHFR gene.

Z NOTE: Research published in *Circulation* found that thyroid hormones also have a profound effect on the heart and blood vessels. A weak or overactive thyroid will cause changes in cardiac contractility and output, blood pressure, and endothelial function. If you are recovering from a heart event and rebuilding yourself to prevent the progression of atherosclerosis, get your thyroid hormones (T3 and T4) evaluated.

The Cancer Terrain

From initial gene dysfunction and uncontrolled cell growth to angiogenesis (blood vessel growth) and metastasis (the spread of cancer from its original site), all stages of cancer development occur due to some disturbance in your physiology—your body's internal terrain. Biomarkers in the blood can give clues to your genetic risk for developing cancer, why you ultimately developed cancer, your prognosis, and the effectiveness of your treatment.

TESTING FOR ONCOGENIC POTENTIAL

Your likelihood of developing cancer is called oncogenic potential. If you are rebuilding after cancer care and looking to prevent recurrence, assessing your continuing oncogenic potential is a must. The following biomarkers provide valuable information regarding your internal terrain and the disrupted physiology that increased your oncogenic potential and set you up for the development of cancer. Oncogenic potential tests include:

- Fasting glucose and insulin, insulin-like growth factor 1 (IGF1), hemoglobin A1c
- Lactulose/mannitol (a urine test to detect dysfunctional intestinal permeability or leaky gut)
- Fecal lactoferrin (a stool test to uncover inflammation in the gut)
- Free radical damage and oxidative stress, including:
  - Lipid peroxides
  - 8-hydroxy-deoxyguanosine (8-OHdG)
  - Isoprostanes
- Steroid hormone analysis and hormone metabolites: estradiol, progesterone, testosterone, 2-hydroxyestrone, 4-hydroxyestrone, and 16-alpha-hydroxyestrone
- Autoantibody testing for autoimmune dysfunction: thyroid peroxidase (TPO), antinuclear antibody (ANA), and antigliadin antibodies for possible celiac disease and gluten intolerance
- 25-hydroxyvitamin D and 1,25 dihydroxyvitamin D
- hs-CRP, TNF-alpha, LpPLA2, galectin-3, and uric acid to assess inflammation
- Antibody testing for *Helicobacter pylori*—to be done only through stool—hepatitis B, hepatitis C, and Epstein-Barr virus
- Cortisol testing associated with immune suppression (tested four times in a day through saliva)

> **CLINICAL NOTE:** Lactulose/mannitol test can be done through Genova Diagnostics (www.gdx.net). I recommend ZRT Laboratory (www.zrtlab .com) for hormone testing and hormone metabolite testing.

TESTING FOR PROGNOSIS AND THE EFFECTIVENESS OF TREATMENT

Biomarkers associated with cancer are usually used to monitor the extent of the disease, determine your prognosis (probable outcome), and evaluate the effectiveness of your treatment. If you are actively going through cancer care, your cancer team should be testing you to monitor your progress to determine how well your treatment is working. The following biomarkers are associated with different types of cancer:

- CA 125—ovarian, lung, and breast cancers
- CA 15–3—breast, pancreatic, ovarian, lung, and colon cancers
- CA 19–9—pancreatic and biliary tract cancers
- CA 27.29—breast cancer
- CEA—colorectal, breast, pancreatic, liver, and stomach cancers
- CYFRA 21–1—lung cancer
- Cyclin E—gastric, colorectal, blood, lung, skin, and genitourinary cancers
- MCM and P16—bladder cancer
- Osteopontin—melanoma, breast, lung, colorectal, stomach, ovarian, and thyroid cancers
- BCL-2—ovarian cancer
- VEGF—vascular endothelial growth factor is a protein that promotes the growth of new blood vessels to tumors
- Alpha-fetoprotein—liver and testicular cancers
- Prostate specific antigen (PSA)—prostate cancer
- Beta 2 microglobulin—multiple myeloma

If you are getting biannual or yearly cancer screenings, consider:

- Papanicolaou test (Pap smear) to detect cervical cancer
- Colonoscopy to examine the large bowel for polyps and colorectal cancer
- Dermatology (skin) screening for skin cancer
- Oral screening for early oral cancer
- Ultrasound and mammogram for breast cancer

Z NOTE: Mammography has been the standard imaging method for detecting breast cancer since the late 1960s. The technology has changed since then, with more advanced machines and much less X-ray exposure. However, current research is now redetermining the best method for imaging breast tissue, and the contenders are mammography, ultrasound, and MRI. Researchers have found that ultrasound is more accurate for dense breast tissue, and mammography is better suited for fatty breast tissue. Data reported in the *American Journal of Surgery* and the *Medical Journal of Malaysia* showed that ultrasound was a more accurate diagnostic method than mammography in the detection of breast cancer in dense breast tissue. Diagnostic ultrasound was also found to be more accurate than mammography in predicting residual tumor size following chemotherapy. A study published in the *American Journal of Roentgenology* found that ultrasound was more accurate than mammography in detecting breast cancer in women forty-five years old and younger. Ultrasound detected 84.9 percent of cancers, while mammography detected 71.7 percent. However, mammography was found to be a better tool at detecting breast cancer in fatty breasts and in women fifty years old and older. If the presence of breast cancer is questionable on both an ultrasound and a mammogram, an MRI is suggested for evaluating residual disease and for detecting the subset of tumors not seen on ultrasound and mammography. Discuss these tests with your doctor to determine which screening method is right for you.

CLINICAL NOTE: The toxicity associated with chemotherapy can be devastating during cancer care and, for many people, long after. Following your chemotherapy regimen, you may develop chronic anemia consisting of low red blood cells, hemoglobin, and hematocrit. You may also be suffering from fatigue, low energy, and general brain fog. If so, get your thyroid tested. The thyroid hormone T3 affects all systems of the body and is also responsible for producing a hormone called erythropoietin (EPO) in the kidneys, which causes bone marrow to make more red blood cells. By increasing your red blood cell mass, you can quickly rebuild from anemia caused by chemotherapy, so making sure your thyroid is functioning optimally is essential.

TESTING FOR GENETIC RISK

If you have a family history of cancer—or are in the throes of cancer care—talk to your doctor to determine which of these genetic tests (if any) you should have done. Remember, genes don't determine whether you develop a disease, but they can indicate if you're *at risk* of developing the disease. Here is a list of genetic markers that can be tested to determine risk of certain cancers:

- KRAS and APC genes (associated with metastatic colorectal cancer)
- HER2 (a protein found on breast cancer cells that controls cancer growth and spread)
- BRCA1 and BRCA2 (the well-known tumor suppressor genes associated with breast cancer)
- Tp53 (a tumor suppressor gene that creates the tumor protein p53, which, in turn, prevents cells from growing out of control and causes a cell to commit suicide [apoptosis] when the DNA in the cell gets damaged)
- BAT26 gene mutation (associated with stomach and colorectal cancer)

You may not need all these genetic tests. However, you may want to discuss them with your doctor to determine which are appropriate for you and your specific cancer.

The Diabetic and Alzheimer's Terrain

Diabetes mellitus is a condition of high blood sugar resulting from either inadequate insulin production (type 1 diabetes) or lack of cellular response to insulin (type 2 diabetes). Alzheimer's disease is also linked to abnormal blood sugar, insulin resistance, and inflammation.

TESTING FOR DIABETES AND YOUR RISK OF ALZHEIMER'S DISEASE

If you are rebuilding from diabetes and/or you want to understand your risk for developing Alzheimer's disease, make sure to have these biomarkers tested:

- Fasting blood glucose
- Fasting insulin
- Hemoglobin A1c
- Comprehensive metabolic panel including BUN/creatinine ratio
- Uric acid
- C-peptide
- TNF-alpha
- hs-CRP
- Insulin growth factor 1 (IGF1)

CLINICAL NOTE: Your fasting blood glucose level must be tested when you have not eaten for at least eight hours. If you do not fast for eight hours prior to the test, your test results will be inaccurate.

The Autoimmune Disease Terrain

Autoimmune diseases are complex dysfunctions of the immune system involving an imbalance of the Th1 and Th2 immune responses. If you are dealing with an autoimmune disease and/or are in active treatment, ask your doctor about testing the balance between your Th1 and Th2 cytokines, along with CD4 and CD8 T lymphocytes. You must also consider looking at a leaky gut. It's vital to eliminate any foods containing gluten from your diet, even if you have no apparent symptoms after eating gluten.

TESTING THE IMMUNE RESPONSE

These tests will give you a more in-depth look at the abnormal immune response:

- Th1 cytokines (IL-2, IL-6, IFN-gamma, TNF-alpha)
- Th2 cytokines (IL-4, IL-6, IL-10, IL-13)
- Th17 cytokine (IL-17)
- Celiac profile, including anti-gliadin antibodies IgA and transglutaminase
- *H. pylori* through stool testing

TESTING FOR CELIAC DISEASE

- Tissue transglutaminase antibodies (tTG-IgA)
- IgA endomysial antibody (EMA)
- HLA DQ2 and DQ8 genes

TESTING FOR LEAKY GUT

- Lactulose and mannitol testing (Genova Diagnostics, www.gdx.net)
- Intestinal antigenic permeability screen (Cyrex Laboratories, www.cyrexlabs.com)

- GI Effects Comprehensive Stool Profile with Zonulin (Genova Diagnostics, www.gdx.net)

> **CLINICAL NOTE:** When testing for celiac or the other diseases associated with gluten and zonulin, don't refrain from eating foods containing gluten. The tTG-IgA antibody test is a sensitive test but will be valid only if you are eating gluten-containing foods. If this test and the others come back positive, you must then give up eating anything containing gluten. Note, however, that not all people who are sensitive to gluten have celiac disease. If you have any symptoms after eating foods containing gluten but your tests come back negative, you must avoid gluten-containing foods anyway.

TESTING FOR PRIMARY BILIARY CIRRHOSIS

- Alanine transaminase (ALT)
- Alkaline phosphatase (ALP)
- Anti-mitochondrial antibody
- Aspartate aminotransferase (AST)
- Gamma-glutamyl transferase (GGT)
- Immunoglobulin M (IgM)
- Liver biopsy

TESTING FOR MULTIPLE SCLEROSIS

- Brain stem and auditory evoked potential tests
- MRI (checking for lesions in the nervous system)
- Spinal tap (invasive procedure to look at spinal fluid)

TESTING FOR RHEUMATOID ARTHRITIS

- 14-3-3 eta
- Anti-citrullinated peptide antibody (ACPA)

- Citrullinated protein
- C-reactive protein
- Rheumatoid factor

TESTING FOR HASHIMOTO'S THYROIDITIS

- Anti-nuclear antibody (ANA)
- Anti-thyroglobulin antibody (TgAb)
- Anti-TPO antibodies
- Double-stranded DNA (dsDNA)
- For Grave's disease or hyperthyroidism:
  - Thyroid-stimulating immunoglobulin (TSI)
  - Thyroid-stimulating hormone receptor antibody (TRAb)
- Free T3
- Free T4
- TSH

The Obesity Terrain

Excessive body fat and visceral fat (fat surrounding the organs) can release hormones, modify your appetite, increase inflammation, and increase your risk for cancer, heart disease, and diabetes. Metabolic syndrome is a state of upper-body (truncal) obesity, high blood pressure, high blood fat (triglycerides), and elevated blood sugar. When rebuilding from obesity and/or metabolic syndrome, consider these tests:

- Adiponectin
- ALT
- AST
- Blood pressure (taken in both arms). Why? Because you have arteries in both arms. Often the blood pressures are different from side to side.

- Body mass index (BMI; see page 234)
- Fasting glucose
- Fasting insulin
- Hemoglobin A1c
- hs-CRP
- Lipid panel including cholesterol, LDL, HDL, triglycerides, Apo B, and Apo A
- Uric acid
- Vitamin D, 25(OH)D
- Waist-to-hip ratio (see page 241)

General Health Profile

If you are looking to rebuild your body because of an unhealthful lifestyle, or you want to stay ahead of the disease train, here is a good overall biomarker panel to assess your internal terrain. If any markers are out of range, further investigation will be needed.

- Complete blood count with white blood cell differential
- Comprehensive metabolic panel
- Lipid panel including cholesterol, LDL, HDL, triglycerides, ApoB, and ApoA
- Fasting glucose
- Hemoglobin A1c
- Uric acid
- Free T3
- Free T4
- Vitamin D, 25(OH)D
- Celiac panel, including tissue transglutaminase antibodies (tTG-IgA) and IgA endomysial antibodies (EMA)
- Consider testing for leaky gut (see page 348)

Note: When looking at anemia, include with the above:

- Folate
- B_{12}
- Serum iron and iron binding capacity
- Ferritin

Record Your Rebuild

As you apply the supportocols in this book, record your initial medical tests and your progress during your personal rebuild. Enter the name of the test and the results in the Medical Tests Report to track your progress. As you move forward with your rebuild, check your current levels with the results from your past tests and note any changes. For example, if you have problems with blood sugar, you would want to check your hemoglobin A1c and fasting glucose. If you have cardiovascular issues, you would check your lipid profile and inflammatory biomarkers. The frequency of testing depends on the severity of your condition. Ask your doctor if you should be retested every twelve or twenty-four weeks.

While you are improving your internal terrain and rebuilding from your current state of health, consider recording the changes in your body composition. We've already covered the instructions for calculating your BMI, total metabolic rate, and body fat percentage, as well as how to take your physical measurements. After your calculations are complete, enter the initial values in the 12-Week Progress Report on page 354. Every four weeks, weigh and measure yourself again, recalculate your BMI and other values, and enter them in the appropriate column. The comparison will provide evidence of your progress.

Here is a sample medical tests report:

MEDICAL TESTS REPORT			
Name of Test	**Start**	**12 Weeks**	**24 Weeks**
Hemoglobin A1c	6.8%	5.3%	5.1%
Glucose	120 mg/dL	97 mg/dL	86 mg/dL

And here is a blank worksheet for you to use:

MEDICAL TESTS REPORT			
Name of Test	**Start**	**12 Weeks**	**24 Weeks**

12-WEEK PROGRESS REPORT				
Name of Test	**Start**	**4 Weeks**	**8 Weeks**	**12 Weeks**
Body Mass Index (BMI)				
Total Metabolic Rate (TMR)				
Basal Metabolic Rate (BMR)				
Body Fat Percentage				
Body Measurements				
Chest				
Waist				
Hips				
Biceps				
Weight				
What other changes have you noticed? Do you have more energy? Are you sleeping better? Has your digestion improved? Make notes about any changes you have noticed regarding any symptoms you may have been having.				
4 Weeks:				
8 Weeks:				
12 Weeks:				

Whether you are recovering from an illness, want to prevent the recurrence of disease, are looking to improve your body composition, or just want information about your state of health, biomarker testing provides information about your internal terrain, and can show you the improvements you've made in your health as you progress through your personal rebuild.

Here's to your victory.

III

Recipes

CONGRATULATIONS! YOU'VE REACHED THE final destination for your rebuild. Before you get started with the delicious recipes, take a look at the following chart to see how flexible they can be. Some recipes work well early in the day, while some are best suited for lunch or dinner. You can mix and match to create more variety. That way, no matter what time of day, you know what you're eating is just right!

RECIPES

KEY: B = Breakfast; L = Lunch; D = Dinner; S = Snack

	B	L	D	S
Ambrosia Fruit Salad	√			√
Asian Red Slaw	√	√	√	√
Beef or Lamb Shank		√	√	
Bison Burgers with Salsa	√	√	√	
Blueberry Smoothie	√			√
Broccoli & Kale Pasta		√	√	
Broccoli Rabe		√	√	
Cabbage & Carrot Soup		√	√	√
Cauliflower & Leek Fritters	√	√		√
Chester's Chili		√	√	
Chicken or Shrimp Stir-Fry		√	√	
Chicken Sausage & Sweet Potatoes		√	√	
Chinese Chicken		√	√	
Chunky Vegetable Soup		√	√	
Cleansing Ginger Cabbage Soup		√	√	√
Cod Oreganato		√	√	
Color-Changing Shrimp Stir-Fry		√	√	
Crispy Cruciferous Salad	√	√	√	√
Curried Chicken Salad	√	√	√	
Devilicious Curried Eggs	√			√
Dr. Z's Fast & Easy Snacks				√

	B	L	D	S
Easy Meatloaf		√	√	
Egg & Avocado on Toast	√			√
Egg & Olive Salad	√	√		√
Eggplant Tapenade				√
Fresh Fruit & Mint Salad	√	√		√
Garlic Spinach				
Grilled Chicken, Beef or Lamb Kebobs		√	√	
Guacamole/Chunky Guacamole	√	√	√	√

"Just Wing It" Salads
  Classic Vinaigrette
  "This Rocks" Salad
  Mediterranean Salad
  Crunchy Cabbage Salad
  Healthy Heart Salad
  Pantry Salad
  Kale Salad
		√	√	

Hearty Navy Bean Soup		√	√	√
Homemade Sports Drink				√
Hummus				√
Jalapeño-Apple Salsa				√
Kale & White Bean Soup		√	√	√
Lemon-Fresh Quinoa with Herbs	√	√	√	√
Mango & Black Bean Salsa	√	√	√	√
Manhattan Clam Chowder		√	√	
Marinated Chicken Kebobs		√	√	
Middle Eastern Burger		√	√	
Muffin Tin Frittatas	√	√		√

	B	L	D	S
Mushroom & Broccoli Frittata	√	√	√	
Orange-Lime Shrimp with Apricot Rice		√	√	
Poached Fish Pouches		√	√	
Power Oatmeal	√			
Quick Lemon Chicken		√	√	
Quinoa Tabouleh	√	√	√	√
Red Cabbage, Onions & Oranges		√	√	
Roasted Brussels Sprouts		√	√	√
Salmon Salad	√	√		√
Sautéed Salmon & Green Beans		√	√	
Scrambled Eggs & Sun-Dried Tomatoes	√			
Scrambled Eggs & Sweet Potatoes	√	√		
Seafood Lettuce Tacos		√	√	
Seasonal Salad		√	√	
Sesame Broccoli		√	√	
Spanish Stuffed Peppers		√	√	
Spiced Sweet Potato Cubes	√	√	√	
Spicy Garlic Hummus				√
String Beans & Tomatoes		√	√	
Summer Fruit Salad	√	√	√	√
Summer Poached Salmon		√	√	
Super-Moist Turkey Meatballs		√	√	√

	B	L	D	S
Sweet Mushroom Salad		√	√	√
Taco-less Taco Salad		√	√	
Tangy Salsa & Eggs	√			
Thai Curried Cod or Chicken		√	√	
Tomato Relish				√
Tomato Soup		√	√	√
Tuna Salad		√	√	√
Turkey & Vegetable Stew		√	√	
Turkey Bolognese		√		
Turkey or Beef Confetti Bowl		√	√	
Tuscan Bean Dip				√
Tuscan Cabbage, Kale & Beans	√	√	√	
Vegetable Stir-Fry		√	√	
Waldorf Salad	√	√		
Zucchini Pancakes	√	√		

	B	L	D	S
Flourless Almond Butter Cookies				√
Gluten-Free Banana Muffins				√

A list of product recommendations and resources, including websites, can be found on page 445. Refer to that list if you are looking for grass-fed meat or wild seafood, or any of the brand-name products I've called for in the recipes.

Breakfast

Cauliflower & Leek Fritters

These fritters can be eaten as a breakfast, snack, or lunch. The herbaceous flavor of leeks and the earthy flavor notes of cauliflower make this a satisfying dish. Cauliflower is loaded with plant-based anti-inflammatories and phytochemicals that stave off disease. Did I mention it is high in vitamin C, a powerful antioxidant needed to prevent free-radical damage in the body? Low in calories, but high in quality protein, eggs contain the antioxidants lutein and zeaxanthin, which are needed to prevent age-related macular degeneration and cataracts.

Serves 6
Calories per serving: 138

4 cups rough-chopped cauliflower (dime-sized)
2 tablespoons avocado oil
1 bunch leeks, white only, split and sliced half inch
4 cloves diced garlic
1 teaspoon sea salt
½ teaspoon fresh ground black pepper

4 eggs (preferably organic or cage free), lightly beaten
½ cup cashew milk
4 tablespoons brown rice flour
1 teaspoon garlic powder
1 teaspoon onion powder
1 teaspoon fennel powder (or ground fennel seeds)
1 pinch sea salt

Wash and chop cauliflower, drain, and set aside. In a large frying pan add oil and leeks; cook on medium heat for 2 minutes. Add garlic, and cook for 2 minutes. Add cauliflower, salt, and pepper. Sauté until cauliflower is tender but not mushy. Set aside to cool.

Combine all remaining ingredients; stir until well mixed. Add leek-and-cauliflower mixture, and stir well. In a large frying pan on medium-high heat, add enough oil to glaze the bottom of the pan. Add a heaping tablespoon of mixture; flatten and shape into a round. Cook until bottom is golden brown, then turn it over and repeat on other side. (Always test one first to make sure the pan is hot enough.) When done, drain on a paper towel to blot excess oil.

Unused mixture can be refrigerated for a couple of days for later use.

Devilicious Curried Eggs

The curry powder, sweet with a little bite, makes this superfood an elegant and healthful protein source for breakfast or as an appetizer. Eggs are an excellent source of protein, contain all nine essential amino acids, and are loaded with other nutrients important for health.

Serves 6 for breakfast, 12 as a snack
Calories per serving (2 eggs/4 halves for breakfast; 1 egg/2 halves as a snack):
267 breakfast; 133 snack

12 large eggs (preferably organic or cage free), hard-boiled
¾ cup mayonnaise or Vegenaise (see Resources), plus more if needed
1 tablespoon spicy mustard (smooth, not grainy)

2 teaspoons hot curry powder
½ teaspoon onion powder
½ teaspoon sea salt (optional)
6 to 8 Spanish olives, pitted and sliced

Slice the hard-boiled eggs in half lengthwise; remove the yolks and set the whites aside. By hand or in a food processor, mash the yolks to a fine consistency. Add the mayonnaise, mustard, curry powder, and onion powder; blend thoroughly until smooth. If necessary, add a little more mayonnaise to get a smooth consistency.

Taste to see if the mixture needs salt. Usually salt is not needed, but that depends on the mustard. Spoon the mixture into a pastry bag and pipe it into the egg whites. (Alternatively, spoon the mixture to a resealable plastic bag and twist the bag to remove air. Snip off a small corner of the bag and pipe the filling into the egg whites.) Garnish each egg with an olive slice.

Variations

SMOKED SALMON EGGS: Omit the mustard, curry powder, salt, and olives. Add ¼ cup finely minced smoked salmon and the zest and juice of ½ lemon to the mashed egg yolks, and garnish with capers.

DILLED EGGS: Omit the mustard, curry powder, and olives. Add 1 tablespoon chopped fresh dill to the mashed egg yolks, and garnish with fresh dill.

SMOKY BACON EGGS: Omit the mustard, curry powder, salt, and olives. Cook 2 slices of naturally cured turkey bacon, let cool, and mince. Add the minced bacon and ¼ teaspoon cayenne pepper (optional) to the mashed egg yolks.

Egg & Avocado on Toast

There is something about the combination of eggs and toast that is most satisfying. The avocado plays well with the egg and the nutty flavor of the brown rice bread to make a most satisfying dish. All at once, you are getting the perfect combination of protein, healthful fat, and carbs to power you through your morning. This one is quick and easy to prepare.

Serves 2
Calories per serving: 265

2 slices brown rice bread (usually found in the frozen-foods section of the grocery)
2 large eggs (preferably organic or cage free)

1 to 2 teaspoons avocado oil
¼ ripe avocado, mashed

Toast the bread to your liking. (Brown rice bread is not chewy like white Italian bread; don't expect that same texture.)

Prepare the eggs the way you like. I like them fried (with avocado oil), scrambled (see Note), or boiled and sliced.

Spread the mashed avocado over the bread and add the eggs on top.

NOTE: If you usually add milk when scrambling eggs, substitute a nondairy milk (unsweetened almond or rice milk). I suggest adding nothing but your favorite seasoning. I like Bragg Organic Sprinkle (see Resources).

Muffin Tin Frittatas

Here you have an Egg McMuffin without the muffin. These fluffy baked egg cups are loaded with protein, immune-enhancing mushrooms, and the earthy taste of cauliflower. These frittatas are easy to create and great on the run. Did I mention kids will love them? These refrigerate well and make for a great breakfast or a snack on the go.

Serves 12
Calories per serving: 44

¼ teaspoon salt
2 cups finely chopped curly kale
2 tablespoons avocado oil to prepare muffin pan
1 tablespoon avocado oil
1 medium onion, diced
2 cups chopped cauliflower (small bite-sized)

½ teaspoon dried oregano
1 teaspoon McCormick Montreal steak seasoning
2 cups chopped portobello or cremini mushrooms
5 eggs (preferably organic or cage free)
1 tablespoon avocado oil for cooking

Preheat oven to 350°F.

In lightly salted water steam kale until tender; drain and set aside.

Prepare non-stick or silicone muffin pan (12 muffins) by placing a bit of avocado oil in each cup. This will ensure no sticking and allow the frittatas to create a solid crusty bottom.

Heat a large skillet to medium heat and add 1 tablespoon avocado oil, onion, cauliflower, oregano, and steak seasoning; cook for 3 minutes. Add mushrooms; cook until tender. Add steamed kale, and mix well. Set aside to cool.

Lightly whisk eggs; add to vegetables and mix well. If mixture is too stiff, add another egg. Do not add liquid; it will make the frittatas too fragile to eat like a muffin. Bake for 15 minutes; check one muffin to see if the bottom is golden brown. Check firmness by pushing the top lightly in the center. Bake for another 5 minutes, if needed. Let cool before removing from pan.

Mushroom & Broccoli Frittata

There is no question that a frittata loaded with broccoli and mushrooms is a perfect food. In one serving, the eggs provide adequate protein, the mushrooms enhance your immune system, and the broccoli goes to work helping the body get rid of toxins. The combination of spices, vegetables, and eggs is big on flavor, and this dish is inexpensive to boot.

Serves 4 to 6
Calories per serving: 210 for 4; 141 for 6

1½ cups chopped broccoli
1 tablespoon plus 1 teaspoon avocado oil
1 bunch scallions, sliced
1 (8-ounce) package cremini mushrooms, sliced
¼ red bell pepper, minced
Sea salt and freshly ground black pepper
1 teaspoon dried oregano
7 large eggs (preferably organic or free range)
1 teaspoon onion powder

Steam the chopped broccoli just until tender; set aside.

In a 10-inch sauté pan, heat 1 tablespoon of the oil over medium heat. Add the scallions, mushrooms, bell pepper, and a little salt and black pepper. Cook, stirring, for a few minutes to reduce the moisture. Add the steamed broccoli, oregano, and a bit more salt and black pepper. Cook for a few minutes to combine the flavors; taste and add more salt if needed. Remove the vegetable mixture from the pan and set aside.

In a medium bowl, combine the eggs, onion powder, and salt and pepper to taste. Mix well with a fork to break the egg yolks.

Coat the same pan with the remaining 1 teaspoon of oil and set the pan over low heat. Pour a small portion of the egg mixture into the pan; add the vegetable mixture in an even layer. Pour the rest of the egg mixture on top. Using a fork, gently push the vegetables to mix in the egg. Cover the pan and cook for about 15 minutes, until the top is set; then set a large plate over the pan and, holding the pan and plate together, carefully flip the frittata onto the plate. Slide the frittata back into the pan and cook on the second side, uncovered, for 5 minutes to eliminate excess moisture.

Power Oatmeal

Why Power Oatmeal? How else would you describe a hearty serving of steel-cut oats? Oatmeal is a gluten-free hot cereal that makes a great pre-workout meal to power you through your training session. Steel-cut oats—not rolled oats—are rich in soluble and insoluble fiber, vitamins, and minerals. The fresh fruit increases the nutrient value; try adding walnuts for a more well-rounded meal. Make sure to buy oats certified as "gluten-free," as some oats are processed in the same facilities as gluten-containing grains, which may result in cross-contamination.

Serves 1
Calories per serving: 400

¾ cup steel-cut oats
½ scoop protein powder (whey, egg white, or rice protein)

¼ cup sliced fresh strawberries
¼ cup fresh blueberries
Ground cinnamon (optional)

Cook the oats as directed on the package. Add the protein powder to the cooked oats; mix thoroughly. Top with berries and a dash of cinnamon.

Variations

BANANA OATMEAL: While the oatmeal cooks, stir in ½ cup mashed banana. Stir in 6 chopped walnuts, ¼ teaspoon sea salt, ½ teaspoon vanilla extract, and 1 teaspoon chia seeds before serving. (Calories per serving: 389)

PUMPKIN OATMEAL: While the oatmeal cooks, stir in ¼ cup canned pure pumpkin puree. Stir in 1 teaspoon pumpkin pie spice (or ground cinnamon), ¼ teaspoon sea salt, 1 teaspoon chia seeds, and 1 tablespoon agave syrup before serving. (Calories per serving: 509)

Scrambled Eggs & Sweet Potatoes

This simple and nutritious dish was a go-to for me while I was going through my cancer care and rebuilding myself back to excellent health. The flavor combination of eggs, sweet potatoes, mushrooms, tomatoes, and greens can't be beat.

Serves 2
Calories per serving: 217

1 to 2 teaspoons avocado oil
1 large egg (preferably organic or
   cage free)
3 egg whites
¼ cup diced cooked sweet potato
¼ cup chopped yellow or white onion
½ cup chopped leafy greens (fresh or
   frozen spinach or leafy greens such
as collard greens, mustard greens,
   or kale)
¼ cup chopped white button
   mushrooms
¼ cup chopped grape tomatoes
Sea salt and freshly ground black
   pepper
Red pepper flakes (optional)

In a medium skillet, heat the oil over medium heat. In a small bowl, lightly beat together the whole egg and the egg whites. When the oil is hot, add the egg mixture. Once the egg mixture starts to solidify, add the sweet potato, onion, greens, mushrooms, and tomatoes and mix well. Cook until the eggs are completely cooked through. Season with salt, black pepper, and, if you like, red pepper flakes. Divide between two plates and serve hot.

Variation

Instead of sweet potato, use ½ cup cooked brown rice. Stir the rice into the eggs when you add the vegetables, or serve the egg mixture over the rice.

Scrambled Eggs & Sun-Dried Tomatoes

Two of my favorite foods are eggs and tomatoes. Eggs are a great source of protein and nutrients, and tomatoes are an excellent source of antioxidants, which can tame the effects of free radicals. Serve with fruit for a complete breakfast.

Serves 2
Calories per serving: 318

2 teaspoons avocado oil
4 large or extra-large eggs
   (preferably organic or cage free)

5 or 6 sun-dried tomatoes packed in
   oil, chopped
Sea salt and freshly ground black
   pepper

This is a quick one. In a medium skillet, heat the oil over medium heat. In a small bowl, whisk together the eggs and tomatoes until thoroughly combined. When the oil is hot, add the egg mixture and cook until the eggs are cooked through.

Season with salt and pepper and serve.

Tangy Salsa & Eggs

What better way to spice up your eggs for breakfast than with a topping of tangy salsa served over a bed of nutty-tasting brown rice? This is another nutrient-dense breakfast that will help you power through your morning.

Serves 1
Calories per serving: 337

½ cup cooked brown rice
½ cup sugar-free salsa
½ teaspoon avocado oil

2 large eggs (preferably organic or
   cage free)
¼ avocado (optional)

In a bowl, mix the brown rice and salsa; set aside.

In a small skillet, heat the oil over medium heat. Add the eggs and fry or scramble to your liking. Add the eggs to the rice-salsa mixture and stir to combine. Serve with ¼ of an avocado to add additional flavors and creaminess.

Zucchini Pancakes

These are not the traditional buttermilk pancakes smothered in Vermont maple syrup that put you to sleep after a short stack. The sweet taste of raisins and coconut, combined with the earthy flavor of zucchini and brown rice, will have you eating more than just one. Zucchini is a summer squash that provides antioxidants, electrolytes, omega-3 fatty acids, zinc, and niacin, and is a good source of the B vitamins needed for optimal health.

Serves 5 to 6 (makes 30 to 36 pancakes)
Calories per serving (6 pancakes): 174

3 cups shredded zucchini
Sea salt
1 cup cooked brown rice
¼ cup unsweetened shredded
    coconut
½ bunch scallions, white and light
    green parts only, sliced
⅓ cup raisins
1 teaspoon grated fresh ginger

1 tablespoon curry powder
2 large eggs (preferably organic or
    cage free), lightly beaten
3 tablespoons brown rice flour, plus
    more if needed
1 (8-ounce) can whole water
    chestnuts, drained and coarsely
    chopped
1 tablespoon avocado oil

Put the shredded zucchini in a colander and sprinkle it with salt. Set the colander in the sink for 30 minutes to drain excess water. Press on the zucchini to extract more moisture, then transfer the drained zucchini to a food processor.

Add the brown rice, coconut, scallions, raisins, ginger, curry powder, and 2 teaspoons salt and process to a grainy consistency.

In a large bowl, whisk the eggs with the brown rice flour. Add the zucchini mixture and water chestnuts; mix well. At this point, the batter can be refrigerated in an airtight container for a few days before cooking. It also freezes well, if divided into several batches.

In a nonstick skillet, heat the oil over medium heat. Form a 2-inch pancake from the zucchini mixture; if it does not hold together, stir another teaspoon of brown rice flour into the batter. Cook a test pancake and taste to see if more salt is needed, then form and cook the remaining pancakes in batches (cook until slightly browned). You should end up with 30 to 36 (2-inch) pancakes.

Lunch

Bison Burgers with Salsa

Bison/buffalo meat has a sweeter and richer flavor than beef. As with all grass-fed meats, bison/buffalo is abundant in fatty acids, vitamin B$_{12}$, and iron. When combined with tangy salsa, the result is a burger that will definitely satisfy your hunger. This burger makes an excellent protein source when you are creating your personal meal plan.

Serves 4
Calories per serving: 337

1 pound ground bison $\frac{1}{3}$ cup sugar-free mild salsa

Heat a grill to low-medium heat or a grill pan over medium heat.

In a medium bowl, combine the bison and salsa; mix thoroughly with clean hands. Form the mixture into 4 patties (about 4 ounces each). Grill to your preference, about 4 minutes on each side for medium doneness. Be careful not to char the meat, as that makes it very toxic.

Variation

With a few tweaks, this recipe also makes a great meat loaf: Preheat the oven to 350°F. In a large bowl, combine 2 pounds ground bison, beef, turkey, or other grass-fed meat with $\frac{1}{2}$ to $\frac{3}{4}$ cup sugar-free mild salsa. Bake for 40 minutes to 1 hour, or until the internal temperature is 160°F.

Cabbage & Carrot Soup

There is something very comforting about a bowl of hot soup. The mild and earthy flavor of the cabbage, the sweetness of the carrot, and the hint of ginger will have you going back for seconds. Cabbage is a cruciferous vegetable that is a powerhouse of phytochemicals, including indole-3-carbinol (I3C), which helps to detoxify drugs and other ingestible toxins, while protecting against heart disease and cancers of the breast, colon, and prostate.

Serves 6
Calories per serving: 90

1 tablespoon sesame oil
1 bunch scallions, sliced
½ head savoy cabbage, sliced into
   ½-inch-thick strips
2 cups ½-inch pieces fresh green
   beans
3 large carrots, sliced
1 green bell pepper, diced
10 cremini mushrooms, thinly sliced
Sea salt and freshly ground black
   pepper

2 to 3 quarts organic low-sodium
   chicken stock
¼ cup coconut liquid aminos
   (see Resources), plus more as
   needed
½ bunch fresh cilantro, coarsely
   chopped
¼ cup thickly sliced fresh ginger
   (make the pieces large enough to
   remove easily)

In a large stockpot, cook the sesame oil and scallions over low to medium heat for a minute to soften the scallions. Add the cabbage, green beans, carrots, bell pepper, and mushrooms; stir together and season with salt and black pepper. Cook for a few minutes to soften the vegetables, then add the stock and raise the heat to medium-high. Bring the mixture to a boil, then reduce the heat to maintain a simmer. Add the coconut liquid aminos, cilantro, and ginger and simmer for 1 hour. Taste; add more salt, black pepper, or coconut liquid aminos as needed.

Before serving, remove and discard the pieces of ginger.

Chunky Vegetable Soup

This soup has all the flavors you can imagine, from sweet and tangy to mild and earthy, salty, and spicy—all of Mother Nature's vegetables provide a full-bodied taste. This is a nutrient-dense soup, providing you with an abundance of antioxidants, phytochemicals, vitamins, minerals, and electrolytes to help you rebuild and recover from any chronic disease. This is a very versatile recipe. Use the recommended ingredients or substitute whatever you have on hand. Frozen vegetables work well in this recipe, too.

Serves 4 to 6
Calories per serving: 182 for 4; 121 for 6

2 to 3 tablespoons avocado oil
1 onion, diced
2 carrots, sliced
2 celery stalks, sliced
4 cups organic low-sodium vegetable broth
1 (15-ounce) can diced tomatoes with their juices
2 garlic cloves, minced, or 1 tablespoon jarred minced garlic

1 cup bite-size pieces of green beans
1 small sweet potato, diced
½ cup fresh or frozen peas
1 cup chopped cabbage, kale, or collard greens
1 tablespoon dried herbs (such as thyme, rosemary, tarragon)
½ cup minced fresh parsley
Sea salt and freshly ground black pepper

In a large soup pot, heat the oil over medium heat. Add the onion, carrots, and celery; cook, stirring, until the vegetables have softened. Add 4 cups water, the broth, tomatoes, garlic, green beans, sweet potato, peas, cabbage, dried herbs, and parsley. Simmer until all the vegetables are soft, about 30 to 45 minutes. Taste and season with salt and pepper.

Crispy Cruciferous Salad

If you like crunch and the distinctive flavor of broccoli, cauliflower, and cabbage, this salad is a must for your personal rebuild. This group of edible plants provides an abundance of nutrients and phytochemicals shown to regulate hormones, as well as reduce inflammation and free radical damage, key factors in the production and progression of all disease. If you aren't a big fan of cruciferous vegetables, adding the sweet and tangy dressing to this salad will certainly improve your taste for these most healthful vegetables.

Serves 6
Calories per serving: 250

Salad
1 large head broccoli (2 pounds), cut into bite-size pieces
¾ head cauliflower, cut into bite-size pieces
2 large carrots, shredded
¼ head red cabbage, finely chopped
5 radishes, sliced

1 cup sliced snap peas or snow peas
½ small red onion, sliced, or 2 scallions, thinly sliced
½ bunch flat-leaf parsley, chopped
½ cup pumpkin seeds or slivered raw almonds

Dressing
¼ cup extra-virgin olive oil
¼ cup rice vinegar or apple cider vinegar
2 teaspoons light agave syrup

Freshly ground black pepper
1 to 2 teaspoons sea salt, plus more as needed
1 sprig lemon thyme, chopped

Salad
In a large bowl, toss all the salad ingredients together.

Dressing
In a small bowl, whisk together all the dressing ingredients.

Add the dressing to the salad; mix well. Taste and add more salt if needed. Cover and refrigerate until chilled before serving. Stir the mixture often while it's chilling; this will release more liquid and marinate the vegetables.

Curried Chicken Salad

If you like the taste of curry, you will love this high-protein salad. On top of the protein-packed chicken, the curry powder is abundant in turmeric, which contains the powerful compound curcumin. Studies show that this yellow-colored curcuminoid helps to fight a wide range of diseases by acting as a powerful antioxidant, anti-inflammatory, and anticancer agent.

Serves 6 to 8
Calories per serving: 367 for 6; 275 for 8

4 large boneless, skinless chicken breasts
½ to ¾ cup mayonnaise or Vegenaise (see Resources)
2 teaspoons dehydrated onion or ½ small red onion, finely chopped
2 tablespoons curry powder

4 celery stalks, sliced lengthwise and cut into ¼-inch pieces
½ to ¾ cup raisins or dried cranberries
Sea salt and freshly ground black pepper
Endive or radicchio, leaves separated, for serving

Rinse chicken and place in a pot fitted with a steamer basket over water. Bring water to a boil, and steam the chicken until juices run clear, about 30 minutes. Remove from the pot and let cool, then cut into bite-size pieces. Set aside in a large bowl.

In a small bowl, combine ½ cup of the mayonnaise, the onion, and the curry powder; stir to combine. Add the mayonnaise mixture to the chicken and mix well. If needed, add the remaining ¼ cup mayonnaise and stir to combine. Add the celery and raisins, season with salt and pepper, and mix well. Serve over a bed of endive or radicchio.

Variation
Roasted turkey breast can be substituted for the chicken. Cut an equivalent amount of cooked turkey into bite-size pieces, and continue as directed above.

Egg & Olive Salad

The light, briny taste of olives makes this salad a real treat. Besides being an excellent source of protein, eggs contain cysteine, an important amino acid needed to detoxify harmful chemicals and drugs.

Serves 1
Calories per serving: 279

2 large eggs (preferably organic or cage free), hard-boiled
2 tablespoons mayonnaise or Vegenaise (see Resources)

¼ teaspoon mustard (Dijon is good, but any mustard will do)
4 to 6 green olives with pimientos, sliced
Freshly ground black pepper

Slice the eggs in an egg slicer, or slice them lengthwise, then crosswise into small cubes. Transfer the eggs to a small bowl, add the remaining ingredients, and stir to combine. Taste and adjust the seasoning. (Because of the olives, you probably will not need to add salt.)

Hearty Navy Bean Soup

Bacon and spices really round out the flavor of this soup. Turkey and beans provide the healthful protein you need, while the carrot, onion, and celery provide an array of disease-fighting nutrients to speed up recovery from any chronic health issue.

Serves 4
Calories per serving: 150

3 (15-ounce) cans organic navy beans or other white beans, undrained
1 tablespoon avocado oil
4 slices naturally cured turkey bacon, halved lengthwise and sliced into ½-inch pieces (see Note)

1 large yellow onion, diced
2 celery stalks, diced
3 carrots, halved lengthwise and sliced ¼ inch thick
2 to 3 teaspoons sea salt, plus a pinch

1 teaspoon freshly ground black
   pepper, plus a pinch
6 cups organic low-sodium chicken
   stock

2 teaspoons onion powder
1 teaspoon dried oregano
1 bay leaf

Pour 1 can of the beans, including their liquid, into a blender; blend until smooth.

In a large stockpot, heat the oil over medium heat. Add the bacon and cook, stirring, until the bacon starts to brown. Add the onion, celery, carrots, and a pinch each of the salt and pepper. Cook for about 5 minutes, until the onion softens a bit. Remove the mixture from the pot and set aside.

In the same pot, combine the blended beans, stock, remaining 2 cans of whole beans (including their liquid), the onion powder, oregano, remaining 1 teaspoon pepper, 2 teaspoons of the salt, and the bay leaf. Cover and bring to a boil; reduce the heat to maintain a simmer. Add the bacon-vegetable mixture; cook, uncovered, over low heat until the beans are smooth in texture and the liquid has thickened to a creamy consistency, about 1 hour. As the soup thickens, taste and add the remaining 1 teaspoon salt as needed.

Remove the bay leaf before serving.

"Just Wing It" Salads

Have you ever wondered how someone can make a mouth-watering meal out of just a few foods and spices, all without measuring or following a recipe? Well, you can, too. The following salad recipes are designed to let you get creative. If you want more romaine lettuce, go for it. If you would rather have more red cabbage than green cabbage, make it your way. Look to see what's in your fridge and use whatever vegetables you have. Mixing different kinds of greens can be tasty; don't be afraid to throw them all together.

You build your own salad. You can't mess this up. Just add and subtract ingredients until you have the salad you want. When making any of these salads, make enough for leftovers. Before adding the dressing, take what you will eat now and then store the rest, well covered, in the refrigerator for another meal. (Pouring dressing over the whole salad will make the leftovers very soggy.)

The recipe for Classic Vinaigrette that follows is perfect for all the salads. Save time by making enough dressing for several salads.

NOTE: When a recipe calls for legumes, fats, grains, or protein, be conscious of serving size. For example, if you add butter beans to a salad, don't add the entire can unless you're making a large salad meant to be eaten for several meals—you shouldn't eat the whole can of beans at one meal.

Classic Vinaigrette

Makes ¼ to ⅓ cup dressing, to serve 2
Calories per serving: 120

2 tablespoons extra-virgin olive oil
1 to 2 tablespoons apple cider vinegar
1 tablespoon balsamic vinegar

⅛ teaspoon sea salt
⅛ teaspoon freshly ground black pepper

Combine the olive oil and both vinegars in a jar or cruet; cover and shake to mix well. Season with the salt and pepper.

NOTE: Adjust the amounts to make more or less dressing. When adding it to your salad, use just enough to wet the leaves; they should look shiny but should not be dripping with oil. This will prevent you from eating too much oil at one meal.

"This Rocks" Salad

This salad does rock, not only for providing a full palate of different tastes but also for its sheer health benefit. It is loaded with protein, essential fatty acids, vitamins, minerals, and phytochemicals to quickly recalibrate your genes for optimal health.

Serves 1
Calories per serving: 73 (without dressing)

Mixed greens
Romaine lettuce, shredded
Grape tomatoes
Cucumber, sliced or chopped
Carrots, sliced or chopped
Butter beans

Black olives
Fresh green peas
White onion, chopped
Red bell peppers, chopped
Hard-boiled egg, if you want protein

Mediterranean Salad

The smooth and buttery texture of artichoke sets this salad apart. Artichoke is loaded with fiber, folate, magnesium, and the antioxidants rutin and quercetin, which are needed for cancer prevention, immune support, and protection against heart disease.

Serves 1
Calories per serving: 219 (without dressing)

Romaine lettuce, shredded
White onion, chopped
Mixed olives, pitted
Sun-dried tomato, chopped

Artichoke hearts, quartered
Butter beans
Red bell pepper, chopped

Crunchy Cabbage Salad

If you like the crunch and earthy taste of cabbage and the sweet taste of snap peas, you will love this healthful salad. Red and green cabbage provide phytochemicals with unique abilities to detoxify and prevent toxic compounds from attaching to DNA, which could lead to cancer. Cabbage and other cruciferous vegetables have also been shown to help promote the production of a less potent form of estrogen. High estrogen is implicated in the development of cancers of the breast, endometrium, uterus, and prostate.

Serves 1
Calories per serving: 131 (without dressing)

Red and green cabbage, shredded
Carrot, sliced or chopped
Snap peas
Red bell pepper, sliced

Cucumber, sliced
Grape tomato
Red onion, chopped

Healthy Heart Salad

Cranberries tickle your palate with sweetness and a touch of tartness, while the broccoli, cauliflower, and jicama give the salad crunch. Not only is it satisfying, but this salad is loaded with antioxidants and phytochemicals needed to combat free radical damage and extinguish inflammation, both of which are responsible for the development and progression of heart disease, cancer, and other chronic conditions.

Serves 1
Calories per serving: 348 (without dressing)

Cauliflower, coarsely chopped
Broccoli, coarsely chopped
Carrot, sliced or chopped
Red onion, chopped

Jicama, chopped (optional)
Dried cranberries (sweetened with
   juice, not sugar)
Sunflower seeds

Pantry Salad

This one varies depending on my mood and what I have in the refrigerator, but I will give you one recipe to use as a starting point. Get creative and follow your own taste buds!

When putting this one together, use more lettuce and spinach. Also use one medium to large carrot. If you don't like a strong onion taste, use a very small onion. Be creative here and use what you have. The nice thing about this salad is that you create your own flavors and textures. Any combination of rainbow-colored vegetables will provide you with all the right nutrients to recover from your chronic health issues.

Serves 1
Calories per serving: 110 (without dressing)

Spring mix lettuce
Spinach
Mushrooms, sliced
Asparagus, sliced
Green beans, sliced
Carrot, chopped

Celery, chopped
Tomato, chopped
Broccoli, chopped
Red or yellow bell pepper, sliced
Red or white onion, sliced
Red cabbage, shredded

Kale Salad

This salad is one of my go-to dishes for several reasons. It takes only a few minutes to make. It features all the right flavors, from the slightly bitter and tangy taste of kale to the satisfying sweetness of cranberries and apple. Walnuts provide crunch to make this salad a real treat. Kale is a popular cruciferous vegetable that is one of the most nutrient-dense foods in existence, providing plenty of beta-carotene, vitamins C and K, and the phytochemicals indole-3-carbinol and sulforaphane, all very important for recovering from chronic disease.

Serves 1
Calories per serving: 331 (without dressing)

Kale, stemmed and chopped
Spinach
Apple, cored and chopped
Walnuts

Carrot, sliced or chopped
Dried cranberries (sweetened with
juice, not sugar)

Kale & White Bean Soup

*A touch of oil and a little garlic and onion are all you need to complement
the sharp flavor of kale. In addition to tomato and carrot, the nutty flavor
and creamy texture of the cannellini beans really round out this soup.
Kale is a superfood rich in disease-fighting compounds, and cannellini
beans are good source of folate and thiamin (vitamin B_1)—both needed to
convert carbohydrates into energy. This soup is a must to help you defeat
your disease.*

Serves 8
Calories per serving: 105

1 cup sliced carrots (from 2 medium
or large)
2 tablespoons avocado oil
1 cup diced yellow onion
4 large garlic cloves, minced, or
equivalent jarred minced garlic
1 (32-ounce) container organic low-

sodium vegetable broth
1 (14.5-ounce) can diced tomatoes,
with their juices
1 (8-ounce) can tomato sauce
6 to 8 cups chopped kale
1 (14-ounce) can cannellini beans,
drained and rinsed

Bring a small saucepan of water to a boil; add the carrots and cook until
soft, then drain and set aside.

In a large soup pot, heat the oil over medium heat. Add the onion and
cook for 3 to 4 minutes. Add the garlic and cook for 2 to 3 minutes more.
Add the broth, diced tomatoes with their juices, tomato sauce, kale, and
cooked carrots and cook until the kale is tender; then stir in the beans.
Turn off the heat and let sit for 2 to 3 minutes.

Serve immediately.

Manhattan Clam Chowder

Bacon . . . need I say more? Bacon makes everything taste better, includ-ing a pot of tender minced clams surrounded by a sea of sweet and tangy crushed tomatoes. The sweet potato cubes add a taste and texture different from the standard white potato typically used in most chowders. If you are concerned about eating a little bacon, don't be. Companies like Applegate and Coleman make bacon without hormones, antibiotics, or preservatives (which make processed pork bacon unhealthful to eat). A serving of this chowder has plenty of protein from the clams and bacon, and the tomatoes add an abundance of the antioxidant lycopene—shown to combat heart disease, cancer, diabetes, and age-related macular degeneration.

Serves 8 to 10
Calories per serving: 205

2 tablespoons avocado oil
1 cup chopped naturally cured pork
   bacon or turkey bacon
1 medium-large onion, chopped
2 cups chopped celery
1 cup sliced carrot
1 cup chopped green bell pepper
6 garlic cloves, minced
1 cup bottled clam juice
2 (14.5-ounce) cans crushed tomatoes

2 medium sweet potatoes, cut into
   small cubes
1 bay leaf
1 teaspoon dried thyme
2 tablespoons chopped fresh parsley
Sea salt and freshly ground black
   pepper
7 or 8 (6.5-ounce) cans chopped or
   minced clams

In a large soup pot, heat the oil over medium heat. Add the bacon and cook, stirring, until browned, 3 to 4 minutes. Add the onion, celery, car-rot, bell pepper, and garlic; cook, stirring, for a few minutes more. Add the clam juice, crushed tomatoes, sweet potatoes, bay leaf, thyme, and parsley and season with salt and black pepper. Simmer until the carrot and sweet potatoes are soft. This can take anywhere from a few minutes to half an hour, depending on how you cut them and how cooked you like them. Try testing them with a fork—the fork should easily go through them. Add the clams and their liquid and simmer for 5 to 10 minutes more. Remove and discard the bay leaf.

Taste and season with salt and black pepper, if needed. Serve immediately.

Middle Eastern Burger

Middle Eastern cuisine is known for its flavorful dishes featuring an array of spices. The aromatic notes of cardamom and the smoky flavor of cumin add a touch of the Middle East to this burger. The spices aid digestion, improve immunity, and help regulate inflammation—the driving force behind chronic disease. Grass-fed beef is abundant in essential fatty acids, B vitamins, and, of course, protein.

Serves 4
Calories per serving: 231

1 small yellow onion, finely diced
1 garlic clove, minced
1 tablespoon tamari
1 teaspoon ground cumin
1 teaspoon ground cardamom
1 teaspoon smoked sea salt
Freshly ground black pepper

Cayenne pepper or diced jalapeño (optional)
1 pound grass-fed organic lean ground beef
Avocado, sliced, or Eggplant Tapenade (page 434), for serving

Heat a grill to medium or a grill pan or skillet over medium heat.

In a large bowl, mix together the onion, garlic, tamari, cumin, cardamom, smoked sea salt, and black pepper to taste. For a spicier (hotter) flavor, add cayenne or jalapeño to your liking. Add the ground beef, mix well with clean hands to combine, and form into four 4-ounce patties. Grill or cook on the stovetop until browned on both sides and cooked to your liking. Be careful not to char the meat, as that makes it very toxic.

Serve with avocado or Eggplant Tapenade.

Quinoa Tabbouleh

Quinoa (pronounced KEEN-wah) is a great source of magnesium, iron, vitamin E, potassium, and fiber. As versatile as rice, quinoa has a rich, nutty flavor. Quinoa is coated with a natural compound call sapo-nin, which some people think has a soapy or slightly bitter taste, which is why you should rinse or soak the quinoa before you eat it.

Serves 4
Calories per serving: 318

Tabbouleh

1 cup uncooked quinoa, rinsed well
1 pint grape tomatoes, sliced
1 small cucumber (see Note), cut into
   bite-size pieces

¾ cup sliced pitted ripe olives
2 cups chopped fresh flat-leaf parsley
   leaves
½ cup chopped fresh mint

Dressing

1 teaspoon lemon zest
¼ cup fresh lemon juice
¼ cup olive oil

1 teaspoon agave syrup (dark or light)
Sea salt and freshly ground black
   pepper

Tabbouleh

In a large saucepan, combine the quinoa and 2 cups water. Bring to a boil, cover, reduce the heat to low, and simmer until all the water has been absorbed, about 15 minutes. Refrigerate, covered, until chilled. This can be done a day ahead of time.

In a large bowl, combine the cooked quinoa, tomatoes, cucumber, olives, parsley, and mint; stir well.

Dressing

In a small bowl, combine the lemon zest, lemon juice, olive oil, and agave syrup. Mix well; season with salt and pepper.

Add the dressing to the tabbouleh and toss well to be sure the dressing is evenly distributed.

This can be refrigerated in an airtight container for 1 to 2 days without losing flavor or texture.

NOTE: Lebanese or Japanese cucumbers are best; they have tender skins and a crunchy texture. English cucumbers are also good. If using a regular cucumber, remove the seeds.

Salmon Salad

I really enjoy eating salmon, a soft and flaky fish with a mild taste created by the fat within the muscle of the fish. Dried dill complements this meaty fish to make this salad an excellent choice for lunch or dinner. Salmon is another one of those foods that provides superior protein, anti-inflammatory omega-3 essential fatty acids, selenium, vitamin B$_{12}$, and vitamin D.

Serves 2
Calories per serving: 186

1 (6-ounce) can wild salmon, or 6 ounces cold poached or grilled fresh salmon
¼ cup diced celery
2 tablespoons mayonnaise or Vegenaise (see Resources)
¼ teaspoon chopped dried dill

Sea salt and freshly ground black pepper
1 teaspoon prepared horseradish (optional)
Cucumber, sliced, for serving
Fresh tomatoes, sliced, for serving

Mix the first six ingredients together in a medium bowl. Serve chilled with sliced cucumber and tomatoes.

Cleansing Ginger Cabbage Soup

The main bioactive compound in ginger is gingerol, responsible for much of its medicinal properties and its spicy and peppery taste. This phyto-nutrient is also a powerful anti-inflammatory and antioxidant. I would be remiss not to mention the soothing effects it has on different conditions of the stomach. Cabbage is a nutrient-powerhouse vegetable, and it also adds a satisfying sweetness to this soup.

Serves 6 to 8
Calories per serving: 110

4 stalks celery, chopped bite-sized
4 carrots, chopped
1 medium red onion, diced
1/2 head cabbage, sliced thin
1/2 yellow bell pepper, diced
2 (28-ounce) cans organic diced
    tomatoes with juice
1 tablespoon freshly grated ginger
1/2 teaspoon ground allspice

1/2 teaspoon ground cloves
1 teaspoon ground coriander
1 teaspoon ground stick cinnamon
1 teaspoon ground cumin
1 teaspoon ground turmeric
1 teaspoon sea salt
1 teaspoon black pepper
1 large sweet potato, coarsely
    shredded

In a stock pot on medium heat, sweat celery, carrots, and onion for 3 minutes with a pinch of salt. Add cabbage, bell pepper, tomatoes, and another pinch of salt and pepper. Add all remaining ingredients but the sweet potato. Simmer for 30 minutes. Add sweet potato, and cook for 10 minutes more. Add salt, if needed.

Taco-less Taco Salad

If you enjoy tacos but don't want the guilt, this salad has it all: crunch, spice, and countless nutrients to help you recover and rebuild. I use organic, non-GMO (genetically modified organism) blue corn chips, as this old variety of corn contains a high level of anthocyanins, the phytochemi-

cal that gives plants a purple or blue color. Anthocyanins help metabolize toxins, enhance glucose metabolism, and reduce inflammation. However, keep in mind that more is not better here, as eating too much corn can affect your blood sugar.

Serves 4 to 6
Calories per serving: 292

Taco Spice

2 teaspoons ground cumin
1 teaspoon Himalayan sea salt
1 teaspoon freshly ground black
  pepper
1 teaspoon paprika

¼ teaspoon onion powder
¼ teaspoon garlic powder
¼ teaspoon red pepper flakes
¼ teaspoon dried oregano
1 tablespoon chili powder

Fillings

1 pound organic grass-fed ground
  beef, bison, or free-range turkey
½ to ¾ (8-ounce) package
  mozzarella-style shredded
  nondairy cheese (such as Daiya)
2 heads romaine lettuce, chopped
2 hearty handfuls of spring mix
  lettuces, chopped
1 large carrot, shredded
¼ medium white onion, diced

½ red bell pepper, diced
½ to ¾ medium-large cucumber,
  diced
¾ cup halved grape tomatoes
10 large black olives, pitted and
  chopped
1 cup sugar-free mild or medium
  salsa
Organic sprouted-grain blue corn
  chips (not taco shells)

Taco Spice

In a small bowl, mix all the spices and set aside.

Fillings

In a large skillet, cook the ground meat over medium heat until browned and cooked through. While still warm, add the taco spice a little at a time, tasting as you go until you like the flavor. Sprinkle the nondairy cheese over the meat so it melts.

In a large bowl, combine the lettuces, carrot, onion, bell pepper, cucumber, tomatoes, and olives. Put the spiced meat on top and top with the salsa. Serve with blue corn chips.

Tomato Soup

Many varieties of tomatoes have numerous health benefits. Their deep red color comes from a pigment called lycopene, a powerful antioxidant that has been shown to improve bone health, reduce low-density lipoprotein (LDL), prevent blood platelet aggregation (clumping), and prevent the oxidation of LDL—a key factor in the formation of coronary artery disease. This sweet and tangy soup is also rich in phytonutrients, needed to combat all chronic health issues.

Serves 8 to 10
Calories per serving: 90 for 8; 70 for 10

1 soup bone from a grass-fed cow
2 (16-ounce) cans organic tomato
   sauce
1 (12-ounce) can tomato paste
2 teaspoons sea salt or pink
   Himalayan salt

½ teaspoon freshly ground black
   pepper
2 organic beef bouillon cubes or
   equivalent bouillon powder (I
   recommend Edward & Sons, which
   is free of MSG and gluten)
4 carrots, chopped
4 celery stalks, chopped

In a large soup pot, combine the soup bone, tomato sauce, and 3 quarts water. Bring to a boil, then reduce the heat to maintain a simmer. To thicken the soup, add the tomato paste a little at a time until you get the consistency you want (you may not use the whole can). Add the salt, pepper, and bouillon cubes or powder. Simmer for 1 hour. Add the carrots and celery. Simmer for another hour, or until the carrots and celery are soft.

Tuna Salad

Growing up, school lunches were always a surprise; I never knew what I was going to pull out of my lunch bag. However, I did look forward to unwrapping the foil around my tuna fish sandwich. The sweet and mild flavor of tuna varies according to its source. Tuna from a can is slightly different from seared tuna. For this reason, try using tuna from different sources to add variety. This fish is a great source of omega-3 fatty acids and the mineral selenium. Selenium is important for a healthy immune system, fertility in both men and women, and cognitive function.

Serves 2
Calories per serving: 232

1 (5-ounce) can white tuna, packed in water (I like American Tuna, which is low in mercury—see Resources)
1 Fuji apple, cored and chopped
¼ cup dried cranberries (sweetened with juice, not sugar)
2 tablespoons mayonnaise or Vegenaise (see Resources)
½ teaspoon mustard, or to taste
Freshly ground black pepper

In a medium bowl, mix together the tuna, apple, and cranberries. In a small bowl, stir together the mayonnaise and mustard; add the mixture to the salad and mix well. Taste and season with pepper.

Vegetable Stir-Fry

You can't beat a vegetable stir-fry when you want a meal loaded with flavor and filling. The liquid aminos give this classic dish the flavor of soy sauce without the unwanted properties of unfermented soy. Stir-fries are so versatile because you can use whatever vegetables you like. Just make sure you add a complete mix of colorful vegetables to ensure you are getting a variety of the vitamins, minerals, fiber, and phytochemicals you need to rebuild.

Serves 2 or 3
Calories per serving: 167 for 2; 111 for 3

1 tablespoon avocado oil
1 large onion, diced
3 garlic cloves, finely chopped
1 teaspoon chopped fresh ginger
1 carrot, sliced
2 celery stalks, cut into ½-inch-thick slices
1 large head broccoli, cut into small pieces
1 (8-ounce) can sliced water chestnuts, drained
1 cup snap peas (whole or sliced)
Sea salt and freshly ground black pepper
1 tablespoon tamari
1 teaspoon sesame oil

In a large skillet, heat the avocado oil over medium heat. Add the onion, garlic, and ginger; cook, stirring continuously to avoid burning, for 1 minute. Add all the vegetables and a pinch each of salt and pepper; cook for 2 minutes. Add the tamari and cook for 2 minutes more. Add the sesame oil and season with salt and pepper; stir well and transfer to a platter to avoid overcooking.

Dinner

Beef or Lamb Shank

Big, beautiful, moist beef or lamb shank swimming in a marinade of garlic, salt, pepper, and stewed tomatoes says "comfort food." If you enjoy beef or lamb—grass-fed and free-range, of course—your palate and appetite will be pleased with this entrée. Both meats are rich in essential fatty acids and protein, and are an excellent source of vitamin B_{12}, important for building blood cells and maintaining healthy nerve function. The zinc found in beef and lamb is needed for proper reproductive and immune function, as well as regulating DNA synthesis and cellular metabolism.

Serves 4
Calories per serving: 325 (with brown rice: 380) (with quinoa: 381)

¾ cup fresh orange juice (from 3 or 4 oranges)
1 tablespoon garlic powder
1 tablespoon onion powder
1 teaspoon pink Himalayan salt, plus more as needed
1 teaspoon freshly ground black pepper, plus more as needed
2 to 4 large beef or lamb shanks

1 (15-ounce) can organic whole stewed tomatoes, sliced, juices reserved
½ cup red wine
1 teaspoon dried thyme
2 bay leaves
1 yellow onion, sliced
4 celery stalks, sliced
3 carrots, sliced
10 large cremini mushrooms, sliced
2 cups cooked brown rice or quinoa (optional)

In a large bowl, combine the orange juice, garlic powder, onion powder, salt, and pepper. Add the meat; stir to be sure all the meat is covered with the marinade. Cover the bowl and marinate for a couple of hours at room temperature.

Preheat the oven to 350°F.

Arrange the shanks in a Dutch oven. Add the marinade, tomatoes with their juices, wine, thyme, and bay leaves. Cover and bake for 1½ hours. Remove from the oven; add the onion, celery, carrots, and mushrooms. Season with salt and pepper; return to the oven and cook for another 1½ hours.

Serve over ½ cup brown rice or quinoa for a more substantial meal.

Broccoli & Kale Pasta

Two of the most nutrient-dense foods all in one. Broccoli and kale both belong to the plant species Brassica oleracea. *These cruciferous vegetables, well-known for their disease-fighting actions, should be at the top of your grocery list if you are rebuilding from any disease or chronic health issue. Consuming these earthy-flavored vegetables can also reduce your risk of developing heart disease, cancer, diabetes, and obesity.*

Serves 4 to 6
Calories per serving: 514 for 4; 343 for 6

1 tablespoon sea salt, plus more as needed
1 large head broccoli, cut into small pieces
1 tablespoon avocado oil
6 to 8 garlic cloves, smashed and chopped
1 bunch scallions, sliced
½ bunch kale, sliced

1 medium zucchini, shredded
2 teaspoons dried basil
1 teaspoon dried oregano
8 ounces cremini mushrooms, sliced
Freshly ground black pepper
1 tablespoon extra-virgin olive oil
1 pound brown rice pasta (I like tricolor fusilli)

In a large pot, bring 6 quarts water to a boil for the pasta; add the salt.

Fit a separate large saucepan with a steamer basket and add water to come just beneath the basket. Bring the water to a boil, add the broccoli to the steamer, and cook until tender, roughly 10 to 15 minutes. Remove from the pot and set aside.

Meanwhile, in a large skillet, heat the avocado oil over medium heat; add the garlic and scallions and cook, stirring, for 1 to 2 minutes. Add the kale, season with salt, and sprinkle with a teaspoon or two of water; cook until the kale is wilted. Add the zucchini, basil, and oregano; cook for 2 minutes. Add the mushrooms and season with salt and pepper; cook, stirring, for 1 minute, then cook undisturbed for 1 minute more. Add the broccoli and olive oil; reduce the heat, and cook until flavors are combined.

Add the pasta to the pot of boiling water. Cook until al dente according to the package directions; do not overcook. Use tongs to scoop the pasta from the boiling water into the sauce; allow some of the pasta water to mix in (this will thicken the sauce and make it silkier). Cook for another minute, then serve immediately.

Chester's Chili

My father has always been known for his skill in the kitchen. Staring at the war zone he creates out of his cooking space, I often wonder how he can combine texture and flavors into an unforgettable meal, especially his spicy and meaty chili. The cayenne pepper used in the recipe is known for its bite, but the compound capsaicin found in cayenne is an effective treatment for arthritis and muscle pain. Capsaicin can also help regulate your blood sugar, reduce inflammation, and act as a natural decongestant. This dish is a perfect meal to warm you up on a cool autumn night. For a twist on the taste, substitute ground bison or turkey for the ground beef.

Serves 6
Calories per serving: 216

1 tablespoon avocado oil
2 medium onions, chopped
1 cup chopped green bell pepper
1 pound grass-fed ground beef
1 (28-ounce) can diced tomatoes, with
 their juices
1 (8-ounce) can tomato sauce

2 teaspoons chili powder
1 teaspoon sea salt
½ teaspoon paprika
⅛ teaspoon cayenne pepper
1 (15-ounce) can red kidney beans,
 drained and rinsed

In a soup pot, heat the oil over medium heat. Add the onions and cook, stirring, until soft. Add the bell pepper and cook for a couple of minutes more. Add the ground beef; cook, stirring, until the meat is cooked through.

Add all the remaining ingredients except the kidney beans and stir. Reduce the heat to medium and simmer for 1 hour, stirring occasionally. Tip the pot slightly to determine the amount of extra water and juices, then skim off extra liquid with a soup ladle.

Turn off heat and add the kidney beans. Mix well and serve.

Chicken Sausage & Sweet Potatoes

The fresh, sweet, and light flavor of fennel complements the flavor of the sweet potatoes and chicken in this dish. Sweet potatoes are inexpensive, readily available, and rich in nutrients. They are high in fiber, vitamin B_6, vitamin C, iron, and magnesium. Magnesium is essential for the health of muscles, arteries, blood, bone, and nerve function. The choline in fennel is a versatile nutrient that can improve memory, sleep, and muscle function. If you love the taste of licorice, lose the package of Twizzlers and cut up a fennel bulb and stem to satisfy your craving.

Serves 6
Calories per serving: 374

3 large sweet potatoes
Sea salt and freshly ground black
  pepper
1 fennel bulb, sliced (optional)
3 tablespoons avocado oil
1 large Vidalia onion, quartered and
  sliced ¼ inch thick

2 teaspoons fennel powder (substitute
  dried oregano, if preferred)
1 to 1½ cups frozen green peas,
  thawed
6 chicken sausage links, sliced into
  ¼ inch thick rounds

Cook the sweet potatoes in the microwave for 8 to 15 minutes, until tender. Cut them in half lengthwise, then set aside until cool enough to handle. Cut them into ½-inch-thick slices, keeping the skin intact. Season the slices with salt and pepper and set aside to cool completely.

Fit a separate large saucepan with a steamer basket and add water to come just beneath the basket. Bring the water to a boil, add the fennel to the steamer, and cook until tender but still firm, roughly 10 minutes. Drain and cut into bite-size pieces. (If you do not like the flavor of fennel, you can skip this.)

In a large skillet, heat 1 tablespoon of the oil over medium heat. Add the onion; cook, stirring frequently, for 3 minutes. Season with salt and pepper. Add the fennel powder and peas; cook, stirring, for 5 minutes more, until the peas and onions are a bit browned. Remove from the pan set aside.

In the same pan, heat the remaining 2 tablespoons oil over medium heat. Add the sausage; cook until browned (this won't take long, as most chicken sausages are precooked). Return the onions and peas to the pan and add the steamed fennel (if using) and sliced sweet potatoes. Toss gently for 3 to 4 minutes, until the flavors combine.

Chicken or Shrimp Stir-Fry

This stir-fry is another favorite of mine, as I really enjoy both chicken and shrimp flavored with a touch of salt from the liquid aminos. Chicken and shrimp are both good sources of protein, and the nutrient-dense vegetables provide a plethora of plant-based compounds to help you recover from your chronic health issue. Despite making your urine smell funny, asparagus should be part of your food plan, as it helps you detoxify from medications and other harmful compounds you may have been exposed to.

Serves 6
Calories per serving: 240 without rice; 349 with rice

2 to 3 tablespoons avocado oil
1 pound boneless, skinless organic chicken, cut into strips, or 1 pound peeled and deveined shrimp
organic tamari
1 medium white onion, chopped
1½ cups chopped asparagus
1½ cups chopped broccoli
1 cup slivered carrots
1 cup chopped zucchini
1 cup chopped mushrooms (button, maitake, or shiitake)

¾ cup chopped snow peas
1 can water chestnuts, roughly chopped
½ to ¾ cup chopped bell peppers (any color)
1 tablespoon minced fresh ginger
1 tablespoon minced garlic
1 teaspoon sesame oil (optional)
3 cups cooked brown rice (optional)

In a 13-inch stainless-steel wok or skillet, heat 1 tablespoon of the avocado oil over medium to high heat. When the oil is hot, add the chicken and a small amount of tamari. Cook, stirring continuously, until the chicken is coated with the sauce but not completely cooked through (it will still be slightly pink on the inside). Remove the chicken from the wok and set aside.

Add the remaining 1 to 2 tablespoons avocado oil and the onion to the wok; cook, stirring, until the onion is soft. Add the asparagus, broccoli, and carrots, along with a splash of tamari. Once the vegetables are soft, add the zucchini, mushrooms, snow peas, water chestnuts, and bell pepper. Cook, stirring frequently, until the vegetables are the consistency you like.

Add the ginger and garlic; Cook, stirring frequently, for 1 to 2 more minutes. If more liquid is needed, add more tamari. Return the chicken to the wok and cook until warmed. At the last minute, stir in the sesame oil for flavor.

Serve the stir-fry on its own, or over 1/2 cup brown rice, if desired, for a more substantial meal.

Chinese Chicken

Ginger and scallion sauce over cooked chicken is a dish I make on the weekends when I'm not racing out the door and can take my time in the kitchen. The combination of ginger and scallions with a touch of oil provides a little bite to this dish. Ginger contains a compound called gingerol, which has powerful medicinal properties. It's a strong anti-inflammatory and antioxidant, and has a long history of success in aiding digestion, reducing nausea, and improving immunity to fight the common cold and the flu.

Serves 4
Calories per serving: 390 without rice; 404 with rice

Chicken
1 (3- to 4-pound) whole plump chicken
2 carrots
1 onion
4 celery stalks

Sea salt
1½ cups uncooked brown jasmine rice

Ginger Sauce
¼ cup chopped fresh ginger
1 bunch scallions, light and dark green parts only, chopped
½ cup avocado oil

Sea salt
¼ cup oyster sauce (thin with water, if desired), for serving

Chicken

Put the chicken, carrots, onion, and celery in a large pot; add enough water to completely submerge them, and season with salt. Cover the pot and bring the water to a boil. Turn off the heat and let stand, covered, for 20 minutes. Repeat this step twice more. Pull one chicken leg back; if it moves easily and the liquid in the joint runs clear, the chicken is done. Remove the chicken from the liquid in the pot (see Notes) and set aside to rest. When it's cooled enough to handle, pull it apart into bite-size pieces.

Meanwhile, cook the rice according to the package directions.

Ginger Sauce

In a food processor, puree the ginger to a fine gritty texture. Add the scallions and oil; process until smooth. Season with salt.

To serve, start with 3/4 cup rice on each plate. Add a bit of oyster sauce; use it sparingly, as it is very strong. Add 3 to 4 ounces chicken (the size of the palm of your hand—see Notes) and top with a little of the ginger sauce. Use the sauce sparingly, as it is high in calories.

NOTES: Use the liquid from cooking the chicken as stock to make the Cabbage & Carrot Soup (page 370), or in any other dish calling for chicken stock. Use the leftover chicken in the soup or to make chicken salad.

Cod Oreganato

Cod has a mild sweet flavor and a tender texture that is pleasing to the palate. A great source of protein, this fish is loaded with phosphorus, vitamin B_{12}, iodine, and selenium. This meal is a must for anyone rebuilding from disease or other chronic health issues.

Serves 8
Calories per serving: 160

2 tablespoons extra-virgin olive oil
2 teaspoon garlic powder
2 teaspoon onion powder
2 teaspoons dried oregano
1 teaspoon sea salt

1 teaspoon freshly ground black
 pepper
2 pounds wild-caught codfish, cut into
 servings
1/4 cup gluten-free bread crumbs
1 cup dry white wine

Preheat oven to 350°F.

In a Pyrex baking dish, drizzle 1 tablespoon extra-virgin olive oil to cover the bottom of the pan. On the surface of the pan where the fish will be placed, sprinkle 1 teaspoon each of garlic powder, onion powder, and oregano; add a pinch of salt and pepper. Place fresh fish on top of seasoning, and add remaining seasonings on top. Add breadcrumbs and top with remaining olive oil. Any breadcrumbs that fall into the dish will serve to thicken the sauce. Carefully pour the wine around the fish, not over it. Add a small amount of water if desired.

Bake for 15 minutes, then turn the broiler to high. Watch the fish carefully; if it splits, that is a sign it is done. About 8 minutes should be enough, but all ovens are different.

Color-Changing Shrimp Stir-Fry

There is nothing magical about this delightful dish besides the distinctive flavors of ginger, cabbage, and sesame oil. Shrimp is low in fat and calories and high in protein. While shrimp are small, they are full of nutrients, including zinc and iodine. Iodine is important for proper thyroid function, and zinc is needed for proper immune function. Why does the shrimp change color? Red cabbage contains a red pigment called anthocyanin; when cooked, the pigment is released and then absorbed by the shrimp, turning them a different color.

Serves 6
Calories per serving: 196

1 tablespoon avocado oil
4 garlic cloves, coarsely chopped
1 bunch scallions, sliced
1 tablespoon chopped or grated fresh
    ginger
1/4 head red cabbage, shredded
3 celery stalks, thinly sliced
1 cup sliced baby carrots

1 (8-ounce) can water chestnuts,
    drained and sliced
1 to 2 tablespoons rice vinegar
1 to 2 tablespoons organic tamari
1 1/2 pounds small shrimp, peeled and
    deveined
1 tablespoon toasted sesame oil
Sea salt

In a large skillet, heat the avocado oil over medium heat. Add the garlic, scallions, and ginger; cook, stirring, for 1 minute. Add the cabbage, celery, carrots, water chestnuts, vinegar, and tamari; cook, stirring, until the vegetables are tender.

In separate pan, cook the shrimp in the sesame oil with a pinch of salt until they are just turning pink, then remove from the pan.

Add the shrimp to the vegetables. Stir as the mixture reheats. The red cabbage will cause the shrimp to turn green.

Easy Meat Loaf

If you're pinched for time and love an abundance of flavor, this meat loaf is the ticket. The type of meat you choose has different flavor notes and textures, so choose the kind that excites your palate. The tangy flavors of salsa really make this meal satisfying. Combining protein from the meat and phytonutrients from vegetables in the salsa makes this a super-healthful meal.

Serves 8
Calories per serving: 288

2 pounds grass-fed beef, turkey, bison, or venison

1 (16-ounce) jar of your favorite salsa
1 teaspoon salt

Preheat oven to 350°F.

In a large bowl blend the meat and salsa until well mixed. Put the mixture into a 9x13 Pyrex dish and form it into a loaf.

Bake in preheated oven for about 40 minutes. Be careful not to overcook, which will dry it out. I recommend using a meat thermometer to determine doneness. You can also use a fork to see if it's cooked through. After taking it out of the oven, sprinkle a pinch of salt and pepper over the loaf for additional seasoning. Let it rest for 10 minutes, then cut and serve.

Serve with a sweet potato and some greens like broccoli rabe or a salad. Save leftovers for lunch, dinner, or a snack.

Grilled Chicken, Beef, or Lamb Kebabs

If you like to grill as much as I do, you will enjoy these succulent kebabs. You can't go wrong with beef, chicken, or lamb, as all three are high in protein and abundant in nutrients. If you haven't tried a grilled lamb kebab, I suggest you do. Lamb is a very flavorful and tender meat that melts in your mouth. Coating the meat and vegetables with this tangy marinade brings out the flavor of whichever meat you choose.

Serves 2
Calories per serving: 270

Marinade

2 tablespoons avocado oil
¼ cup white wine vinegar
1 tablespoon onion powder
2 teaspoons garlic powder

2 teaspoons steak seasoning
Sea salt and freshly ground black
  pepper

Kebabs

8 ounces chicken, beef, or lamb
1 large red onion, cut into pieces
1 pint cherry tomatoes
1 bell pepper, cut into pieces

1 tablespoon avocado oil, plus more
  for the grill grates
Sea salt and freshly ground black
  pepper

Marinade

In a medium bowl, combine all the marinade ingredients. Mix thoroughly.

Kebabs

Cut the meat into even-sized cubes. Place in a large resealable bag or a flat-bottomed container. Add the marinade and stir well to be sure all the meat is covered; seal the bag or cover the container. Cover and marinate for 2 to 3 hours at room temperature or overnight in the fridge.

In a large bowl, toss together the onion, tomatoes, bell pepper, and oil and season with salt and black pepper.

Heat a grill to medium heat.

I recommend using long skewers to assemble the kebabs. (If using wooden skewers, soak them in water for 30 minutes beforehand.) Skewer 4 or 5 cubes of meat per kebab, alternating the meat with the three vegetables.

Lightly coat the grill grates with oil to prevent sticking. Grill the kebabs for 3 to 4 minutes on each side. Check frequently to avoid overcooking.

Marinated Chicken Kebabs

Why offer two kebab recipes? For one thing, they are easy and quick to prepare. For another, why not? If you are an all-season grill master, this is another recipe that provides an excuse to fire up the Weber. The refreshing citrus and notes of garlic and herbs help to create a mouth-watering protein source that works well with a healthful salad or side of your favorite greens.

Serves 4 to 6
Calories per serving: 535 for 4; 357 for 6

¼ cup avocado oil, plus more for the grill grates
½ cup fresh orange juice (from 2 or 3 oranges)
Juice of 1 lemon
4 garlic cloves, crushed
2 scallions, sliced
1 teaspoon dried oregano
1 teaspoon dried thyme
1 teaspoon sea salt
Freshly ground black pepper
4 to 6 boneless and skinless chicken breasts, cut into uniform cubes

In a large flat container or resealable bag, combine all the ingredients except the chicken to create a marinade. Add the chicken cubes, cover the container or seal the bag, and marinate in the refrigerator for several hours or up to overnight. Stir several times to be sure all the meat is covered.

Heat a grill to low or medium heat.

If using wooden skewers, soak them in water for 30 minutes before assembling the kebabs. Skewer the chicken cubes; allow a little space between cubes to ensure proper cooking.

Lightly coat the grill grates with oil. Grill the kebabs for a few minutes on each side, turning them halfway through cooking. They cook quickly, so keep an eye on them.

Orange-Lime Shrimp with Apricot Rice

The sweetness of apricots, as well as the fruity and tangy flavor of orange, makes this a favorite of mine. Both oranges and apricots are loaded with carotenoids—phytochemicals known for their disease-fighting properties. Besides being low in calories, shrimp is loaded with protein, selenium, vitamin B_{12}, and iodine, all vital nutrients for the body.

Serves 4
Calories per serving: 298

Orange-Lime Shrimp

Juice of 1 orange
Juice of 1 lime
2 tablespoons fresh chopped cilantro
1 teaspoon ground coriander
1/4 green bell pepper, chopped
2 scallions, sliced from white until end of light green

1 tablespoon fresh ginger, minced
1/2 teaspoon sea salt
1/2 teaspoon ground black pepper
25 large fresh raw shrimp, cleaned and deveined
2 tablespoons coconut oil

Apricot Rice

2 cups uncooked brown rice
4 tablespoons coconut oil
1 tablespoon minced fresh ginger
1/2 bunch scallions, sliced from white to edge of dark green
3/4 cup sliced Turkish dried apricots (or any type without preservatives)

1 can water chestnuts, drained and sliced
1 ear of corn, kernels removed (or 1 cup frozen corn)
1 teaspoon sea salt
1/2 teaspoon ground black pepper
1 tablespoon cilantro, chopped

Shrimp

Mix together all ingredients except shrimp and coconut oil. Add shrimp and marinate for at least 1 hour. Remove shrimp, and set aside the marinade to create the sauce.

Add 2 tablespoons of coconut oil to a large skillet on medium-high heat. Cook half the shrimp until pink, about 1 minute on each side. Do not overcook. Repeat this for the other half of the shrimp. Set shrimp aside, and add the marinade to the skillet. Cook on medium-low heat for 1 to 2 minutes, add the shrimp and cook for another 3 minutes.

Rice

The rice can be made ahead of time, even the day before. Cook rice according to instructions on the package; always add about 1 tablespoon salt to the water.

In a skillet large enough to hold all the rice, add 2 tablespoons of the coconut oil, the ginger, and the scallions; sauté for 2 minutes, stirring often. Add the apricots, water chestnuts, corn, salt, and pepper; cook for a few minutes until the corn begins to smell a bit nutty. Add the cilantro and cook for 1 more minute. Add the remaining 2 tablespoons coconut oil and the rice. Stir continually until all ingredients are mixed well and the rice sizzles a bit. Salt to taste, if needed.

Plate and serve with the shrimp.

Poached Fish Pouches

Who would have thought cooking fish in a pouch could produce such a moist and tender entrée? The fish pouch is a simple way to get more flavorful fish into your diet. From the cleansing flavor of cilantro to the heat of the gingery marinade, this mixture is sure to please your palate. The small fish fillets are just the right amount of protein to be included in your daily meal planning and personal rebuild.

Serves 2
Calories per serving: 245 with rice, 245 with quinoa

1 celery stalk, thinly sliced
1 teaspoon fresh ginger, grated
¼ yellow bell pepper, thinly sliced
1 scallion, thinly sliced
1 teaspoon extra-virgin olive oil
Sea salt and freshly ground black pepper

2 (4-ounce) fresh (not frozen) fish fillets (sole, haddock, or trout)
Zest and juice of 1 lemon
2 pinches of minced fresh cilantro or parsley
1 cup cooked wild rice or quinoa

Preheat the oven to 350°F.

In a bowl, toss the celery, ginger, bell pepper, and scallion with the olive oil and a pinch each of salt and black pepper.

Tear off a piece of aluminum foil about 12 x 14 inches for each fillet. Lay the foil flat and, if you like, cover each piece with a slightly smaller piece of parchment paper. Place one fillet lengthwise on each piece. Sprinkle with a pinch each of salt and black pepper, and add the lemon zest and juice. Divide the vegetables in half and place on top of the fish. Add a pinch of cilantro or parsley on top of each.

To seal the pouches, begin by pulling up the long sides and folding them together at the very top. Fold the ends in to make the pouch airtight. The goal is to create a well-sealed tent-like pouch with room inside for steam. Set the pouches on a baking sheet and transfer to the oven.

Bake for 10 to 15 minutes, depending on the thickness of the fish.

Serve each fillet with ½ cup wild rice or quinoa. Be careful of escaping steam when opening the pouch.

Quick Lemon Chicken

The lemon juice and zest combined with the yellow onion create a refreshing and most satisfying flavor. Lemon zest is an excellent source of vitamin C, calcium, beta-carotene, potassium, and magnesium. It also contains the compounds limonene and salvestrol Q40, both of which help to fight cancerous cells, thereby reducing the risk of developing skin, colon, and breast cancers. I recommend using boneless, skinless chicken thighs, which are more tender and tastier than white meat.

Serves 8
Calories per serving: 180

Sea salt and freshly ground black pepper
2 pounds boneless, skinless chicken thighs
1 tablespoon avocado oil
2 large yellow onions, halved and thinly sliced

1 clove garlic, coarsely chopped
1 tablespoon dried or fresh rosemary
2 teaspoons agave syrup (dark or light)
Zest and juice of 1 large lemon

Preheat the oven to 350°F.

Sprinkle salt and pepper on both sides of the chicken thighs; lay them flat in a large baking dish.

In a medium skillet, heat the oil over medium heat. Add the onions and garlic; cook for a few minutes. Add the rosemary, agave syrup, salt and pepper to taste, and the lemon juice. Cook, stirring, until the vegetables have softened; pour the mixture over the chicken.

Bake for about 40 minutes. Midway through the cooking process, sprinkle the chicken with the lemon zest and spoon the pan juices over the top a few times. The onions and garlic will create a smooth texture, and the zesty taste of lemon will brighten the flavors.

Sautéed Salmon & Green Beans

Do you have 20 to 25 minutes to make a satisfying and healthful meal? Perfect. If you like the taste and texture of salmon and enjoy the combination of lemon, salt, and dill, your palate won't be disappointed. The nutrient composition of wild-caught salmon is off the charts; it is high in protein; omega-3 fatty acids; vitamins B_3, B_6, B_{12}, and D; selenium; and iodine. If you are recovering from heart disease, cancer, diabetes, auto-immune disease, or some other chronic illness, sautéed salmon and green beans should be a dish in your personal rebuild.

Serves 2
Calories per serving: 287

Salmon
1 tablespoon avocado oil
2 (4-ounce) wild salmon fillets, skin on
1 teaspoon fresh lemon juice
½ teaspoon chopped fresh dill
Sea salt and freshly ground black
  pepper

Green Beans
1 tablespoon avocado oil
8 ounces green beans
1 tablespoon fresh lemon juice

Salmon

In a medium skillet, heat the oil over low heat. When the oil is hot, add the salmon, skin-side down, and cook, turning often, for about 10 minutes. When the salmon is almost done, sprinkle with the lemon juice and dill. Remove from the heat and season with salt and pepper.

Green Beans

In a large skillet, heat the oil over medium heat. When it is hot, add the green beans and cook, stirring continuously, for 1 to 2 minutes. Do not let the beans burn.

When the beans are hot—and very slightly browned—add the lemon juice and cover the pan. Reduce the heat and steam the beans for 2 to 3 minutes, depending on how crisp you like them. Check them frequently.

Season the beans with salt and pepper, and serve immediately with the salmon.

Seafood Lettuce Tacos

If you are trying to cut back on carbs, but not on taste, these seafood tacos are a good choice. The fresh lime and cilantro are a flavorful way to complement the moist and flaky tuna and salmon. Both fish are excellent sources of protein, anti-inflammatory omega-3 fatty acids, iodine, and other essential nutrients that will help you quickly restore your health.

Serves 5
Calories per serving: 275

10 large lettuce leaves (Bibb or
 romaine hearts)
1 teaspoon ground coriander
1/2 teaspoon chili powder
1 teaspoon garlic powder
2 teaspoons plus 2 tablespoons
 avocado oil
1 teaspoon sea salt

Juice of 1 lime (if using fresh tuna;
 1/2 lime if using canned tuna)
1 teaspoon chopped fresh cilantro
1 small onion, very thinly sliced
8 ounces wild salmon, cut into cubes
8 ounces wild tuna (see Note), cut into
 cubes

Wash and dry each lettuce leaf very well. Refrigerate until ready to use to keep them crisp. To shorten romaine leaves, cut off some of the white at the bottom.

In a large bowl, combine the coriander, chili powder, garlic powder, 2 teaspoons of the oil, the salt, lime juice, cilantro, and onion to create the marinade. Add the cubed fish, cover, and marinate at room temperature for 1 hour, stirring often.

In a large skillet, heat the remaining 2 tablespoons of oil. Once the oil is hot, remove the fish from the marinade and add the cubes to the skillet. Cook for 5 to 7 minutes.

Fill each lettuce leaf with the fish just as you would a taco. Top with hot sauce, sugar-free salsa, red onion, cilantro, lime juice, pico de gallo, pickled jalapeños, or whatever you prefer. Chunky Guacamole (page 435) is a good accompaniment.

NOTE: For a quick and inexpensive alternative to the fresh fish used in this recipe, use two 5-ounce cans of solid white tuna (packed in water) and two 5-ounce cans of wild salmon. Drain the fish before marinating.

Spanish Stuffed Peppers

This is a perfectly balanced and satisfying meal all in one beautifully colored bell pepper. Briny olives, sweet tomatoes, and fresh cilantro balance out the flavors of turkey and brown rice. Red, yellow, orange, and green bell peppers are abundant in colorful carotenoids, powerful antioxidants that prevent cellular damage by the onslaught of unwanted free radicals.

Serves 6 to 8
Calories per serving: 326 for 6; 245 for 8

6 to 8 large bell peppers (any color)
1 pound ground organic, free-range turkey
Smoked sea salt (such as Maldon; see Resources)
Freshly ground black pepper
1 tablespoon avocado oil
1 medium red onion, diced
4 garlic cloves, crushed
10 cremini mushrooms, chopped

1 (14.5-ounce) can organic diced tomatoes, without juices
2 teaspoons dried oregano
2 tablespoons chopped fresh cilantro
Pinch of saffron (optional)
½ cup uncooked brown jasmine rice
½ cup uncooked wild rice
1 cup thinly sliced Spanish olives (optional)
1 (8-ounce) can organic tomato puree

Preheat the oven to 350°F.

Cut the tops off the peppers and clean out the insides. Stand them upright in a baking dish. Chop 2 of the pepper tops to add to the filling. Set the remaining tops around the peppers to help keep them upright. Set aside.

In a large deep skillet, brown the turkey; season with smoked salt and black pepper. Remove from the pan and set aside.

In the same pan, heat the oil over medium heat. Add the onion and garlic. Cook for 2 minutes, stirring often. Do not let the garlic brown. Add the chopped bell pepper tops and mushrooms, and season with salt and black pepper. After it cooks down a bit, add the diced tomatoes, oregano, cilantro, and saffron (if using). When heated, add the turkey and both rices; stir well and simmer for a minute or two. Add the olives (if using), and mix well.

Stuff the peppers very full with the filling. Top each pepper with a few spoonfuls of tomato puree to add moisture. Cover with foil; bake for 40 minutes. Uncover and bake for 30 minutes more, or until the peppers are tender.

Summer Poached Salmon

Despite the title of this recipe, this light and satisfying dish can and should be enjoyed all year round. The tender salmon is met with the clean flavors of cucumber, lemon, and dill to create a most delicious entrée. Pair this nutrient-dense dish with wild rice and your favorite side vegetable to send the perfect blend of gene-regulating information to your cells.

Serves 4
Calories per serving: 359

Dressing

1 small cucumber, peeled, seeded, and minced
Sea salt and freshly ground black pepper

1 tablespoon minced fresh dill
½ cup mayonnaise or Vegenaise (see Resources)
1 lemon, quartered

Poached Salmon

3 to 5 celery stalks

1 large wild salmon fillet (1½ pounds)
   or 4 wild salmon steaks

1 to 2 teaspoons onion powder

Sea salt

Lemon pepper or freshly ground
   black pepper

1 lemon, sliced

1 bunch fresh dill (leave intact for
   easy removal)

Dressing

Prepare the dressing first, so the flavors can combine. Put the minced cucumber in a mesh strainer and lightly salt it. Set the strainer in the sink to drain for roughly 30 minutes. Press on the cucumbers with a paper towel to remove excess water.

In a medium bowl, combine the dill, mayonnaise, salt and pepper to taste, and a squeeze of lemon. When the minced cucumber is drained, stir it in. Set aside to serve at room temperature.

Poached Salmon

Arrange the celery stalks over the bottom of a large skillet with a lid. Place the fish on the celery to raise it off the pan. Season with onion powder, salt, and pepper. Top with the lemon slices and whole sprigs of dill. Add water to reach the bottom edge of the fish; *do not submerge the fish*. Bring the water to a boil over medium heat, then gently cook for about 15 minutes. When the thickest part of the fish is still a bit darker, turn off heat, cover, and let sit for another 5 minutes.

Remove the salmon from the pan, discard the dill sprigs, and top with the dressing.

Super-Moist Turkey Meatballs

There is only one description I can give these meatballs: mouth-watering. The combination of rice, zucchini, and egg makes these meatballs super moist and rich in nutrients. Adding zucchini to the meat is a great way to sneak in vegetables if you are dealing with picky eaters—young or old. Dropping these meatballs into a simmering cauldron of chunky tomato sauce allows them to soak up more flavors and become the highlight of your next brown rice pasta meal. Turkey is a great source of tryptophan, an amino acid needed to produce serotonin and melatonin, which you need to get a good night's sleep.

Makes 45 meatballs, to serve 9
Calories per serving (5 meatballs): 280

1 cup shredded zucchini (about 1 medium zucchini)
1 teaspoon sea salt, plus more as needed
¾ cup cooked brown rice
¼ cup chopped fresh parsley
1 tablespoon ground or whole fennel seeds
½ teaspoon freshly ground black pepper
2 large eggs (preferably organic or cage free), lightly beaten
1 tablespoon minced dried onion
2 pounds ground organic, free-range turkey

Preheat the oven to 400°F.

Place the shredded zucchini in a colander and sprinkle with salt. Set the colander in the sink to drain. After about 30 minutes, press on the zucchini to remove excess liquid.

Transfer the zucchini to a food processor. Add the rice, parsley, fennel, salt, and pepper; pulse until finely minced. Add eggs and dried onion, and pulse to combine. Add the ground turkey and pulse to mix thoroughly.

Roll the mixture into 1-inch balls and set them on a baking sheet; the consistency will be soft and somewhat mushy. They will not hold a nice round shape, but they taste great. Bake for 20 minutes, then switch the oven to broil on high and broil until the meatballs are browned.

Serve with tomato sauce, or alongside sweet potatoes and vegetables. These meatballs also make a good snack. They keep very well in the freezer; be sure to wrap them carefully in sealed freezer bags. To defrost, move them to the refrigerator overnight, place them in a sealable bag in a bowl of cold water for about 30 minutes, or use the defrost setting in the microwave. Once defrosted, reheat in the oven or in a skillet with tomato sauce.

Thai Curried Cod or Chicken

Curry paste adds plenty of spicy heat to this dish, while sweet coconut milk smooths out the flavor. Coconut is highly nutritious and rich in B vitamins, vitamin C, iron, calcium, magnesium, and phosphorous. The combination of cod, coconut milk, and rice create a well-balanced meal that provides the right amount of protein, fat, and carbs to help you recover, rebuild, and prevent recurrence.

Serves 4
Calories per serving: 188 for fish; 230 for chicken (add 85 calories if serving with rice)

2 tablespoons coconut oil
1 tablespoon grated fresh ginger
2 garlic cloves, crushed
1/2 bunch scallions, thinly sliced
1 medium red onion, halved and thinly sliced
1 tablespoon green curry paste (or red, if you prefer milder spice)
1 teaspoon sea salt
1/2 green bell pepper, thinly sliced
1/2 red bell pepper, thinly sliced

2 carrots, cut into thin matchsticks
1 (8-ounce) can water chestnuts, drained and sliced
1 (14.5-ounce) can light coconut milk
4 (4-ounce) cod fillets, or 4 (3-ounce) boneless, skinless chicken breasts, cut into strips
2 cups cooked wild rice (optional)
1 tablespoon chopped fresh cilantro (optional)

In a large sauté pan, heat 1 tablespoon of the coconut oil over low to medium heat. Add the ginger, garlic, scallions, and onion. Cook for 2 minutes, stirring continuously. Add the curry paste and cook for another 2 minutes. If using chicken, add it to the pan and cook, stirring occasionally, for 3 to 4 minutes, or until it is no longer pink. Add the remaining 1 tablespoon coconut oil, the salt, bell peppers, carrots, and water chestnuts. Cook for 4 minutes. Add the coconut milk and simmer for a few minutes.

If using cod, add it now and cover the pan. Cook for 5 minutes; uncover and cook for 5 more minutes.

Serve with 1/2 cup wild rice per person and sprinkled with fresh cilantro, if desired.

Turkey & Vegetable Stew

This hearty stew is the perfect dish to serve during Sunday-afternoon football or when you're catching up with friends after a long workweek. This healthful mix can be eaten as is, or served in an edible bowl made from a half-baked squash. Eating the inside flesh of the squash adds a serving of carbohydrate and just the right amount of fiber and nutrients.

Serves 5
Calories per serving: 332

3 tablespoons avocado oil
1 medium onion, chopped
3 garlic cloves, minced, or more or
  less to taste
8 ounces white button or cremini
  mushrooms, cleaned and chopped
1 large bell pepper, chopped
1/4 cup organic low-sodium chicken
  broth
Sea salt and freshly ground black
  pepper

1 pound ground organic, free-range
  turkey
1 teaspoon celery seed
1 teaspoon dried basil
1 (28-ounce) can diced tomatoes, with
  their juices
1 medium to large zucchini, diced
1 (8-ounce) can black olives, drained
  and sliced
1 teaspoon umeboshi vinegar
  (optional; see Note)

In a large skillet, combine 2 tablespoons of the oil and the onion; cook over medium heat, stirring, until soft, 2 to 3 minutes. Add the garlic and cook until the onion is translucent, 2 to 3 more minutes; do not let the garlic burn. Add the mushrooms, bell pepper, and stock; cook for about 5 minutes. Season with salt and black pepper. Remove the mixture from the pan and set aside.

In the same skillet, heat the remaining 1 tablespoon avocado oil over medium heat. Add the turkey and cook, breaking up the meat so it cooks uniformly, until browned. Add the celery seed and basil; cook, stirring, until the meat is cooked through, about 5 minutes. Reduce the heat and return the vegetable mixture to the pan. Add the tomatoes and their juices. Mix well; taste and adjust the seasoning with salt and black pepper. While the mixture simmers, add the zucchini; it will cook as the liquid reduces. Immediately add the olives and vinegar (if using); simmer for about 10 minutes more to reduce the liquid. Just before serving, taste and adjust the seasoning one more time.

NOTE: Umeboshi vinegar (or ume plum vinegar) is available in most specialty groceries. It is used often in Japanese dishes and brightens flavors with a mildly salt/citrus note.

Turkey Bolognese

Simple on prep, bold on flavor. This is one of my go-to recipes when I am short on time and crave a filling meat sauce. Add a side of salad to dish this to make it a complete meal.

If you're watching your carbs, use zucchini noodles in place of pasta. Remember: When buying prepared pasta sauce, read the label and avoid brands with added sugar.

Serves 5
Calories per serving: 248

2 to 3 teaspoons avocado oil
1 pound ground organic, free-range
  turkey

1 (25-ounce) jar organic sugar-free
  tomato sauce
6 medium zucchini, stems removed
2 teaspoons sea salt

In a skillet, heat 2 teaspoons of the oil over medium heat. Add the turkey and cook, stirring to break up the meat, until evenly cooked. Stir in the tomato sauce and cook until the sauce is hot. Reduce the heat to keep the sauce warm while you prepare the noodles.

To manually cut the zucchini, use a mandoline on the thinnest setting. Cut the resulting wide noodles into any size you want. Alternatively, use a spiralizer to create very thin spaghetti-like noodles.

Add the salt to the zucchini noodles; mix well. Salt will extract water from the zucchini. Drain for 30 to 60 minutes.

Mix the drained noodles into the sauce and cook over medium heat for 3 minutes. Serve immediately.

Turkey or Beef Confetti Bowl

The earthy flavors of the brown rice and the turkey make for a comforting meal any time of the year. The corn and zucchini add a touch of sweetness while the jalapeño gives it a little bite. The ingredients provide a healthful combination of protein, carbs, and plant-based foods. Turkey is a great source of dietary tryptophan, which is used to make the neurotransmitter serotonin and the hormone melatonin. Serotonin is most well known for its role in the brain, where it helps balance mood. Melatonin functions to regulate our sleep cycles. Perhaps this is why we get relaxed and sleepy after eating a meal containing turkey.

Serves 6
Calories per serving: 285

2 medium zucchini, shredded
Sea salt
1 large red onion, cut into chunks
1 red bell pepper, cut into chunks
1 pound ground organic, free-range
    turkey or grass-fed ground beef
Freshly ground black pepper

1 tablespoon avocado oil
1 jalapeño, seeded and chopped
    (optional)
3 cups cooked wild rice
Kernels from 1 ear fresh corn, or
    1 cup frozen corn
5 large fresh basil leaves, chopped

Put the shredded zucchini in a colander and sprinkle with salt. Set the colander in the sink to drain for 30 to 60 minutes. Press on the zucchini to remove excess moisture.

In a food processor, pulse the onion to chop it into smaller, uniform pieces; set aside. Repeat with the bell pepper. (This can also be done by hand.)

In large, deep skillet, brown the meat over medium heat and season with 1 teaspoon salt and black pepper. Remove from the pan and set aside.

In the same skillet, heat the oil over medium heat. Add the onion and a pinch of salt. Cook until the onion is soft, then add the bell pepper, drained zucchini, and jalapeño (if using). Cook for about 10 minutes. Add the cooked rice, meat, corn, and basil; cook for 5 minutes to combine the flavors. Taste and adjust the salt and black pepper as needed.

Side Dishes

Asian Red Slaw

This is a great twist on the typical coleslaw served at the neighborhood barbecue. The Asian-inspired flavors of sesame oil, coconut aminos, and rice vinegar with the sweet note of agave syrup really wake up this crunchy salad. Packed full of antioxidants and phytochemicals from the red cabbage, this is the perfect accompaniment to grilled meats. Red cabbage helps to offset any hazardous compounds created when meat is charred by cooking at high temperatures.

Serves 6
Calories per serving: 187

Dressing

1 tablespoon sesame oil
1 tablespoon extra-virgin olive oil
1 tablespoon Bragg Coconut Liquid
  Aminos
¼ cup rice vinegar
1 tablespoon agave syrup

Salad

1 small head red cabbage, shredded
½ head savoy cabbage, shredded
1 (8-ounce) can water chestnuts,
  drained and sliced
1 or 2 large carrots, shredded
2 scallions, thinly sliced
3 tablespoons toasted sesame seeds
¼ cup slivered almonds

Dressing

In a jar, combine all the dressing ingredients. Shake vigorously to mix well; set aside.

Salad

In a large bowl, combine all vegetables until evenly distributed.

To preserve the crunchy texture, add the dressing just before serving. Garnish with toasted sesame seeds and slivered almonds.

Broccoli Rabe

There is something about the flavors of broccoli rabe sautéed with garlic and onion that go so well together. Whether you are serving it as a side or mixed into pasta, it will be the perfect addition. For those whose taste for broccoli rabe is still developing, the sweetness of the raisins cuts the mild bitterness this cruciferous vegetable can have. Broccoli rabe is a superfood, providing phytonutrients that will assist you in rebuilding from cancer, heart disease, diabetes, and other chronic illnesses.

Serves 2 or 3
Calories per serving: 139 for 2; 93 for 3

1 bunch broccoli rabe
Sea salt and freshly ground black
   pepper
1 tablespoon extra-virgin olive oil,
   plus more if needed

2 shallots or 1 small onion,
   finely diced
½ clove garlic, smashed and coarsely
   chopped
¼ cup raisins (optional)
Pinch of red pepper flakes (optional)

Wash the broccoli rabe very well, leaving some water on the leaves. Cut away the lower half of the stems and cut the bunch into three sections.

In a large skillet, combine the broccoli rabe and 1 cup water and sprinkle with salt. Steam over medium heat until just tender and still bright green; do not overcook. Transfer the broccoli rabe and cooking liquid to a bowl and set aside.

In the same skillet, heat the oil over medium heat. Add the shallots and garlic; cook until light golden. Do not burn; add a bit more oil if needed. Add the broccoli rabe with its cooking liquid and the raisins (if using); cook for 2 minutes. Season with salt and black pepper and finish with the red pepper flakes, if desired.

Fresh Fruit and Mint Salad

Sweet, clean, and refreshing, this nutrient-dense side dish works well with breakfast, lunch, or dinner. Berries are low on the glycemic index and dense with disease-fighting antioxidants and phytochemicals that should be part of your daily meal plan.

Serves 6
Calories per serving: 105

1 pint fresh blueberries
8 ounces fresh strawberries, sliced
1/2 pint fresh raspberries
3 ripe kiwifruits, peeled and sliced
  into rounds

1 cup sliced red grapes
Juice of 1/2 lime
4 fresh mint leaves, cut into
  chiffonade

In a large bowl, mix the fruit with the lime juice and mint leaves.

Garlic Spinach

This versatile dish is a great addition to almost any meal. For breakfast, top it with a poached egg. Garlic contains allicin, a compound that has potent medicinal properties. Besides warding off vampires, garlic has been proven to improve immune function, reduce blood pressure, and reduce free radical damage to the body; it's also a potent detoxifier. Regarding spinach, Popeye was onto something: spinach is loaded with flavonoids, nutrients with anticancer and anti-inflammatory properties.

Serves 4
Calories per serving: 115

3 tablespoons avocado oil
6 large garlic cloves, chopped
2 shallots, minced, or 1 tablespoon
  dried minced onion

Juice of 1 lemon
Sea salt and freshly ground black
  pepper
1 (16-ounce) bag organic baby spinach

In a large skillet, heat the oil over medium heat; add the garlic and shallots. Cook, stirring, until the garlic and shallots are lightly browned, which will produce a nutty fragrance. Reduce the heat to low. Stir in the lemon juice, salt, and pepper. Add the fresh spinach and toss to get all the leaves coated and gently cooked. In order to preserve the fresh green color, be sure not to overcook the spinach.

Lemon-Fresh Quinoa with Herbs

Prep time for this is determined by how quickly you can chop parsley and slice tomatoes. The lemon works well with the earthy flavor of the quinoa and the mildly bitter taste of parsley. Quinoa is a good source of fiber, iron, magnesium, and vitamin B_2. Make sure you rinse the quinoa to get rid of the bitter saponins, which can interrupt the absorption of nutrients contained in this funny-looking grain.

Serves 4
Calories per serving: 278

1 cup uncooked quinoa, rinsed well
Zest and juice of 1 lemon
1 scallion, light and dark green parts only, thinly sliced
$1/2$ cup chopped fresh parsley
$1 1/2$ cups sliced grape tomatoes
$1/4$ cup extra-virgin olive oil
Sea salt and freshly ground black pepper

Cook the quinoa according to the package directions. Set aside to cool.

In a bowl, mix together the remaining ingredients; stir them into the quinoa. Serve chilled or at room temperature.

Red Cabbage, Onions & Oranges

If you enjoy grilling meat as much as I do, you must include this side with your next meat entrée. Sweet cabbage and onion, combined with the bright citrus flavor of orange zest, work well with any type of meat you cook. Cooking meat at high temperatures, as you do when grilling, causes the production of toxic compounds called heterocyclic amines. Research shows that the anthocyanins found in red cabbage neutralize the harmful effects of these damaging toxins.

Serves 4 to 6
Calories per serving: 148 for 4; 98 for 6

1 tablespoon avocado oil
1 large red onion, thinly sliced
1 large yellow onion, thinly sliced
Sea salt and freshly ground black
  pepper

1 medium red cabbage, halved and
  thinly sliced
Zest and juice of 1 large orange
1 tablespoon fresh or dried tarragon

In a large skillet, heat the oil over medium heat. Add the onions and season with salt and pepper; cook for a few minutes. Add the cabbage and cook for 10 minutes, stirring often.

Once the cabbage has cooked down a bit, add the orange juice and tarragon. Stir well, reduce the heat to low, and cook for 5 minutes. Taste and add more salt and pepper, if needed.

In the last minute of cooking, add the orange zest and stir well.

Roasted Brussels Sprouts

Roasted Brussels sprouts are the first appetizer to disappear during our holiday parties. Shallots and fennel add a burst of flavor to this cruciferous vegetable. As with the other crucifers, these sprouts contain sulforaphane and indole-3-carbinol, both of which have been shown to regulate hormones, protect cellular DNA, and offer cancer-preventive components against different types of cancer.

Serves 4
Calories per serving: 72

4 cups halved Brussels sprouts
2 small shallots, sliced
1 tablespoon avocado oil
2 tablespoons ground fennel seed

1 teaspoon onion powder
2 teaspoons sea salt
Freshly ground black pepper

Preheat the oven to 350°F.

In a large bowl, stir all the ingredients together; be sure all the sprouts are coated with seasoning. Spread the sprouts on a rimmed baking sheet and bake for about 40 minutes, tossing the pan a few times so the sprouts are caramelized on both sides.

Seasonal Salad

Whether you are preparing meat, pasta, or seafood, this salad is a flavor-packed side that can become a main dish with the addition of your favorite protein. Plant-based foods are the most important foods to eat when you're rebuilding from a disease or chronic health issue, or getting rid of toxic fat. Make sure you eat plenty of plant-based foods, including this salad, throughout the day to ensure that you're getting the proper amount of disease-preventing nutrients.

Serves 4
Calories per serving: 370

Easy Balsamic Dressing

3 tablespoons extra-virgin olive oil
1 to 1½ tablespoons balsamic vinegar
½ teaspoon garlic powder

½ teaspoon Italian seasoning
¼ teaspoon sea salt
Freshly ground black pepper

Salad

1 romaine heart
2 cups mesclun salad mix
1 carrot, shredded
1 cup sliced snap peas
½ cup halved grape tomatoes
½ cup sliced black olives
½ cup chopped yellow or red bell pepper

½ bunch flat-leaf parsley, coarsely chopped
3 or 4 sprigs dill, coarsely chopped
4 fresh basil leaves, cut into chiffonade
¼ cup slivered or sliced almonds
¼ cup pumpkin seeds

Easy Balsamic Dressing

In a small bowl, whisk together all the dressing ingredients.

Salad

In a large bowl, combine all the salad ingredients. Add the dressing and toss well to make sure dressing is thoroughly distributed.

Sesame Broccoli

Adding the nutty flavor of toasted sesame oil to the earthy flavor of these little green trees makes them the perfect side for any entrée. Chew the broccoli well, as this will release the disease-preventing nutrients needed for your recovery from your current health issues.

Serves 6
Calories per serving: 123

2 tablespoons toasted sesame oil
½ bunch scallions, sliced, plus more for garnish
2 garlic cloves, crushed
1 carrot, thinly sliced
½ red bell pepper, diced

Sea salt
2 pounds broccoli florets, halved
2 tablespoons mirin (Japanese rice wine)
1 tablespoon toasted sesame seeds

In a large skillet, heat the oil over medium heat. Add the scallions and garlic; cook for 1 minute. Add the carrot, bell pepper, and a little salt. Cook for a few more minutes, then add the broccoli. Stir well to be sure all the vegetables are coated with the oil. Add the mirin and cook, stirring, for 3 minutes. Stir in the sesame seeds.

Garnish with additional scallions.

Spiced Sweet Potato Cubes

Sweet potatoes with a bite—love them. Sweet potatoes are rich in the antioxidant beta-carotene, the precursor to vitamin A. Consuming beta-carotene in sufficient amounts can lower your risk of developing coronary artery disease, stroke, and macular degeneration, as well as prevent their recurrence. This is a smooth and sweet complement to any dish, including your morning omelet or frittata.

Serves 6
Calories per serving: 78

2 large sweet potatoes, cut into cubes
2 tablespoons extra-virgin olive oil
1 teaspoon ground cumin
1 teaspoon sea salt
¼ teaspoon paprika
¼ teaspoon cayenne pepper

Preheat the oven to 400°F.

In a large bowl, combine the sweet potato with the olive oil; mix thoroughly so the cubes are evenly coated with the oil. Stir in the spices so they are evenly spread throughout the mixture. Spread the cubes on a baking sheet and bake until soft, 35 to 45 minutes.

String Beans & Tomatoes

Green beans and tomatoes smothered in mint and tarragon make for a refreshing dish with a satisfying crunch. It takes only minutes to prepare and is a bountiful source of vitamins K, C, and A. Green beans also contain folate, vitamin B_1, and iron, making them a perfect choice to add to your daily diet. After all, who doesn't like green beans?

Serves 6
Calories per serving: 73

2 pounds green beans, trimmed and halved
Sea salt and freshly ground black pepper
1 tablespoon avocado oil

1 bunch scallions, sliced
2 cups halved grape tomatoes
1 teaspoon chopped fresh tarragon
1 teaspoon chopped fresh mint (see Note)

Put the beans in a large skillet and add water to come halfway up the beans. Season with salt. Bring the water to a boil; remove from the heat, cover, and steam for 5 minutes, or until tender. Drain the green beans and set aside.

In the same skillet, heat the oil over medium heat. Add the scallions, a little salt and pepper, the grape tomatoes, and the tarragon. Cook for a minute; add the green beans and fresh mint, and season with salt and pepper. Cook until the tomatoes break down to a creamy consistency.

NOTE: For a more Italian flavor, use fresh basil instead of mint and tarragon.

Sweet Mushroom Salad

The title says it all. The savory, meaty flavor of cremini mushrooms is sweetened with a touch of agave syrup. Of the many medicinal properties of mushrooms, enhanced immune function is at the top of the list. The compounds in mushrooms can modulate and regulate the immune response in autoimmune diseases and allergies, and support the defense against cancer.

Serves 4
Calories per serving: 60

Juice of ½ lime
½ scallion, light and dark green parts only, thinly sliced
1 teaspoon coriander seeds
1 teaspoon cardamom seeds
1 teaspoon agave syrup

1 tablespoon extra-virgin olive oil
Sea salt and freshly ground black pepper
1 pound firm cremini mushrooms, very thinly sliced

Combine the lime juice, scallion, coriander, cardamom, agave syrup, oil, and salt and pepper in a jar; seal and shake well to blend. Pour over the mushrooms in a bowl, and toss well. Marinate in the refrigerator, stirring often, for at least 30 minutes before serving (but in a pinch, they can be eaten immediately).

Tuscan Cabbage, Kale & Beans

This is a tasty and satisfying main dish that can also be served as a side with beef, lamb, or poultry. It's also great with a poached egg for breakfast. Cabbage and kale offer an array of powerful phytonutrients that will allow for a quick recovery and rebuild.

Serves 6
Calories per serving: 334

2 tablespoons avocado oil
1 clove garlic, coarsely chopped
1 tablespoon sea salt
1 teaspoon freshly ground black pepper
2 teaspoons dried oregano
2 (8-ounce) cans organic great northern beans, or 1 pound cooked navy beans, with their liquid

1 medium yellow onion, quartered and sliced
1 head savoy cabbage, quartered and sliced ¼ inch thick
½ bunch kale, stemmed and finely chopped
1 teaspoon red pepper flakes (optional)

In a small saucepan, heat 1 tablespoon of the avocado oil and all the garlic; cook until tender. Add a pinch of salt, pepper, oregano, and both cans of beans, including their liquid. Cook over low heat, uncovered, for 10 minutes; cover and cook for 10 minutes more, until the beans are tender. Add more salt for flavor if needed. This mixture will supply most of the flavor in the recipe.

In a large sauté pan, heat the remaining 1 tablespoon oil over medium heat. Add the onion, salt, and pepper; cook until tender. Add all the cabbage and kale; sprinkle lightly with water to create steam. Stir, cover, and cook for 1 minute; repeat those steps until the cabbage is tender but not too soft. Add the bean mixture; stir well and cover. Remove from the heat and set aside to allow the flavors to combine. Season with red pepper flakes, if desired, and serve.

Waldorf Salad

This light and creamy apple and walnut salad pairs well with any main dish. There is a lot of truth to the saying "An apple a day keeps the doctor away." Apples are high in antioxidants and fiber. They are also abundant in flavonol, a polyphenol that can reduce your risk of coronary artery disease, stroke, and high blood pressure. This phytochemical can also lower C-reactive protein, a biomarker for chronic inflammation.

Serves 6
Calories per serving: 183

2 red apples, such as Pink Lady or Gala, cored and cut into bite-size pieces
2 cups halved red grapes
4 celery stalks, sliced ¼ inch thick

½ small red onion, thinly sliced
½ cup coarsely chopped walnuts
Juice of 1 lemon
¼ cup mayonnaise or Vegenaise (see Resources)

In a large bowl, combine all the ingredients except the mayonnaise. Add the mayonnaise and mix well.

Variations
Make this salad a main dish by adding steamed or grilled chicken.

Vary the flavor by adding fresh tarragon or mint.

Snacks

Blueberry Smoothie

This is an excellent pre- or post-workout snack. Blueberries are high in antioxidants, which combat the free radicals produced in muscles after resistance exercise.

Serves 1
Calories per serving: 157

½ small banana
1 cup blueberries
1 scoop powdered greens (see Note)

1 scoop protein powder (whey, egg
white, or rice protein)

Put all the ingredients and 1 cup water in a high-speed blender (such as a Vitamix) and blend until the desired consistency is reached. If it's too thick, use a little more water. If it's too watery, use less water.

NOTE: nutraMetrix Complete Greens can be ordered from my website. Depending on the grams of protein per scoop, you may have to add more protein powder. I use a micro-filtered whey protein or pea-and-rice protein; both are available as Perfect Protein made by a division of Metagenics. (Perfect Protein can be ordered from my website.) One scoop has 16 grams of protein. I usually use 1½ scoops after my workout.

Homemade Sports Drink

Instead of reaching for unhealthful drinks that claim to contain electrolytes, consider making your own. You need citrus fruits, water, nutrient-dense salt, and a natural sweetener. When using salt, you need only a few shakes; don't overdo it.

8 ounces water
1/2 orange
1/2 lemon
1/4–1/2 grapefruit

2–3 shakes of sea salt, pink Himalayan salt, or Celtic sea salt
1 teaspoon organic honey or agave syrup

Combine all ingredients. Shake well and drink during your workout.

DR. Z'S FAST AND EASY SNACKS

These combinations provide one serving of two or three food groups.

1 hard-boiled egg
1 medium apple
Calories: 155

1 apple, sliced
2 tablespoons almond butter
Calories: 180

1/4 cup hummus
1 medium carrot
Calories: 135

1/4 cup hummus
8 rice crackers
Calories: 206

1/4 cup blueberries
1/2 cup strawberries
Calories: 80

1/2 to 3/4 cup broccoli
1/4 cup hummus
Calories: 115

8 brown rice crackers
1 serving non starchy vegetable
1 apple
Calories: 176

4 or 5 brown rice crackers
1/4 cup Guacamole (page 435)
Calories: 145

4 or 5 brown rice crackers
1/4 cup Jalapeño-Apple Salsa (page 436)
Calories: 100

4 or 5 brown rice crackers
1/4 cup Mango & Black Bean Salsa (page 437)
Calories: 110

4 or 5 brown rice crackers
1/4 cup Tomato Relish (page 438)
Calories: 110

Eggplant Tapenade

This is a versatile recipe. Use the tapenade as a spread with rice crackers, a filling for steamed kale leaves, or a side dish with chicken or fish. Eggplant has a creamy-white flesh that can be both sweet and bitter. Besides being beautiful in color, eggplant is rich in caffeic and chlorogenic acids, phenolic compounds that have anticancer, antimicrobial, and antiviral properties.

Serves 6
Calories per serving: 110

1 large eggplant, cut into ¾-inch dice
1 large red onion, cut into ¾-inch dice
1 large red bell pepper, cut into ¾-inch dice
3 tablespoons avocado oil
1 teaspoon Italian seasoning
2 tablespoons balsamic vinegar
6 garlic cloves, coarsely chopped (optional)
10 kalamata or Italian green olives, pitted
1 to 2 tablespoons olive brine (optional)
Pinch of dried oregano
Sea salt and freshly ground black pepper
Red pepper flakes (optional)

Preheat the oven to 400°F. Line a baking sheet with aluminum foil.

In a large bowl, combine the eggplant, onion, and bell pepper. Add the oil, Italian seasoning, vinegar, garlic (if using), olives, olive brine (if using), and oregano. Season with salt, black pepper, and red pepper flakes (if using). Toss to coat the vegetables evenly with the seasonings. Spread the mixture on the prepared baking sheet and bake until the vegetables are roasted to a creamy texture; this can take up to 1 hour. Stir every 20 minutes to ensure even roasting.

For a rustic texture, serve it just as it is. For a smoother texture, puree in a food processor (this version is often called "eggplant caviar").

Guacamole

Avocado, a hint of lime, salt, and mustard combine to create a flavor profile that goes well with organic blue corn chips. Avocado is a superior source of poly- and monounsaturated fats that prevent the oxidation of LDL.

Serves 4 to 6 (makes about 1½ cups)
Calories per serving (based on 6 servings): 107

2 ripe medium avocados, halved and
  pitted
1 tablespoon fresh lime juice
1 garlic clove, minced, or 1 teaspoon
  jarred minced garlic

¾ teaspoon sea salt or pink
  Himalayan salt
Pinch of mustard powder
1 teaspoon onion powder
1 small tomato, chopped

Scoop the avocado flesh into a bowl and add the lime juice and spices. Add the chopped tomato and mix. Serve immediately.

Chunky Guacamole

This variation is for those who want guacamole with added texture. You'll love it.

Serves 4
Calories per serving: 95

1 large avocado, halved and pitted
1 scallion, thinly sliced
Juice of 1 lime
1 tablespoon chopped fresh cilantro
¼ red bell pepper, finely diced
1 cup quartered grape tomatoes

1 teaspoon ground cumin
1 teaspoon garlic powder
1 teaspoon extra-virgin olive oil
1 teaspoon sea salt
Hot sauce

Cut the avocado flesh into cubes and drop them in a medium bowl. Add the remaining ingredients and mix well. Press plastic wrap directly against the surface of the guacamole and refrigerate until chilled before serving.

Hummus

When I work with patients one-on-one to create a personal meal plan, this creamy Middle Eastern dip made from chickpeas is a popular healthful snack. Chickpeas are high in fiber, which your body needs to maintain regular digestion. Hummus is a satisfying dip for raw vegetables, including broccoli, cauliflower, carrots, and green beans. It can also help you avoid unhealthful snacks.

Serves 6
Calories per serving (¼ cup): 95

2 garlic cloves, chopped
1 (15-ounce) can no-salt-added
    chickpeas, drained and rinsed
2 tablespoons tahini
3 tablespoons fresh lemon juice

½ teaspoon organic tamari
½ teaspoon ground cumin
½ teaspoon ground coriander
1 tablespoon finely chopped fresh
    parsley (optional)

In a food processor, puree the garlic to a creamy consistency. Add the chickpeas, tahini, lemon juice, tamari, cumin, coriander, and ¼ cup water; process until very smooth. Transfer to a bowl and chill for an hour or two. Before serving, garnish with the parsley, if desired.

Jalapeño-Apple Salsa

Although small in size, jalapeños are big in flavor and nutrition. They are high in vitamin C and the compound capsaicin, which acts as an anti-inflammatory by regulating NF-kB, the orchestrator of inflammation. Capsaicin can also regulate the dilation of arteries. If you have high levels of unwanted body fat, eating foods containing capsaicin can help you burn it off by increasing your energy expenditure.

Serves 6
Calories per serving: 49

3 crisp apples, cored and finely diced
½ red bell pepper, finely diced
Juice of 1 lime
1 tablespoon agave syrup
½ jalapeño, seeded and finely diced

½ scallion, light and dark green parts
  only, thinly sliced
2 tablespoons grated fresh ginger
Sea salt

In a bowl, combine all the ingredients; taste and adjust the seasoning. Serve chilled with rice crackers or as a sauce for fish or chicken.

Mango & Black Bean Salsa

I really love the sweetness and texture of fresh, ripe mango combined with the flavors of black beans, cilantro, and jalapeños. Black beans are prized for their fiber, protein, folate, iron, and magnesium. The nutrients in these dark-colored legumes help support digestion and regulate appetite. This salsa is a tasty accompaniment to fish or a poached egg.

Serves 6
Calories per serving: 85

1 large semi-ripe mango (see Note),
  diced
1 (15.5-ounce) can black beans,
  drained and rinsed
¼ red bell pepper, finely diced
1 or 2 scallions, thinly sliced

1 tablespoon chopped fresh cilantro
Dash of extra-virgin olive oil
Sea salt and freshly ground black
  pepper
Hot sauce or diced jalapeño (optional)

Mix all the ingredients together. Adjust the seasoning with salt, pepper, hot sauce, or jalapeño to taste.

NOTE: Mango is a high-glycemic fruit, so eat it sparingly.

Spicy Garlic Hummus

Creamy hummus with some heat—need I say more? Serve it as a snack with rice crackers or vegetables—try celery, broccoli, zucchini, and cauliflower.

Serves 12
Calories per serving (¼ cup): 95

2 (15-ounce) cans organic chickpeas, drained, liquid reserved, and rinsed
4 large garlic cloves
¼ cup tahini
Zest and juice of 1 lemon
½ teaspoon cayenne pepper
1 teaspoon sea salt
1 tablespoon extra-virgin olive oil

In a food processor, blend all the ingredients until smooth. Add reserved liquid from the chickpeas, if necessary, to get a smooth consistency.

Tomato Relish

This is a favorite snack of mine, as I really enjoy tomatoes and red bell peppers. The sweetness of these bright red vegetables with basil and black pepper makes for a satisfying appetizer, a snack with rice crackers, or a sauce for chicken or fish. The red carotenoids in the tomatoes and peppers reduce oxidative stress in the body, which can lead to the development of chronic disease.

Serves 5
Calories per serving (¼ cup): 55

2 tablespoons extra-virgin olive oil
1 large red onion, halved and sliced
1 teaspoon dried oregano
Sea salt and freshly ground black pepper
½ red bell pepper, finely diced
1 (15-ounce) can organic diced tomatoes, drained
8 large fresh basil leaves, cut into chiffonade

In a large skillet, heat the oil over medium heat. Add the onion and oregano, season with salt and black pepper, and cook for 2 minutes. Add the bell pepper and cook for another 10 minutes. Reduce the heat to low, add the tomatoes, and cook until the flavors are combined and the onion is tender. Stir in the basil and cook for just a bit more.

Tuscan Bean Dip

White beans, garlic, and olive oil all contribute to the creamy texture and powerful flavor of this dip. White beans are a great source of fiber needed for healthy digestive function and maintaining healthy gut flora. Serve with rice crackers or gluten-free toasted bread cut into triangles. Both will add to the calories, so check labels carefully. Avoid rice crackers that contain added sugar or potato starch.

Serves 6
Calories per serving (¼ cup): 78

1 tablespoon extra-virgin olive oil
8 large garlic cloves, smashed and coarsely chopped
2 teaspoons crushed dried oregano

Sea salt and freshly ground black pepper
1 (15-ounce) can small white beans, drained, liquid reserved, and rinsed
Red pepper flakes (optional)

In a saucepan, heat the oil over low heat. Add the garlic, oregano, and salt to taste. Cook very slowly until the garlic is soft and golden in color. Add the beans and ½ cup of the liquid from the can. (Water or vegetable broth can be substituted for the can liquid.) Cook until the liquid thickens. Season with salt, black pepper, and red pepper flakes, if desired.

NOTE: To increase the recipe, just add a second can of beans.

Desserts

Ambrosia Fruit Salad

Sweet fruit with coconut and pecans makes for a decadent dessert after any meal. Both fruit and pecans are nutrient-dense, offering healthful phytonutrients that regulate inflammation and oxidation.

Serves 4
Calories per serving: 188

¼ cup fresh orange juice
2 tablespoons unsweetened shredded
  coconut
1 large orange, segmented and
  broken into bite-size chunks

1 small banana, sliced lengthwise,
  then crosswise
1 cup sliced green grapes
½ cup chopped raw pecans

Combine the orange juice and shredded coconut; set aside until the coconut softens, about 30 minutes.

In a bowl, combine the orange segments, banana, grapes, and pecans. Drain the shredded coconut, discarding the orange juice, and mix it into the fruit salad.

NOTE: Drinking the excess orange juice will increase the calorie count. Pure fruit juice is high in sugar.

Flourless Almond Butter Cookies

Once in a while, when I just need to satisfy my sweet tooth, I reach for one of these almond butter cookies. These delectable treats are made with palm sugar, a healthier alternative to refined white sugar, and almond butter. Be careful—it's hard to eat just one.

Makes about 20 cookies
Calories per serving (1 cookie): 119

¾ cup coconut palm sugar
½ teaspoon baking soda
¼ teaspoon sea salt
1 cup creamy natural, no-sugar-added almond butter

1 large egg (preferably organic or cage free), lightly beaten
¾ cup raw almonds, chopped
¼ cup unsweetened shredded coconut (optional)

Preheat the oven to 350°F. Line a baking sheet with parchment paper.

In a large bowl, mix together the coconut palm sugar, baking soda, and salt. Add the almond butter and beaten egg; stir until well combined. Add the almonds and shredded coconut (if using); stir until evenly distributed.

With wet hands, roll about 1 tablespoon of the dough into a ball and place it on the prepared baking sheet. Do the same with the rest of the dough, spacing the cookies about 1½ inches apart on the baking sheet.

Bake for about 15 minutes, until the cookies are slightly puffed and have a cracked look on top. Cool for 5 minutes on the baking sheet; any longer will cause them to overcook. Transfer the cookies to a wire rack to finish cooling. Cool to room temperature and store them in an air-tight container.

Variation

FLOURLESS PEANUT BUTTER COOKIES: Substitute 1 cup creamy natural, no-sugar-added peanut butter for the almond butter and ¾ cup roasted salted peanuts, chopped, for the chopped raw almonds. Space the cookies about 1 inch apart on the baking sheet; these do not spread much as they bake.

Gluten-Free Banana Muffins

The use of almond flour and coconut flour makes these muffins a health-ful alternative to the processed, refined baked goods loaded with white sugar, butter, and fat. Combined with ripe banana and coconut oil, almond flour's healthful fat ensures a flavorful and moist baked treat. Enjoy one of these muffins with a hot cup of coffee or your favorite tea.

Makes 12 muffins
Calories per serving (1 muffin): 208

2 cups almond flour
1 cup coconut flour
$1\frac{1}{2}$ teaspoons baking soda
3 large eggs (preferably organic or cage free)
$\frac{1}{2}$ teaspoon vanilla extract
$\frac{1}{2}$ teaspoon sea salt
2 tablespoons coconut oil, melted, plus more for greasing

2 tablespoons agave syrup
2 cups mashed ripe bananas
1 cup fresh or frozen blueberries (optional)
1 cup coarsely chopped walnuts (optional)
$\frac{3}{4}$ cup bittersweet chocolate chips (optional)

Preheat the oven to 350°F. Grease a 12-cup muffin tin with coconut oil.

In a large bowl, mix the flours and baking soda. In a separate bowl, whisk together the eggs, vanilla, salt, agave, and coconut oil. Add the egg mixture to the flour mixture and mix until smooth. Fold in the mashed bananas until evenly incorporated.

Add any of the optional ingredients, if desired, and mix well.

Fill each well of the prepared muffin tin to the rim; the muffins will not rise very much. Bake for 35 minutes. Insert a knife or toothpick into the center of a few muffins; if it comes out clean, they are done. If not, bake for 10 minutes more and check again.

Cool the muffins before removing them from the tin. Store them in an air-tight container.

Summer Fruit Salad

Fresh berries and mint make a sweet treat with a refreshing twist. Straw-berries and blueberries have a nutritional profile that far surpasses other fruits. The dark purple and bright red pigments of these soft and sweet berries aid in preventing heart disease, cancer, and neurological disor-ders linked to damage caused by free radicals.

Serves 2
Calories per serving: 87

1 cup sliced strawberries
1 cup blueberries
1 peach, pitted and chopped

5 or 6 fresh mint leaves, chopped
¼ cup lime juice, fresh squeezed

Combine all the ingredients in a large bowl. Set aside for 30 minutes to allow the flavors to mingle. Serve at room temperature. If making this ahead, refrigerate, covered, until 30 minutes before serving. The fruits are more flavorful if served at room temperature.

Resources

THROUGHOUT THIS BOOK, YOU will occasionally see recommendations for certain products that I find beneficial and superior in some way. Here I have described those products and provided information of where to locate them.

Primal Kitchen Mayo—A healthful alternative to regular mayonnaise, this is made from avocado oil, organic cage-free eggs, organic vinegar, sea salt, and organic rosemary extract. It is available in most natural-food stores and online at www.primalkitchen.com.

Vegenaise—This is a vegan mayonnaise substitute made without artificial ingredients. It has a very pleasant "clean" flavor. Some think it tastes more like homemade mayonnaise than commercial brands. It is available in most natural-food stores and some supermarkets, as well as online at www.followyourheart.com.

Organic Coconut Aminos—Coconut aminos, from the nutrient-rich sap of the coconut tree, is a delicious non-GMO, gluten-free alternative to soy sauce. This product can be found in most natural-food stores and online at www.coconutsecret.com.

Bragg Organic Sprinkle—This all-natural blend of 24 herbs and spices adds great flavor to most recipes, meals, and snacks. Bragg Organic Sprinkle can be found in most grocery stores and natural markets. You can also find it online at www.bragg.com

Daiya Non-Dairy Cheese—This is the only dairy-free cheese I have found that does not contain traces of casein, a milk protein. It can be found in natural-food stores, some supermarkets, and online at www.daiya foods.com.

Nuts—Organic raw nuts that have been soaked and gently dried are much easier to digest and have greater health benefits than nuts usually found in stores. The best online source is www.livingnutz.com.

Wild Seafood—I recommend that you eat only wild seafood, available at many natural-food stores and some supermarkets. The website www .vitalchoice.com has a complete selection, as well as other organic foods.

Grass-Fed Meats—Like seafood, the type of meat you eat is very important for your health. I recommend only grass-fed, naturally raised meat, available at www.uswellnessmeats.com, as well as natural-food stores and some supermarkets.

Grass-Fed Beef Sticks—Organic grass-fed beef sticks are a great snack when you are on the go. I really enjoy these between meals, after time on the slopes, and after a day on the motorcycle. To order these, check online at www.thenewprimal.com and www.chomps.com.

American Tuna—Pole-and-line caught, this young tuna is low in mercury. High in omega-3 essential fatty acids and protein, American Tuna is an excellent source of tuna for your favorite recipes. It is available at natural-food stores and some supermarkets.

Smoked Sea Salt—Maldon smoked sea salt adds a unique flavor to fish, meat, poultry, sauces, salsas, soups, and marinades. There is no substitute for this soft and flaky salt. Available at natural-food stores and some supermarkets, it is also found online at www.maldonsalt .co.uk.

Nutritional Supplements—For further information on advanced, science-based nutritional supplements to help you rebuild, please go to my online store at www.drzembroski.com.

References

Abdel-Latif, M. M., Raouf, A. A., Sabra K., et al. (2005). Vitamin C enhances chemosensitization of esophageal cancer cells in vitro. *Journal of Chemotherapy, 17* (5), 539–49.

Abe, Y., Iwai, W., Lijima, K., et al. (2013). Gastric hypochlorhydria is associated with an exacerbation of dyspeptic symptoms in female patients. *Journal of Gastroenterology, 48* (2), 214–21.

Adamsen, L., Quist, M., Andersen, C., et al. (2009). Effect of a multimodal high-intensity exercise intervention in cancer patients undergoing chemotherapy: A randomized controlled trial. *British Medical Journal, 339*, b3410.

Alexander, D. D., & Cushing, C. A. (2011). Red meat and colorectal cancer: A critical summary of prospective epidemiologic studies. *Obesity Reviews, 12*, e472–e493.

Alexander, D. D., Weed, D. L., Cushing, C. A., et al. (2011). Meta-analysis of prospective studies of red meat consumption and colorectal cancer. *European Journal of Cancer Prevention, 20* (4), 293–307.

Allison, M. A., Jensky, J., Marshall, S. J., et al. (2012). Sedentary behavior and adiposity-associated inflammation the multiethnic study of atherosclerosis. *American Journal of Preventive Medicine, 42* (1), 8–13.

American Autoimmune Related Disorders Association. Retrieved from www.aarda.org.

American Heart Association. (2010). Heart disease and stroke statistics: 2010 update at a glance. *Circulation, 121*, e46–e215.

American Heart Association. (2013). Heart disease and stroke statistics: 2013 update. *Circulation, 127*, e6–e245.

Ames, B. N. (2001). DNA damage from micronutrient deficiencies is likely to be a major cause of cancer. *Mutation Research, 475* (1–2), 7–20.

Anderson, G., & Horvath, J. (2004). The growing burden of chronic disease in America. *Public Health Reports, 119*, 263–70.

Andrews, N., Prasad, A., & Quyyumi, A. (2001). N-acetylcysteine improves coronary and peripheral vascular function. *Journal of the American College of Cardiology, 37* (1), 117–23.

Anikhovskaya, I. A., Kubatiev, A. A., Yakovlev, M. Y. (2015). Endotoxin theory of atherosclerosis. *Human Physiology, 41* (1), 89–97.

Antoni, M. H., Lutgendorf, S. K., Cole, S. W., et al. (2006). The influence of bio-behavioral factors on tumour biology: Pathways and mechanisms. *Nature Reviews, 6*, 240–48.

Báez, R., Lopes, M. T., Salas, C. E., et al. (2007). In vivo antitumoral activity of stem pineapple (Ananas comosus) bromelain. *Planta Medica, 73* (13), 1377–83.

Barclay, G., & Shiraev, T. (2012). Clinical benefits of high-intensity interval training. *Australian Family Physician, 41* (12), 960–62.

Bilz, S., Ninnis, R., & Keller, U. (1999). Effects of hypoosmolality on whole-body lipolysis in man. *Metabolism, 48* (4), 472–76.

Björntorp, P. (2001). Do stress reactions cause abdominal obesity and comorbidities? *Obesity Reviews, 2,* 73–86.

Borek, C. (2004). Antioxidants and radiation therapy. *Journal of Nutrition, 134* (11), 3207S–209S.

Bouziana, S. D., & Tziomalos, K. (2011). Malnutrition in patients with acute stroke. *Journal of Nutrition and Metabolism,* Article ID 167898.

Boyd, B. D. (2003). Insulin and cancer. *Integrative Cancer Therapies, 2* (4), 315–29.

Britton, E., & McLaughlin, J. T. (2013). Ageing and the gut. *Proceedings of the Nutrition Society, 72,* 173–77.

Brugger, P., Marktl, W., & Herold, M. (1995). Impaired nocturnal secretion in coronary heart disease. *Lancet, 345* (8962), 1408.

Burg, M. M., Jain, D., Soufer, R., et al. (1993). Role of behavioral and psychological factors in mental stress-induced silent left ventricular dysfunction in coronary artery disease. *Journal of the American College of Cardiology, 22* (2), 440–48.

Bytzer, P., Dahlerup, J. F., Eriksen, J. R., et al. (2011). Diagnosis and treatment of *Helicobacter pylori* infection. *Danish Medical Bulletin, 58* (4), C4271.

Cappuccio, F. P., Cooper, D., D'Elia, L., et al. (2011). Sleep duration predicts cardiovascular outcomes: A systematic review and meta-analysis of prospective studies. *European Heart Journal, 32,* 1484–92.

Centers for Disease Control and Prevention. Chronic diseases: The leading causes of death and disability in the United States. Retrieved from www.cdc.gov/chronicdisease/overview/#ref2.

Centers for Disease Control and Prevention. Iron deficiency. Retrieved from www.cdc.gov.

Centers for Disease Control and Prevention. *National Health and Nutrition Examination Survey, 2009–2010.* Retrieved from wwwn.cdc.gov/nchs/nhanes/search/nhanes09_10.aspx.

Cesarone, M., Renzo, A., Errichi, S., et al. (2008). Improvement in circulation and in cardiovascular risk factors with a proprietary isotonic bioflavonoid formula OPC-3®. *Angiology, 59,* 408.

Chakraborti, C. K. (2011). Vitamin D as a promising anticancer agent. *Indian Journal of Pharmacology, 43* (2), 113–20.

Chandan, C. (2013). Evaluation of immunoregulatory activities of green tea (camelia sinensis) in Freund's adjuvant arthritis model. *Journal of Pharmacognosy and Phytochemisty, 1* (2), 26–29.

Chen, S. M., Tsai, Y. S., Lee, S. W., et al. (2014). Astragalus membranaceus modulates Th 1/2 immune balance and activates PPARγ in murine asthma model. *Biochemistry and Cell Biology, 92* (5), 397–405.

Chiang, A. C., & Massagué, J. (2008). Molecular basis of metastasis. *New England Journal of Medicine, 259,* 2814–23.

Chiang, C. D., Song, E. J., Yang, V. C., et al. (1994). Vitamin C (ascorbic acid) reverse chemoresistance of human non-small lung-cancer cells. *Biochemical Journal, 301* (Pt 3), 759–64.

Chi-Fung Chan, G., Keung Chan, W., & Man-Yuen Sze, D. (2009). The effects of β-glucan on human immune and cancer cells. *Journal of Hematology & Oncology,* 2, 25.

Chiodini, I., Adda, G., Scillitani, A., et al. (2007). Cortisol secretion in patients with type 2 diabetes. *Diabetes Care,* 30, 83–88.

Chiru, Z., Popescu, C. R., & Gheorghe, D. C. (2014). Melatonin and cancer. *Journal of Medicine and Life,* 7 (3), 373–74.

Coder, D. E. (2011). Worldwide increasing incidences of cutaneous malignant melanoma. *Journal of Skin Cancer,* Article ID 858425.

Cohen, S., Frank, E., Rabin, B. S., et al. (1998). Types of stressors that increase susceptibility to the common cold in health adults. *Health Psychology,* 17 (3), 214–23.

Coker, R. H., Williams, R. H., Kortebein, P. M., et al. (2009). Influence of exercise intensity on abdominal fat and adiponectin in elderly adults. *Metabolic Syndrome and Related Disorders,* 7, 363–68.

Cordain, L. (1999). Cereal grains: Humanity's double-edged sword. *World Review of Nutrition and Dietetics,* 84, 19–73.

Couch, F. J., DeShano, M. L., Blackwood, M. A., et al. (1997). BRCA1 mutations in women attending clinics that evaluate the risk of breast cancer. *New England Journal of Medicine,* 336, 1409–15.

Cover, C. M., Hsieh, S. J., Cram, E. J., et al. (1999). Indol-3-carbinol and tamoxifen cooperate to arrest the cell cycle of MCF-7 human breast cancer cells. *Cancer Research,* 59, 1244–51.

Cover, C. M., Hsieh, S. J., Tran, S. H., et al. (1998). Indole-3-carbinol inhibits the expression of cyclindependent kinase-6 and induces a G1 cell cycle arrest of human breast cancer cells independent of estrogen receptor signaling. *Journal of Biological Chemistry,* 273 (7), 3838–47.

Dalgard, C., Weihe, P., Petersen, M. S., et al. (2011). Vitamin D status in relation to glucose metabolism and type 2 diabetes in septuagenarians. *Diabetes Care,* 34, 1284–88.

Dall, M., Calloe, K., Haupt-Jorgensen, M., et al. (2013). Gliadin fragments and a specific gliadin 33-mer peptide close katp channels and induce insulin secretion in ins-1e cells and rat islets of Langerhans. *PLOS ONE,* 8 (6), e66474.

De Backer, I. C., Van Breda, E., Vreugdenhil, A., et al. (2007). High-intensity strength training improves quality of life in cancer survivors. *Acta Oncologica,* 46, 1143–51.

De Feo, P., Di Loreto, C., Ranchelli, A., et al. (2006). Exercise and diabetes. *Acta Biomedica,* 77 (Suppl. 1), 14–17.

DeCensi, A., & Gennari, A. (2010). Insulin breast cancer connection: Confirmatory data set the stage for better care. *Journal of Clinical Oncology,* 29 (10), 7–10.

Deeb, K. K., Trump, D. L., & Johnson, C. (2007). Vitamin D signaling pathways in cancer: Potential for anticancer therapeutics. *Nature Reviews Cancer,* 7, 684–700.

DeFelice, F. G., & Lourenco, M. V. (2015). Brain metabolic stress and neuroinflammation at the basis of cognitive impairment in Alzheimer's disease. *Frontiers in Aging Neuroscience,* 7 (94), 9.

Dekker, M. J., Koper, J. W., Van Aken, M. O., et al. (2008). Salivary cortisol is related to atherosclerosis of carotid arteries. *Journal of Clinical Endocrinology and Metabolism, 93* (10), 3741–47.

Del Rios, B., Pedrero, J. M., Martinez-Campa, J. C., et al. (2004). Melatonin, an endogenous-specific inhibitor of estrogen receptor alpha via calmodulin. *Journal of Biological Chemistry, 279* (37), 38294–302.

Dessi, M., Noce, A., Bertucci, P., et al. (2013). Atherosclerosis, dyslipidemia, and inflammation: The significant role of polyunsaturated fatty acids. *ISRN Inflammation,* Article ID 191823.

Devi, K. R., Kusumlatha, C., Reddy, K. D., et al. (2012). Ascorbic acid supplementation prevents Adriamycin induced genotoxicity in male mice. *Journal of Pharmaceutical and Biomedical Sciences. 17* (15), 1–4.

DeVol, R., & Bedroussian, A. (2007). *An unhealthy America: The economic burden of chronic disease.* Santa Monica, CA: Milken Institute.

Diaz, M. N., Frei, B., Vita, J. A., & Keaney, J. F. Jr. (1997). Antioxidants and atherosclerotic heart disease. *New England Journal of Medicine, 337* (6), 408–16.

Dominguez-Rodriquez, A. (2013). Melatonin and the heart: A tool for effective therapy in the cardiovascular disease? *Cardiovascular Pharmacology, 2,* e109.

Dong, J.-Y., Xun, P., He, K., & Qin, L.-Q. (2011). Magnesium intake and risk of type 2 diabetes. *Diabetes Care, 34,* 2116–22.

Donohoe, C. L., Doyle, S. L., & Reynolds, J. V. (2011). Visceral adiposity, insulin resistance, and cancer risk. *Diabetology and Metabolic Syndrome, 3* (12), 12.

Drake, M. T., Maurer, M. J., & Link, B. K. (2010). Vitamin D insufficiency and prognosis in non-Hodgkins's lymphoma. *Journal of Clinical Oncology, 28,* 4191–98.

Dunn, A. J., Swiergiel, A. H., & de Beaurepaire, R. (2005). Cytokines as mediators of depression: What can we learn from animal studies? *Neuroscience and Biobehavioral Reviews, 29,* 891–909.

Enseleit, F., Sudano, I., Périeat, D., et al. (2012). Effects of Pycnogenol® on endothelial function in patients with stable coronary artery disease: A double-blind, randomized, placebo-controlled, cross-over study. *European Heart Journal, 33,* 1589–97.

Epel, E. S., McEwen, B., Seeman, T., et al. (2000). Stress and body shape: Stress-induced cortisol secretion is consistently greater among women with central fat. *Psychosomatic Medicine, 62,* 623–32.

Fairfield, K. M., & Fletcher, R. H. (2002). Vitamins for chronic disease prevention in adults: Scientific review. *Journal of the American Medical Association, 287,* 23.

Farshchi, H. R., Taylor, M. A., & MacDonald, I. A. (2005). Deleterious effects of omitting breakfast on insulin sensitivity and fasting lipid profiles in healthy lean women. *American Journal of Clinical Nutrition, 81,* 388–96.

Ferro, R., Parvathaneni, A., Patel, S., & Cheriyath, P. (2012). Pesticides and breast cancer. *Advances in Breast Cancer Research, 1,* 30–35.

Feskanich, D., Willett, W. C., Stampfer, M. J., & Colditz, G. A. (1997). Milk, dietary calcium, and bone fractures in women: A 12-year prospective study. *American Journal of Public Health, 87,* 992–97.

Fink, M. (2011). Vitamin D deficiency is a cofactor of chemotherapy-induced mucocutaneous toxicity and dysgeusia. *Journal of Clinical Oncology, 29* (4), e81–e82.

Ford, E. S., Bergmann, M. M., Kröger, J., et al. (2009). Healthy living is the best revenge: Findings from the European Prospective Investigation into Cancer and Nutrition-Potsdam study. *Archives of Internal Medicine, 169* (15), 1355–62.

Gallaher, C. M., & Meliker, J. R. (2007–2008). Mercury and thyroid autoantibodies in U.S. women, NHANES 2007–2008. *European Journal of Clinical Nutrition, 61,* 691–700.

Garland, C. F., Gorham, E. D., Mohr, S. B., & Garland, F. C. (2009). Vitamin D for cancer prevention: Global perspective. *Annals of Epidemiology, 19* (7), 468–83.

Gaurav, K., Goel, R. K., Shukla, M., et al. (2012). Glutamine: A novel approach to chemotherapy-induced toxicity. *Indian Journal of Medical and Paediatric Oncology, 33* (1), 13–20.

Gebauer, S. K., Chardigny, J., Jakobsen, M. U., et al. (2011). Effects of ruminant trans fatty acids on cardiovascular disease and cancer: A comprehensive review of epidemiological, clinical, and mechanistic studies. *Advances in Nutrition, 2,* 332–54.

Ghiadoni, L., Donald, A. E., Cropley, M., et al. (2000). Mental stress induces transient endothelial dysfunction in humans. *Circulation, 102,* 2473–78.

Ginde, A. A., Liu, M. C., & Camargo, C. A. (2009). Demographic differences and trends of vitamin D insufficiency in the US population, 1988–2004. *Archives of Internal Medicine, 169* (6), 626–32.

Ginter, E. (2007). Chronic vitamin C deficiency increases the risk of cardiovascular diseases. *Bratislava Medical Journal, 108* (9), 417–21.

Giovannucci, E. (2001). Insulin, insulin-like growth factors and colon cancer: A review of the evidence. *Journal of Nutrition, 131,* 3109s–120s.

Glaser, R., & Kiecolt-Glaser, J. K. (2003). Stress-induced immune dysfunction: Implications for health. *Nature Reviews, 5,* 243.

Goel, A., & Aggarwal, B. B. (2010). Curcumin, the golden spice from Indian saffron, is a chemosensitizer and radiosensitizer for tumors and chemoprotector and radioprotector for normal organs. *Nutrition and Cancer, 62,* (7), 919–30.

Gottlieb, D. J., Punjabi, N. M., Newman, A. B., et al. (2005). Association of sleep time with diabetes mellitus and impaired glucose tolerance. *Archives of Internal Medicine, 165,* 863–68.

Gregg, E. W., Chen, H., Wagenknecht, L. E., et al. (2012). Association of an intensive lifestyle intervention with remission of type 2 diabetes. *Journal of the American Medical Association, 308* (23), 2498–96.

Gross, L. S., Li, L., Ford, E. S., & Liu, S. (2004). Increased consumption of refined carbohydrates and the epidemic of type 2 diabetes in the United States: An ecological assessment. *American Journal of Clinical Nutrition, 79,* 774–79.

Grube, B. J., Eng, E. T., Kao, Y.-C., et al. (2001). White button mushroom phytochemicals inhibit atomatase activity and breast cancer cell proliferation. *Journal of Nutrition, 131,* 3288–93.

Grün, F., & Blumberg, B. (2006). Environmental obesogens: Organotins and endocrine disruption via nuclear receptor signaling. *Endocrinology, 147,* s50–s55.

Guerrero-Romero, F., & Rodriguez-Moran, M. (2011). Magnesium improves the beta-cell function to compensate variation of insulin sensitivity: Double-blind, randomized clinical trial. *European Journal of Clinical Investigation, 41* (4), 405–10.

Häussinger, D., Roth, E., Lang, F., & Gerok, W. (1993). Cellular hydration state: An important determinant of protein catabolism in health and disease. *Lancet, 22,* 341.

Hagiwara, A., Yoshino, H., Ichihara, T., et al. (2002). Prevention by natural food anthocyanins,purple sweet potato color and red cabbage color, of 2-amino-1-methyl-6-phenylimidazo[4,5-b] pyridine-associated colorectal carcinogenesis in rats initiated with 1,2-dimethylhydrazine. *Journal of Toxicological Sciences, 27* (1), 57–68.

Hansson, G. K. (2005). Inflammation, atherosclerosis, and coronary artery disease. *New England Journal of Medicine, 352,* 1685–95.

Hassanain, E., Silverberg, J. I., Norowitz, K. B., et al. (2010). Green tea suppresses b cell production of IgE without inducing apoptosis. *Annals of Clinical and Laboratory Science, 40* (2), 135–43.

He, K., Zhao, L., Daviglus, M. L., et al. (2008). Association of monosodium glutamate intake with overweight in Chinese adults: The INTERMAP study. *Obesity, 16,* 1875–80.

Helmich, I., Latini, A., Sigwalt, A., et al. (2010). Neurobiological alterations induced by exercise and their impact on depressive disorders. *Clinical Practice & Epidemiology in Mental Health, 6,* 115–25.

Hemminki, K. (1994). DNA adducts, mutations, and cancer. *Carcinogenesis, 14* (10), 2007–12.

Higashi, Y., Sasaki, S., Kurisu, S., et al. (1999). Regular aerobic exercise augments endothelium dependent vascular relaxation in normotensive as well as hypertensive subjects: Role of endothelium derived nitric oxide. *Circulation, 100,* 1194–1202.

Hoffman, J. R., & Falvo, M. J. (2004). Protein—which is best? *Journal of Sports Science and Medicine, 3,* 118–30.

Hollander, D. (2002). Crohn's disease, TNF-alpha, and the leaky gut. The chicken or the egg? *American Journal of Gastroenterology, 97* (8), 1867–68.

Houssami, N., Irwig, L., Simpson, J. M., et al. (2003). Sydney breast imaging accuracy study: Comparative sensitivity and specificity of mammography and sonography in young women with symptoms. *American Journal of Roentgenology, 180* (4), 935–40.

Houston, M. C. (2014). The role of mercury in cardiovascular disease. *Journal of Cardiovascular Diseases and Diagnosis, 2,* 5.

Inoue, A., Kodama, N., & Nanba, H. (2002). Effect of maitake (grifola frondosa) D-fraction on the control of the T lymph node Th1/Th2 proportion. *Biological and Pharmaceutical Bulletin, 25* (4), 536–40.

Ip, M. S. M., Lam, B., Ng, M. M. T., et al. (2002). Obstructive sleep apnea is independently associated with insulin resistance. *American Journal of Respiratory and Critical Care Medicine, 165,* 670–76.

Irwin, M. R., Carrillo, C., & Olmstead, R. (2010). Sleep loss activates cellular markers of inflammation: Sex differences. *Brain, Behavior, and Immunity, 24* (1), 54–57.

Irwin, M. R., Wang, M., Campomayor, C. O., et al. (2006). Sleep deprivation and activation of morning levels of cellular and genomic markers of inflammation. *Archives of Internal Medicine, 166,* 1756–62.

Irwin, M. R., Wang, M., Ribeiro, D., et al. (2008). Sleep loss activates cellular inflammatory signaling. *Biological Psychiatry,* 64, 538–40.

James, J. T. (2013). A new, evidence-based estimate of patient harms associated with hospital care. *Journal of Patient Safety,* 9, 122–28.

Jayawardena, R., Ranasinghe, P., Galappatthy, P., et al. (2012). Effects of zinc supplementation on diabetes mellitus: A systematic review and meta-analysis. *Diabetology & Metabolic Syndrome, 4,* 13.

Johnstone, A. M., Horgan, G. W., Murison, S. D., et al. (2008). Effects of a high-protein ketogenic diet on hunger, appetite, and weight loss in obese men feeding ad libitum. *American Journal of Clinical Nutrition, 87,* 44–55.

Kaminski, S., Cieoelinska, A., & Kostyra, E. (2007). Polymorphism of bovine beta-casein and its potential effect on human health. *Journal of Applied Genetics, 18* (3), 189–98.

Kanaley, J. A., Weltman, J. Y., Veldhuis, J. D., et al. (1997). Human growth hormone response to repeated bouts of aerobic exercise. *Journal of Applied Physiology, 83,* 1756–61.

Kang, B. Y., Song, J. Y., Kim, K. M., et al. (1999). Curcumin inhibits Th1 cytokine profile in CD4 T cells by suppressing interleukin-12 production in macrophages. *British Journal of Pharmacology, 12* (8), 380–84.

Kang, S., & Min, H. (2012). Ginseng, the "immunity boost": The effects of panax ginseng on the immune system. *Journal of Ginseng Research, 36* (4), 354–68.

Keller, U., Szinnai, G., Bilz, S., & Berneis, K. (2003). Effects of changes in hydration on protein, glucose and lipid metabolism in man: Impact on health. *European Journal of Clinical Nutrition, 57* (Suppl. 2), S69–S74.

Kennedy, D. D., Tucker, K. L., Ladas, E. D., et al. (2004). Low antioxidant intakes are associated with increases in adverse effects of chemotherapy in children with acute lymphoblastic leukemia. *American Journal of Clinical Nutrition, 79* (6), 1029–36.

Keune, J., Jeffe, D., Schootman, M., et al. (2010). Accuracy of ultrasound and mammography in predicting pathologic response after neoadjuvant chemotherapy for breast cancer. *American Journal of Surgery, 199* (4), 477–84.

Khan, N., & Mukhtar, H. (2010). Cancer and metastasis: Prevention and treatment by green tea. *Cancer and Metastasis Reviews, 29* (3), 435–45.

Khan, S., Malik, F., & Suri, K. A., (2009). Molecular insight into the immune up-regulatory properties of the leaf extract of ashwagandha and identification of Th1 immunostimulatroy chemical entity. *Vaccine, 27* (43), 6080–87.

Kiecolt-Glaser, J. K., Marucha, P. T., Malarkey, W. B., et al. (1995). Slowing of wound healing by psychological stress. *Lancet, 346,* 1194–96.

Kim, K. H., Lee, Y. S., Jung, I. S., et.al. (1998). Acidic polysaccharide from panax ginseng, ginsan, induces Th1 cell and macrophage cytokines and generates LAK cell in synergy with rIL-2. *Planta Medica, 64* (2), 110–15.

Kim, K. K., Singh, A. P., Singh, R. K., et al. (2012). Anti-angiogenic activity of cranberry proanthocyanidins and cytotoxic properties in ovarian cancer cells. *International Journal of Oncology, 40* (1), 227–35.

Kiu, K., Zhou, R., Wang, B., et al. (2013). Effect of green tea on glucose control and insulin sensitivity: A meta-analysis of 17 randomized controlled trials. *American Journal of Clinical Nutrition, 98* (2), 340–88.

Klein, I., & Danzi, S. (2007). Thyroid disease and the heart. *Circulation, 116,* 1725–35.

Klevay, L. M. (2006). Heart failure improvement from a supplement containing copper. *European Heart Journal, 27* (1), 117.

Kris-Etherton, P., Harris, W., & Appel, L. (2002). Fish consumption, fish oil, omega-3 fatty acids, and cardiovascular disease. *Circulation, 106,* 2747–57.

Kurahashi, N., Sasazuki, S., Iwasaki, M., et al. (2008). Green tea consumption and prostate cancer risk in Japanese men: A prospective study. *American Journal of Epidemiology, 167* (1), 71–77.

Kurahashi, N., Inoue, M., Iwasaki, M., et al. (2008). Dairy product, saturated fatty acid, and calcium intake and prostate cancer in a prospective cohort of Japanese men. *Cancer Epidemiology, Biomarkers & Prevention, 17,* 930–37.

Lambert, G. P. (2009). Stress-induced gastrointestinal barrier dysfunction and its inflammatory effects. *Journal of Animal Science, 87,* E101–E108.

Lambert, G. P., Broussard, L. J., Mason, B. L., et al. (2001). Gastrointestinal permeability during exercise: Effects of aspirin and energy-containing beverages. *Journal of Applied Physiology, 90* (60), 2075–80.

Lanou, A. J., Berkow, S. E., & Barnard, N. D. (2005). Calcium, dairy products, and bone health in children and young adults: A reevaluation of the evidence. *Pediatrics, 115,* 3.

Lee, J., Nam, D. E., Kim, O. K., et al. (2014). Pycnogenol attenuates the symptoms of immune dysfunction through restoring a cellular antioxidant status in low micronutrient-induced immune deficient mice. *Nutrition Research and Practice, 8* (5), 533–38.

Libby, P., Ridker, P. M., & Maseri, A. (2002). Inflammation and atherosclerosis. *Circulation, 105,* 1135–43.

Lira, F. S., Carnevali, L. C., Jr., Zanchi, N. E., et al. (2012). Exercise intensity modulation of hepatic lipid metabolism. *Journal of Nutrition and Metabolism, 2012* (3), 809576.

Liu, C., Huang, C., Huang, L., et al. (2014). Effects of green tea extract on insulin resistance and glucagon-like peptide 1 in patients with type 2 diabetes and lipid abnormalities: A randomized, double-blinded and placebo-controlled trial. *PLOS ONE, 9,* 3.

Liu, D.-Y., Sie, B.-S., Liu, M.-L., et al. (2009). Relationship between seminal plasma zinc concentration and spermatozoa-zona pellucida binding and the ZP-induced acrosome reaction in subfertile men. *Asian Journal of Andrology, 11,* 499–507.

Lockwood, C. M., Moon, J. R., Tobkin, S. E., et al. (2008). Minimal nutrition intervention with high-protein/low-carbohydrate and low-fat, nutrient-dense food supplement improves body composition and exercise benefits in overweight adults: A randomized controlled trial. *Nutrition & Metabolism, 5,* 11.

Lu, Y., Qin, W., Shen, T., et al. (2011). The antioxidant N-acetylcysteine promotes atherosclerotic plaque stabilization through suppression of rage, MMPS and NF-kB in apoe-deficient mice. *Journal of Atherosclerosis and Thrombosis, 18* (11), 998–1008.

Lull, C., Wichers, H., & Savelkoul, H. (2005). Antiinflammatory and immunomodulating properties of fungal metabolites. *Mediators of Inflammation, 2005* (2), 63–80.

Luo, T., Wang, J., Yin, Y., et al. (2010). Epigallocatechin gallate sensitizes breast cancer cells to paclitaxel in a murine model of breast carcinoma. *Breast Cancer Research, 12,* R8.

Ma, Y., Trump, D. L., & Johnson, C. S. (2010). Vitamin D in combination cancer treatment. *Journal of Cancer, 1,* 101–17.

Manini, T. M., Clark, B. C., Nalls, M. A., et al. (2007). Reduced physical activity increases intermuscular adipose tissue in healthy young adults. *American Journal of Clinical Nutrition, 85* (2), 377–84.

Marucha, P. T., Kiecolt-Glaser, J. K., & Favagehi, M. (1998). Mucosal wound healing is impaired by examination stress. *Psychosomatic Medicine, 60,* 362–65.

Mason, C., & Doneen, A. (2012). Niacin: A critical component to the management of atherosclerosis (contemporary management of dyslipdemia to prevent, reduce, or reverse atherosclerotic cardiovascular disease). *Journal of Cardiovascular Nursing, 27* (4), 303–16.

May, J., & Qu, Z. (2010). Ascorbic acid prevents increased endothelial permeability caused by oxidized low density lipoprotein. *Free Radical Research, 44* (11), 1359–68.

McGinnis, J. M., & Foege, W. H. (1993). Actual causes of death in the United States. *Journal of the American Medical Association, 270* (18), 2207–12.

McTiernan, A., Tworoger, S. S., Ulrich, C. M., et al. (2004). Effect of exercise on serum estrogens in postmenopausal women: A 12-month randomized clinical trial. *Cancer Research, 64,* 2923–28.

Miller, A. H., Maletic, V., & Raison, C. L. (2009). Inflammation and its discontents: The role of cytokines in the pathophysiology of major depression. *Biological Psychiatry, 65* (9), 732–41.

Milton, K. (2003). The critical role played by animal source foods in human (homo) evolution. *Journal of Nutrition, 133,* 3886S–92S.

Mokdad, A. H., Mark, J. S., Stroup, D. F., et al. (2004). Actual causes of death in the United States, 2000. *Journal of the American Medical Association, 291* (10), 1238–45.

Mooren, F. C., Kruger, K., Volker, K., et al. (2011). Oral magnesium supplementation reduces insulin resistance in non-diabetic subjects: A double-blind, placebo-controlled, randomized trial. *Diabetes, Obesity and Metabolism, 13* (3), 281–84.

Moss, R. (2007). Do antioxidants interfere with radiation therapy for cancer? *Integrative Cancer Therapies, 6* (3), 281–92.

Mozaffarian, D., Rimm, E. B., King, I. B., et al. (2004). Trans fatty acids and systemic inflammation in heart failure. *American Journal of Clinical Nutrition, 80* (6), 1521–25.

Mullington, J. M., Simpson, N. S., Meier-Ewert, H. K., et al. (2010). Sleep loss and inflammation. *Best Practice & Research Clinical Endocrinology, 24* (5), 775–84.

Nabekura, T. (2010). Overcoming multidrug resistance in human cancer cells by natural compounds. *Toxins, 2,* 1207–24.

Nagy, B., Mucsi, I., Molnar, J., et al. (2003). Chemosensitizing effect of vitamin C in combination with 5-fluorouracil in vitro. *In Vivo, 17* (3), 289–92.

Nandakumar, V., Vaid, M., & Katiyar, S. K. (2011). Epigallocatechin-3-gallate reactivates silenced tumor suppressor genes, Cip1/p21 and p16INK4a, by reducing DNA methylation and increasing histones acetylation in human skin cancer cells. *Carcinogenesis, 32* (4), 537–44.

Naugler, W. E., & Karin, M. (2008). The wolf in sheep's clothing: The role of interleukin-6 in immunity, inflammation and cancer. *Trends in Molecular Medicine, 14* (3), 109–19.

Nedeltcheva, A. V., Kilkus, J. M., Imperial, J., et al. (2009). Sleep curtailment is accompanied by increased intake of calories from snacks. *American Journal of Clinical Nutrition, 89,* 126–33.

Neuwirt, H., Arias, M. C., Puhr, M., et al. (2008). Oligomeric proanthocyanin complexes (OPC) exert anti-proliferative and pro-apoptotic effects on prostate cancer cells. *Prostate, 68* (15), 1647–54.

O'Donovan, P. J., & Livingston, D. M. (2010). BRCA1 and BRCA2: Breast/ovarian cancer susceptibility gene products and participants in DNA double-strand break repair. *Carcinogenesis, 31* (6), 961–67.

O'Dwyer, S. T., Michie, H. R., Ziegler, T. R., et al. (1988). A single dose of endotoxin increases intestinal permeability in healthy humans. *Archives of Surgery, 123* (12), 1459–64.

Ormsbee, M. J., Thyfault, J. P., Johnson, E. A., et al. (2007). Fat metabolism and acute resistance exercise in trained men. *Journal of Applied Physiology, 102,* 1767–72.

Outwater, J. L., Nicholson, A., & Barnard, N. (1997). Dairy products and breast cancer: The estrogen and bGH hypothesis. *Medical Hypothesis, 48,* 453–61.

Owen, N., Healy, G. N., Matthews, C. E., & Dunstan, D. W. (2010). Too much sitting: The population health science of sedentary behavior. *Exercise and Sports Sciences Reviews, 38* (3), 105–13.

Patel, S. R., Zhu, X., Storfer-Isser, A., et al. (2009). Sleep duration and biomarkers of inflammation. *Sleep, 32* (2), 200–204.

Pedersen, B. K., & Hoffman-Goetz, L. (2000). Exercise and the immune system: Regulation, integration, and adaptation. *Physiological Reviews, 80* (3), 1055–81.

Pedersen, B. K., & Saltin, B. (2006). Evidence for prescribing exercise as therapy in chronic disease. *Scandinavian Journal of Medicine & Science in Sports, 16* (Suppl. 1), 3–63.

Pendyala, S., Walker, J. M., & Holt, P. R. (2012). A high-fat diet is associated with endotoxemia that originates from the gut. *Gastroenterology, 142* (5), 1100–1101.

Pfeifer, G. P., Denissenko, M. F., Olivier, M., et al. (2002). Tobacco smoke carcinogens, DNA damage and p53 mutations in smoking-associated cancers. *Oncogene, 21,* 7435–51.

Phil Kim, S., Park Ok, S., Jong Lee, S., et al. (2014) A polysaccharide isolated from the liquid culture of lentinus edodes (shiitake) mushroom mycelia containing black rice bran protects mice against salmonellosis through upregulation of the Th1 immune reaction. *Journal of Agricultural and Food Chemistry, 62* (11), 2384–91.

Pittas, A. G., Dawson-Hughes, B., Li, T., et al. (2006). Vitamin D and calcium intake in relation to type 2 diabetes in women. *Diabetes Care, 29,* 650–56.

Pittas, A. G., Lau, F., Hu, F. B., et al. (2007). The role of vitamin D and calcium in type 2 diabetes: A systematic review and meta analysis. *Journal of Clinical Endocrinology & Metabolism, 92* (6), 2017–29.

Punjabi, N. M., & Polotsky, V. Y. (2005). Disorders of glucose metabolism in sleep apnea. *Journal of Applied Physiology, 99* (5), 1998–2007.

Ranelletti, F. O., Maggiano, N., Serra, F. G., et al. (2000). Quercetin inhibits p21-RAS expression in human colon cancer cell lines and in primary colorectal tumors. *International Journal of Cancer, 85* (3), 438–45.

Reyes-Esparza, J., Gonzaga Morales, A. I., González-Maya, L. (2015). Epigallocatechin-3-gallate modulates the activity and expression of P-glycoprotein in breast cancer cells. *Journal of Pharmacology & Clinical Toxicology, 3* (2), 1044.

Richards, M. P. (2002). A brief review of the archaeological evidence for palaeolithic and neolithic subsistence. *European Journal of Clinical Nutrition, 56* (12), 1270–78.

Ridker, P. M., Danielson, E., Francisco, A. H., et al. (2008). Rosuvastatin to prevent vascular events in men and women with elevated C-reactive protein. *New England Journal of Medicine, 359*, 21.

Rissanen, T. H., Voutilainen, S., Nyyssönen, K., et al. (2003). Serum lycopene concentrations and carotid atherosclerosis: The Kuopio Ischaemic Heart Disease Risk Factor Study. *American Journal of Clinical Nutrition, 77*, 133–38.

Rivlin, R. S. (1994). Magnesium deficiency and alcohol intake: Mechanisms, clinical significance and possible relation to cancer development (a review). *Journal of the American College of Nutrition, 13* (5), 416–23.

Robert Wood Johnson Foundation. (2010). Chronic care: Making the case for ongoing care. February. Retrieved from www.rwjf.org/content/dam/farm/reports/reports/2010/rwjf54583.

Roman, A., Kreiner, G., & Nalepa, I. (2013). Macrophages and depression—a misalliance or well-arranged marriage? *Pharmacological Reports, 65* (6), 1663–72.

SanGiovanni, J. P., Chew, E. Y., Clemons, T. E., et al. (2007). The relationship of dietary carotenoid and vitamin A, E, and C intake with age-related macular degeneration in a case-control study. *Archives of Ophthalmology, 125* (9), 1225–32.

Santarelli, R. L., Pierre, F., & Corpet, D. E. (2008). Processed meat and colorectal cancer: A review of epidemiologic and experimental evidence. *Nutrition and Cancer, 60* (2), 131–44.

Sarkar, F. H., & Li, Y. (2006). Using chemopreventive agents to enhance the efficacy of cancer therapy. *Cancer Research, 66* (7), 3347–50.

Schafer, Z. T., & Brugge, J. S. (2007). IL-6 involvement in epithelial cancers. *Journal of Clinical Investigation, 117*, 3660–63.

Schuenke, M. D., Mikat, R. P., & McBride, J. M. (2002). Effect of an acute period of resistance exercise on excess post-exercise oxygen consumption. *European Journal of Applied Physiology, 86*, 411–17.

Sethi, G., Sung, B., & Aggarwal, B. B. (2008). TNF: A master switch for inflammation to cancer. *Frontiers in Bioscience, 13* (13), 5094–107.

Sewerynek, E. (2002). Melatonin and the cardiovascular system. *Neuroendocrinology Letters, 23* (1), 79–83.

Shearer, W. T., Reuben, J. M., Mullington, J. M., et al. (2001). Soluble TNF-alpha receptor 1 and IL-6 levels in humans subjected to the sleep deprivation model of spaceflight. *Journal of Allergy and Clinical Immunology, 107* (1), 165–70.

Sheps, D. S., McMahon, R. P., Becker, L., et al. (2002). Mental stress–induced ischemia and all-cause mortality in patients with coronary artery disease. *Circulation, 105,* 1780–84.

Sherman, M. H., Yu, R. T., Engle, D. D., et al. (2014). Vitamin D receptor-mediated stromal reprogramming suppresses pancreatitis and enhances pancreatic cancer therapy. *Cell, 159* (1), 80–93.

Shively, C. A., Register, T. C., & Clarkson, T. B. (2009). Social stress, visceral obesity, and coronary artery atherosclerosis: Product of a primate adaptation. *American Journal of Primatology, 71* (9), 742–51.

Silverstone, A. E., Rosenbaum, P. F., Weinstock, R. S., et al. (2012). Polychlorinated biphenyl (PCB) exposure and diabetes: Results from the Anniston Community Health Survey. *Environmental Health Perspectives, 120,* 5.

Simone, C. B., Simone, N. L., Simone, V., et al. (2007). Antioxidants and other nutrients do not interfere with chemotherapy or radiation therapy and can increase kill and increase survival, part 1. *Alternative Therapies, 13* (1), 22–28.

Smith, C. D., Herkes, S. B., Behrns, K. E., et al. (1993). Gastric acid secretion and vitamin B_{12} absorption after vertical Roux-en-Y gastric bypass for morbid obesity. *Annals of Surgery, 218* (1), 91–96.

Sola, S., Mir, M., Cheema, F., et al. (2005). Irbesartan and lipoic acid improve endothelial function and reduce markers of inflammation in the metabolic syndrome. *Circulation, 111* (3), 343–48.

Somers, E. C., Ganser, M. A., Warren, J. S., et al. (2015). Mercury exposure and antinuclear antibodies among females of reproductive age in the United States: NHANES. *Environmental Health Perspectives, 123* (8), 792–98.

Song, Y., Dai, Q., & He, K. (2013). Magnesium intake, insulin resistance, and type 2 diabetes. *North American Journal of Medicine and Science, 6* (1), 9–15.

Steen, E., Terry, B. M., Rivera, E. J., et al. (2005). Impaired insulin and insulin-like growth factor expression and signaling mechanisms in Alzheimer's disease—is this type 3 diabetes? *Journal of Alzheimer's Disease, 7,* 63–80.

Stocker, R., Bowry, V., & Frei, B. (1991). Ubiquinol-10 protects human low-density lipoprotein more efficiently against lipid peroxidation that does alpha-tocopherol. *Proceedings of the National Academy of Sciences, 88* (5), 1646–50.

Stojanovich, L. (2010). Stress and autoimmunity. *Autoimmunity Reviews, 9,* A271–A276.

Stojanovich, L., & Marisavljevich, D. (2008). Stress as a trigger of autoimmune disease. *Autoimmune Reviews, 7,* 209–13.

Sun, C. L., Yuan, J. M., Koh, W. P., et al. (2006). Green tea, black tea and breast cancer risk: a meta-analysis of epidemiological studies. *Carcinogenesis, 27* (7), 1310–15.

Syal, S. K., Kapoor, A., Bhatia, E., et al. (2012). Vitamin D deficiency, coronary artery disease, and endothelial dysfunction: Observations from a coronary angiographic study in Indian patients. *Journal of Invasive Cardiology, 24* (8), 385–89.

Talanian, J. L., Galloway, S. D. R., Heigenhauser, G. J. F., et al. (2007). Two weeks of high-intensity aerobic interval training increases the capacity for fat oxidation during exercise in women. *Journal of Applied Physiology, 102* (1), 439–47.

Tan, K. C. B., Chow, W. S., Ai, V. H. G., et al. (2002). Advanced glycation end products and endothelial dysfunction in type 2 diabetes. *Diabetes Care, 25* (6), 1055–59.

Tan, K. P., Azlan, Z. M., Choo, M. Y., et al. (2014). The comparative accuracy of ultrasound and mammography in the detection of breast cancer. *Medical Journal of Malaysia, 69* (2), 79–85.

Tandon, R. K., & Bhatia, V. (2005). Stress and the gastrointestinal tract. *Journal of Gastroenterology and Hepatology, 20,* 332–39.

Tarcin, O., Yavuz, D. G., Ozben, B., et al. (2009). Effect of vitamin D deficiency and replacement on endothelial function in asymptomatic subjects. *Journal of Clinical Endocrinology and Metabolism, 94* (10), 4023–30.

Taylor, A., Villines, T., Stanek, E., et al. (2009). Extended-release niacin or ezetimibe and carotid intima-media thickness. *New England Journal of Medicine, 361.*

Teitelbaum, S. L., Gammon, M. D., Britton, J. A., et al. (2007). Reported residential pesticide use and breast cancer risk on Long Island, New York. *American Journal of Epidemiology, 165,* 643–51.

Tengattini, S., Reiter, R. J., Tan, D., et al. (2008). Cardiovascular diseases: Protective effects of melatonin. *Journal of Pineal Research, 44,* 16–25.

Thompson, C. L., & Li, L. (2012). Association of sleep duration and breast cancer oncotypedx recurrence score. *Breast Cancer Research and Treatment, 134* (3), 1291–95.

Tjønna, A. E., Lee, S. J., Rognmo, Ø., et al. (2008). Aerobic interval training versus continuous moderate exercise as a treatment for metabolic syndrome. *Circulation, 118* (4), 346–54.

Tomasian, D., Keaney, J., & Vita, J. (2000). Antioxidants and the bioactivity of endothelium-derived nitric oxide. *Cardiovascular Research, 47* (3), 426–35.

Tomiyama, A. J., Mann, T., Vinas, D., et al. (2010). Low calorie dieting increases cortisol. *Psychosomatic Medicine, 72* (4), 357–64.

Tremblay, A., Simoneau, J.-A., & Bouchard, C. (1994). Impact of exercise intensity on body fatness and skeletal muscle metabolism. *Metabolism, 43,* 814–18.

Triantafilou. M., Gamper, F. G. J., Lepper, P. M., et al. (2007). Lipopolysaccharides from atherosclerosis-associated bacteria antagonize TLR4, induce formation of TLR2/1/CD36 complexes in lipid rafts and trigger TLR2-induced inflammatory responses in human vascular endothelial cells. *Cellular Microbiology, 9* (8), 2030–39.

Tricker, A. R., & Preussmann, R. (1991). Carcinogenic n-nitrosamines in the diet: Occurrence, formation, mechanisms and carcinogenic potential. *Mutation Research, 259* (93–94), 277–89.

Ungar, P. S., Grine, F. E., & Teaford, M. F. (2006). A review of the evidence and a new model of adaptive versatility. *Annual Review of Anthropology, 35,* 209–28.

Van der Pols, J. C., Bain, C., Gunnell, D., et al. (2007). Childhood dairy intake and adult cancer risk: 65-y follow-up of the Boyd Orr Cohort. *American Journal of Clinical Nutrition, 86,* 1722–29.

Van Immerseel, F., Ducatelle, R., De Vos, M., et al. (2017). Butyric acid-producing anaerobic bacteria as a novel probiotic treatment approach for inflammatory bowel disease. *Journal of Medical Microbiology, 12,* 32–55.

Verrax, J., & Calderon, P. B. (2008). The controversial place of vitamin C in cancer treatment. *Biochemical Pharmacology, 76,* 1644–52.

Versini, M., Jeandel, P. Y., Rosenthal, E., et al. (2014). Obesity in autoimmune diseases: Not a passive bystander. *Autoimmunity Reviews, 13,* 981–1000.

Virtanen, S., Läärä, E., Hyppönen, E., et al. (2000). Cow's milk consumption, HLA-DQB1, genotype, and type 1 diabetes. *Diabetes, 49* (9), 1617.

Vissoci Reiche, E. M., Vargas Nunes, S. O., & Morimoto, H. K. (2004). Stress, depression, the immune system, and cancer. *Lancet Oncology, 5,* 617–25.

Vita, J., Keany, J., Raby, K., et al. (1998). Low plasma ascorbic acid independently predicts the presence of an unstable coronary syndrome. *Journal of the American College of Cardiology, 31,* 980–86.

Vojdani, A., & Tarash, I., (2013). Cross-reaction between gliadin and different food and tissue antigens. *Food and Nutrition Sciences, 4,* 20–32.

Wallace, T. C. (2011). Anthocyanins in cardiovascular disease. *Advances in Nutrition, 2,* 1–7.

Wang, G., Liu, C., Wang, Z., et al. (2006). Effects of astragalus membranaceus in promoting T-helper cell type 1 polarization and interferon-γ production by up-regulating T-bet expression in patients with asthma. *Chinese Journal of Integrative Medicine, 12,* 262.

Wang, Q., Yang, W., Uytingco, M. S., et al. (2000). 1,25-Dihyrdoxyvitamin D3 and All-*trans*-Retinoic acid sensitize breast cancer cells to chemotherapy-induced cell death. *Cancer Research, 60,* 2040–48.

Wang, X. M., & Lehky, T. J., (2012). Discovering cytokines as targets for chemotherapy-induced painful peripheral neuropathy. *Cytokine, 59* (1), 3–9.

Warren, T. Y., Barry, V., Hooker, S. P., et al. (2010). Sedentary behaviors increase risk of cardiovascular disease mortality in men. *Medicine & Science in Sports & Exercise, 42* (5), 879–85.

Wei, Y., Zhao, X., Kariya, Y., et al. (1994). Induction of apoptosis by quercetin: Involvement of heat shock protein. *Cancer Research, 54,* 4952–57.

Weickert, M. O., & Pfeiffer, A. F. H. (2008). Metabolic effects of dietary fiber consumption and prevention of diabetes. *Journal of Nutrition, 138,* 439–42.

Wesa, K. M., Segal, N. H., Cronin, A. M., et al. (2015). Serum 25-hydroxy vitamin D and survival in advanced colorectal cancer: A retrospective analysis. *Nutrition and Cancer, 67* (3), 424–30.

Wiseman, R. A. (2000). Breast cancer hypothesis: A single cause for the majority of cases. *Journal of Epidemiology Community Health, 54,* 851–58.

Wu, D., Wang, J., Pae, M., et al. (2012). Green tea ECGC, T cells, and T cell-mediated autoimmune diseases. *Molecular Aspects of Medicine, 33* (1), 107–18.

Yamada, K., Hung, P., Park, T. K., et al. (2011). A comparison of the immunostimulatory effects of the medicinal herbs Echinacea, ashwagandha, and brahmi. *Journal of Ethnopharmacology, 137* (1), 231–35.

Yan, M., & Nuriding, H. (2014). Reversal effect of vitamin D on different multidrug-resistant cells. *Genetics and Molecular Research, 13* (3), 6239–47.

Yang, G., Shu, X. O., Li, H., et al. (2007). Prospective cohort study of green tea consumption and colorectal cancer risk in women. *Cancer Epidemiology, Biomarkers & Prevention, 16* (6), 1219–23.

Yang, I., Shin, J., & Cho, S. (2014). Pycnogenol induces nuclear translocation of apoptosis-inducing factor and caspase-independent apoptosis in MC-3 human mucoepidermoid carcinoma cell line. *Journal of Cancer Prevention, 19,* 265–72.

Yoo, S., Kim, J. S., Kwon, S. U., et al. (2008). Undernutrition as a predictor of poor clinical outcomes in acute ischemic stroke patients. *Archives of Neurology, 65* (1), 39–43.

Yoshioka, M., Doucet, E., St-Pierre, S., et al. (2001). Impact of high-intensity exercise on energy expenditure, lipid oxidation, and body fatness. *International Journal of Obesity, 25,* 332–39.

Yusuf, S., Hawken, S., Ounpuu, S., et al. (2004). Effect of potentially modifiable risk factors associated with myocardial infarction in 52 countries (the INTERHEART Study): Case-control study. *Lancet, 365* (9438), 937–52.

Zhang, M., Deng, C. S., Zheng, J. J., et al. (2006). Curcumin regulated shift from Th1 to Th2 in trinitrobenzene sulphonic acid-induced chronic colitis. *Acta Pharmacologica Sinica, 27* (8), 1071–77.

Zhu, W., Cai, D., Wang, Y., et al. (2013). Calcium plus vitamin D3 supplementation facilitated fat loss in overweight and obese college students with very-low calcium consumption: A randomized controlled trial. *Nutrition Journal, 12* (8).

Acknowledgments

I would like to express my deepest gratitude to Dr. Jeffrey Bland for providing the world a new way of thinking, as well as the new approach to health care that has allowed me to rebuild myself back to excellent health. His work has encouraged me to help countless others recover from their unresolved chronic health issues.

My very grateful appreciation to Christine "Misty" Barth, my practice manager and dear friend, for helping me make this book a reality. Her impeccable editing skills, attention to detail, and patience through the writing process are admirable. I can't thank Misty enough for her willingness to go the extra step and give her time so generously.

I thank my wife, Holly Bliss, for her loving and unwavering support over the last few years while writing this book. Your encouragement when times got rough is much appreciated. I also appreciate your gifted coaching skills, as evidenced by your contributions to the book. I look forward to our two-wheeled "Rebuild across America" tour!

Loving thanks to my family for your caring and support during my cancer ordeal. I hope one day I can return the same acts of kindness to you all.

My grateful thanks to Dave and Peg Bliss for their ideas, encouragement, and support during the writing process. I cannot express enough thanks to Dave for his time, enthusiasm, unwavering support, creative ideas, and, most of all, his help with bringing this work to life.

A huge thanks to Yve Novotny for the countless hours and effort she spent creating healthful and delicious recipes! Yve shows us that eating healthfully can be fun, flavorful, and full of variety; it doesn't have to be boring and restrictive. Yve is the only cook I know who can make a mouthwatering masterpiece out of whatever is in the fridge.

My heartfelt gratitude to my close friend, Mike Mammana, not only for his friendship and support but also for his enthusiastic efforts to help me get this information in front of the many who need it.

My sincere appreciation is extended to Rui Weidt for his outstanding and creative work, and to Susan Kunin for her commitment and support since this writing journey began.

A deep heartfelt thanks to those patients who allowed the use of their personal stories, and for allowing me to help them rebuild from their chronic health issues.

Finally, many thanks to the exceptional publishing team at Harper Wave. To my publisher, Karen Rinaldi, thank you for having the vision to undertake this project and for recognizing the need for it. Big thanks to editors Sarah Murphy and Hannah Robinson, the creative team, and all those who have helped to create a beautiful book inside and out.

Index

About the Author

DR. ROBERT ZEMBROSKI is a specialist in functional medicine, a clinical nutritionist, and a transformational speaker. Twenty-four years in private practice enabled Dr. Zembroski to become an expert in health topics from heart disease, diabetes, obesity, cancer, and hormone-related issues. Years ago, Dr. Zembroski's own diagnosis of non-Hodgkin's lymphoma led to several courses of toxic chemotherapy, as well as surgery, to remove a five-inch tumor from his chest. Through the use of nutritional support, targeted supplementation, and other lifestyle modifications, he is not only cancer-free, but has returned to excellent health. That experience inspired him to create the Cancer Victor® Protocol—a research-based set of protocols that augments the function of chemotherapy and radiation treatments while reducing their toxic side effects, allowing the patient to stay active and engaged in life. Currently, Dr. Zembroski is the director of the Darien Center for Functional Medicine in Darien, Connecticut. He lives in Wilton, Connecticut, with his wife while pursuing his passions of skiing, biking, hiking, and motorcycling.

www.drzembroski.com/